Nazi Human Experimentation

Contents

Chapter 1

Nazi human experimentation

Nazi human experimentation was a series of medical experiments on large numbers of prisoners (including children), largely Jews from across Europe, but also Romani, Sinti, ethnic Poles, Soviet POWs and disabled Germans, by Nazi Germany in its concentration camps mainly in the early 1940s, during World War II and the Holocaust.

Prisoners were forced into participating; they did not willingly volunteer and no consent was given for the procedures. Typically, the experiments resulted in death, trauma, disfigurement or permanent disability, and as such are considered as examples of medical torture.

At Auschwitz and other camps, under the direction of Eduard Wirths, selected inmates were subjected to various hazardous experiments that were designed to help German military personnel in combat situations, develop new weapons, aid in the recovery of military personnel who had been injured, and to advance the Nazi racial ideology.[1] Aribert Heim conducted similar medical experiments at Mauthausen. Carl Værnet is known to have conducted experiments on homosexual prisoners in attempts to "cure" homosexuality.

After the war, these crimes were tried at what became known as the Doctors' Trial, and revulsion at the abuses perpetrated led to the development of the Nuremberg Code of medical ethics.

1.1 Experiments

According to the indictments at the Subsequent Nuremberg Trials,[2][3] these experiments included the following:

1.1.1 Experiments on twins

Experiments on twin children in concentration camps were created to show the similarities and differences in the genetics of twins, as well as to see if the human body can be unnaturally manipulated. The central leader of the experiments was Josef Mengele, who from 1943 to 1944 performed experiments on nearly 1,500 sets of imprisoned twins at Auschwitz. About 200 people survived these studies.[4] The twins were arranged by age and sex and kept in barracks between experiments, which ranged from injection of different dyes into the eyes of twins to see whether it would change their color to sewing twins together in attempts to create conjoined twins.[5][6]

1.1.2 Bone, muscle, and nerve transplantation experiments

From about September 1942 to about December 1943 experiments were conducted at the Ravensbrück concentration camp, for the benefit of the German Armed Forces, to study bone, muscle, and nerve regeneration, and bone transplantation from one person to another. Sections of bones, muscles, and nerves were removed from the subjects without use of anesthesia. As a result of these operations, many victims suffered intense agony, mutilation, and permanent disability.

1.1.3   Head injury experiments

In mid-1942 in Baranowicze, occupied Poland, experiments were conducted in a small building behind the private home occupied by a known Nazi SD Security Service officer, in which "a young boy of eleven or twelve [was] strapped to a chair so he could not move. Above him was a mechanized hammer that every few seconds came down upon his head." The boy was driven insane from the torture.[7]

1.1.4   Freezing experiments

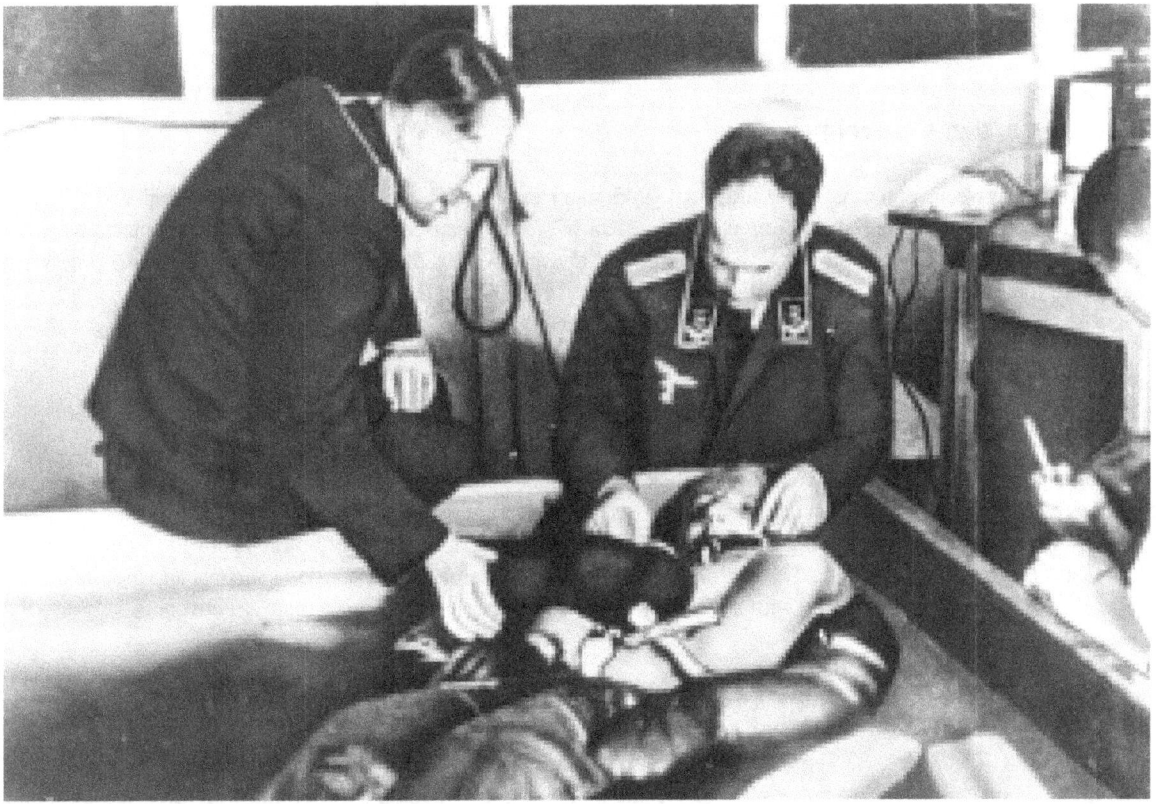

A cold water immersion experiment at Dachau concentration camp presided over by Professor Ernst Holzlöhner (left) and Dr. Sigmund Rascher (right). The subject is wearing an experimental Luftwaffe garment

In 1941, the *Luftwaffe* conducted experiments with the intent of discovering means to prevent and treat hypothermia. There were 360 to 400 experiments and 280 to 300 victims indicating some victims suffered more than one experiment.[8]

Another study placed prisoners naked in the open air for several hours with temperatures as low as −6 °C (21 °F). Besides studying the physical effects of cold exposure, the experimenters also assessed different methods of rewarming survivors.[10] *"One assistant later testified that some victims were thrown into boiling water for rewarming."*[8]

The freezing/hypothermia experiments were conducted for the Nazi high command to simulate the conditions the armies suffered on the Eastern Front, as the German forces were ill-prepared for the cold weather they encountered. Many experiments were conducted on captured Russian troops; the Nazis wondered whether their genetics gave them superior resistance to cold. The principal locales were Dachau and Auschwitz. Dr Sigmund Rascher, an SS doctor based at Dachau, reported directly to Reichsführer-SS Heinrich Himmler and publicised the results of his freezing experiments at the 1942 medical conference entitled "Medical Problems Arising from Sea and Winter".[11] Approximately 100 people are reported to have died as a result of these experiments.[12]

1.1.5 Malaria experiments

From about February 1942 to about April 1945, experiments were conducted at the Dachau concentration camp in order to investigate immunization for treatment of malaria. Healthy inmates were infected by mosquitoes or by injections of extracts of the mucous glands of female mosquitoes. After contracting the disease, the subjects were treated with various drugs to test their relative efficiency. Over 1,000 people were used in these experiments and more than half died as a result.

1.1.6 Immunization experiments

At the German concentration camps of Sachsenhausen, Dachau, Natzweiler, Buchenwald, and Neuengamme, scientists tested immunization compounds and serums for the prevention and treatment of contagious diseases, including malaria, typhus, tuberculosis, typhoid fever, yellow fever, and infectious hepatitis.[13]

1.1.7 Mustard gas experiments

At various times between September 1939 and April 1945, many experiments were conducted at Sachsenhausen, Natzweiler, and other camps to investigate the most effective treatment of wounds caused by mustard gas. Test subjects were deliberately exposed to mustard gas and other vesicants (e.g. Lewisite) which inflicted severe chemical burns. The victims' wounds were then tested to find the most effective treatment for the mustard gas burns.[14]

1.1.8 Sulfonamide experiments

From about July 1942 to about September 1943, experiments to investigate the effectiveness of sulfonamide, a synthetic antimicrobial agent, were conducted at Ravensbrück.[15] Wounds inflicted on the subjects were infected with bacteria such as *Streptococcus*, *Clostridium perfringens* (the causative agent in gas gangrene) and *Clostridium tetani*, the causative agent in tetanus.[16] Circulation of blood was interrupted by tying off blood vessels at both ends of the wound to create a condition similar to that of a battlefield wound. Infection was aggravated by forcing wood shavings and ground glass into the wounds. The infection was treated with sulfonamide and other drugs to determine their effectiveness.

1.1.9 Sea water experiments

From about July 1944 to about September 1944, experiments were conducted at the Dachau concentration camp to study various methods of making sea water drinkable. At one point, a group of roughly 90 Roma were deprived of food and given nothing but sea water to drink by Dr. Hans Eppinger, leaving them gravely injured.[11] They were so dehydrated that others observed them licking freshly mopped floors in an attempt to get drinkable water.[17]

1.1.10 Sterilization experiments

The Law for the Prevention of Genetically Defective Progeny was passed on 14 July 1933, which legalized the involuntary sterilization of persons with diseases claimed to be hereditary: weak-mindedness, schizophrenia, alcohol abuse, insanity, blindness, deafness, and physical deformities. The law was used to encourage growth of the Aryan race through the sterilization of persons who fell under the quota of being genetically defective.[18] 1% of citizens between the age of 17 to 24 had been sterilized within 2 years of the law passing. Within 4 years, 300,000 patients had been sterilized.[19] From about March 1941 to about January 1945, sterilization experiments were conducted at Auschwitz, Ravensbrück, and other places by Dr. Carl Clauberg.[14] The purpose of these experiments was to develop a method of sterilization which would be suitable for sterilizing millions of people with a minimum of time and effort. These experiments were conducted by means of X-ray, surgery and various drugs. Thousands of victims were sterilized. Aside from its experimentation, the Nazi government sterilized around 400,000 people as part of its compulsory sterilization program.[20] Intravenous injections of solutions speculated to contain iodine and silver nitrate were successful, but had unwanted side effects such

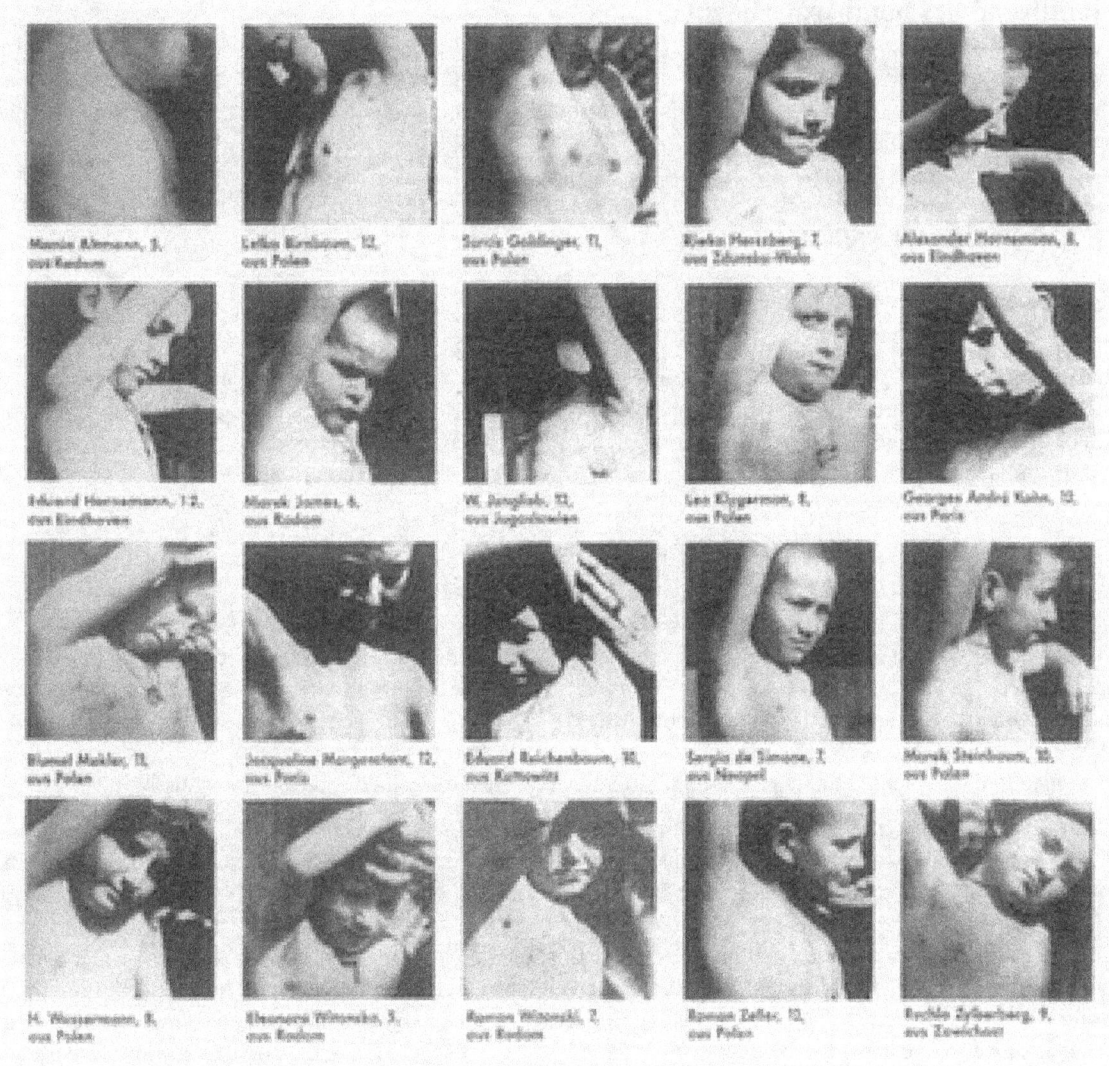

Child victims of Nazi experimentation show incisions where axillary lymph nodes had been surgically removed after they were deliberately infected with tuberculosis at Neuengamme concentration camp. They were later executed.

as vaginal bleeding, severe abdominal pain, and cervical cancer.[21] Therefore, radiation treatment became the favored choice of sterilization. Specific amounts of exposure to radiation destroyed a person's ability to produce ova or sperm. The radiation was administered through deception. Prisoners were brought into a room and asked to complete forms, which took two to three minutes. In this time, the radiation treatment was administered and, unknown to the prisoners, they were rendered completely sterile. Many suffered severe radiation burns.[22]

1.1.11   Experiments with poison

Somewhere between December 1943 and October 1944, experiments were conducted at Buchenwald to investigate the effect of various poisons. The poisons were secretly administered to experimental subjects in their food. The victims died as a result of the poison or were killed immediately in order to permit autopsies. In September 1944, experimental subjects were shot with poisonous bullets, suffered torture and often died.[14]

1.1.12 Incendiary bomb experiments

From around November 1943 to around January 1944, experiments were conducted at Buchenwald to test the effect of various pharmaceutical preparations on phosphorus burns. These burns were inflicted on prisoners using phosphorus material extracted from incendiary bombs.[14]

1.1.13 High altitude experiments

Further information: Hubertus Strughold

In early 1942, prisoners at Dachau concentration camp were used by Sigmund Rascher in experiments to aid German pilots who had to eject at high altitudes. A low-pressure chamber containing these prisoners was used to simulate conditions at altitudes of up to 20,000 m (66,000 ft). It was rumored that Rascher performed vivisections on the brains of victims who survived the initial experiment.[23] Of the 200 subjects, 80 died outright, and the others were executed.[11]

1.2 Aftermath

Many of the subjects died as a result of the experiments conducted by the Nazis, while many others were executed after the tests were completed to study the effects *post mortem*.[24] Those who survived were often left mutilated, suffering permanent disability, weakened bodies, and mental distress.[11][25] On 19 August 1947, the doctors captured by Allied forces were put on trial in *USA vs. Karl Brandt et al.*, commonly known as the Doctors' Trial. At the trial, several of the doctors argued in their defense that there was no international law regarding medical experimentation.

The issue of informed consent had previously been controversial in German medicine in 1900, when Dr. Albert Neisser infected patients (mainly prostitutes) with syphilis without their consent. Despite Neisser's support from most of the academic community, public opinion, led by psychiatrist Albert Moll, was against Neisser. While Neisser went on to be fined by the Royal Disciplinary Court, Moll developed "a legally based, positivistic contract theory of the patient-doctor relationship" that was not adopted into German law.[26] Eventually, the minister for religious, educational, and medical affairs issued a directive stating that medical interventions other than for diagnosis, healing, and immunization were excluded under all circumstances if "the human subject was a minor or not competent for other reasons", or if the subject had not given his or her "unambiguous consent" after a "proper explanation of the possible negative consequences" of the intervention, though this was not legally binding.[26]

In response, Drs. Leo Alexander and Andrew Conway Ivy drafted a ten-point memorandum entitled *Permissible Medical Experiment* that went on to be known as the Nuremberg Code.[27] The code calls for such standards as voluntary consent of patients, avoidance of unnecessary pain and suffering, and that there must be a belief that the experimentation will not end in death or disability.[28] The Code was not cited in any of the findings against the defendants and never made it into either German or American medical law.

1.2.1 Modern ethical issues

The results of the Dachau freezing experiments have been used in some modern research into the treatment of hypothermia, with at least 45 publications having referenced the experiments since the Second World War.[29] This, together with the recent use of data from Nazi research into the effects of phosgene gas, has proven controversial and presents an ethical dilemma for modern physicians who do not agree with the methods used to obtain this data.[17] Some object on an ethical basis, and others have rejected Nazi research purely on scientific grounds, pointing out methodological inconsistencies. In an often-cited review of the Dachau hypothermia experiments, Berger states that the study has "all the ingredients of a scientific fraud" and that the data "cannot advance science or save human lives."[29]

Controversy has also risen from the use of results of biological warfare testing done by the Imperial Japanese Army's Unit 731.[30] The results from Unit 731 were kept classified by the United States until the majority of doctors involved were given pardons.[31]

1.3   See also

- Erwin Ding-Schuler

- Guatemala syphilis experiment

- Herta Oberheuser

- Henry K. Beecher

- Human experimentation in North Korea

- Human radiation experiments

- Japanese human experimentations

- Jewish skeleton collection

- Karl Genzken

- Karl Gebhardt

- List of medical eponyms with Nazi associations

- Nazi eugenics

- Project MKUltra (CIA)

- Shiro Ishii

- Unethical human experimentation in the United States

1.4   References

[1] "Nazi Medical Experimentation". *US Holocaust Memorial Museum*. Retrieved 23 March 2008.

[2] "Medical Experiment". *Jewish Virtual Library*. Retrieved 23 March 2008.

[3] "The Doctors Trial: The Medical Case of the Subsequent Nuremberg Proceedings". *United States Holocaust Memorial Museum*. Retrieved 23 March 2008.

[4] Josef Mengele and Experimentation on Human Twins at Auschwitz, *Children of the Flames; Dr. Josef Mengele and the Untold Story of the Twins of Auschwitz*, Lucette Matalon Lagnado and Sheila Cohn Dekel, and *Mengele: the Complete Story* by Gerald Posner and John Ware.

[5] Black, Edwin (2004). *War Against the Weak: Eugenics and America's Campaign to Create a Master Race*. United States: Thunder's Mouth Press. ISBN 1-56858-258-7. Retrieved 14 April 2008.

[6] Berenbaum, Michael (1993). *The world must know: the history of the Holocaust as told in the United States Holocaust Memorial Museum*. Boston: Little, Brown. pp. 194–5. ISBN 0-316-09134-0.

[7] Small, Martin; Vic Shayne. "Remember Us: My Journey from the Shtetl through the Holocaust", Page 135, 2009.

[8] Berger, Robert L. (May 1990). "Nazi Science — the Dachau Hypothermia Experiments". *New England Journal of Medicine* **322** (20): 1435–40. doi:10.1056/NEJM199005173222006. PMID 2184357.

[9] *The Dachau Concentration Camp, 1933 to 1945*. Comite International Dachau. 2000. p. 183. ISBN 978-3-87490-751-4.

[10] Bogod, David. "The Nazi Hypothermia Experiments: Forbidden Data?", *Anaesthesia*, Volume 59 Issue 12 Page 1155, December 2004.

[11] Tyson, Peter. "Holocaust on Trial: The Experiments". *NOVA Online*. Retrieved 23 March 2008.

[12] Neurnberg Military Tribunal, Volume I · Page 200

[13] "Nazi Medical Experiments". *ushmm.org*.

[14] "Introduction to NMT Case 1: U.S.A. v. Karl Brandt et al.". *Harvard Law Library, Nuremberg Trials Project: A Digital Document Collection*. Retrieved 23 March 2008.

[15] Schaefer, Naomi. *The Legacy of Nazi Medicine, The New Atlantis*, Number 5, Spring 2004, pp. 54–60.

[16] Spitz, Vivien (2005). *Doctors from Hell: The Horrific Account of Nazi Experiments on Humans*. Sentient Publications. ISBN 1-59181-032-9.

[17] Cohen, Baruch C. "The Ethics Of Using Medical Data From Nazi Experiments". *Jewish Law: Articles*. Retrieved 23 March 2008.

[18] Gardella JE. The cost-effectiveness of killing: an overview of Nazi "euthanasia." Medical Sentinel 1999;4:132-5

[19] Dahl M. [Selection and destruction-treatment of "unworthy-to-live" children in the Third Reich and the role of child and adolescent psychiatry], Prax Kinderpsychol Kinderpsychiatr 2001;50:170-91.

[20] Piotrowski, Christa (21 July 2000). "Dark Chapter of American History: U.S. Court Battle Over Forced Sterilization". *CommonDreams.org News Center*. Retrieved 23 March 2008.

[21] Meric, Vesna (27 January 2005). "Forced to take part in experiments". *BBC News*.

[22] "Medical Experiments at Auschwitz". *Jewish Virtual Library*. Retrieved 23 March 2008.

[23] Cockburn, Alexander (1998). *Whiteout:The CIA, Drugs, and the Press*. Verso. ISBN 1-85984-139-2.

[24] Rosenberg, Jennifer. "Mengele's Children – The Twins of Auschwitz". *about.com*. Retrieved 23 March 2008.

[25] "Sterilization Experiments". *Jewish Virtual Library*. Retrieved 23 March 2008.

[26] Vollman, Jochen; Rolf Winau. "Informed consent in human experimentation before the Nuremberg code". *BMJ*. Archived from the original on 4 March 2008. Retrieved 8 April 2008.

[27] "The Nuremberg Code". *United States Holocaust Memorial Museum*. Retrieved 23 March 2008.

[28] "Regulations and Ethical Guidelines: Reprinted from *Trials of War Criminals before the Nuremberg Military Tribunals under Control Council Law No. 10, Vol. 2, pp. 181–182*". *Office of Human Subjects Research*. Washington, D.C.: U.S. Government Printing Office. 1949. Retrieved 23 March 2008.

[29] Robert L. Berger, M.D. (1990). "Nazi Science — The Dachau Hypothermia Experiments". *The New England Journal of Medicine* **20** (322): 1435–1440. doi:10.1056/NEJM199005173222006. PMID 2184357.

[30] "Unit 731: Japan's biological force". *BBC News*. 1 February 2002. Retrieved 27 March 2008.

[31] Reilly, Kevin; Stephen Kaufman; Angela Bodino (2003). *Racism: A Global Reader*. M.E. Sharpe. ISBN 0-7656-1059-0. Retrieved 27 March 2008.

1.5 Further reading

- Annas, George J. (1992). *The Nazi Doctors and the Nuremberg Code: Human Rights in Human Experimentation*. Oxford University Press. ISBN 0195101065.

- Baumslag, N. (2005). *Murderous Medicine: Nazi Doctors, Human Experimentation, and Typhus*. Praeger Publishers. ISBN 0-275-98312-9

- Michalczyk, J. (Dir.) (1997). *In The Shadow Of The Reich: Nazi Medicine*. First Run Features. (video)

- Nyiszli, M. (2011). "3". *Auschwitz: A Doctor's Eyewitness Account*. New York: Arcade Publishing.

- Rees, L. (2005). *Auschwitz: A New History*. Public Affairs. ISBN 1-58648-357-9

- Weindling, P.J. (2005). *Nazi Medicine and the Nuremberg Trials: From Medical War Crimes to Informed Consent*. Palgrave Macmillan. ISBN 1-4039-3911-X

- USAF School of Aerospace Medicine (1950). *German Aviation Medicine, World War II*. United States Air Force.

1.6   External links

- The Infamous Medical Experiments from Holocaust Survivors and Remembrance Project: "Forget You Not"

- United States Holocaust Memorial Museum – Online Exhibition: Doctors Trial

- United States Holocaust Memorial Museum – Online Exhibition: Deadly Medicine: Creating the Master Race

- United States Holocaust Memorial Museum – Library Bibliography: Medical Experiments

- Jewish Virtual Library: Medical Experiments Table of Contents

1.6.1   Controversy regarding use of findings

- Campell, Robert. "Citations of shame; scientists are still trading on Nazi atrocities.", *New Scientist*, 28 February 1985, 105(1445), p. 31.

- "Citing Nazi 'Research': To Do So Without Condemnation Is Not Defensible"

- "On the Ethics of Citing Nazi Research"

- "Remembering the Holocaust, Part 2"

- "The Ethics Of Using Medical Data From Nazi Experiments"

Chapter 2

Wilhelm Beiglböck

Prof. Dr. **Wilhelm Franz Josef Beiglböck** (born October 10, 1905 in Hochneukirchen, Lower Austria, Austria – November 22, 1963 in Buxtehude, Lower Saxony, Germany) was an internist and held the title of Consulting Physician to the German Luftwaffe during World War II.

He was a member of the NSDAP and member of the SA (SA Obersturmbannführer). He performed medical tests involving seawater on inmates at Dachau concentration camp.

Beiglboeck was a defendant in the Nuremberg Doctor's Trial. He was convicted of war crimes and crimes against humanity, and sentenced to 15 years imprisonment. His sentence was commuted to 10 years and from 1952 - 1963 he served as the chief physician at Hospital of Buxtehude.

2.1 See also

- Ex-Nazi

2.2 References

- Alexander Mitscherlich / Fred Mielke: *Medizin ohne Menschlichkeit - Dokumente des Nürnberger Ärzteprozesses*, Lamberg und Schneider, Heidelberg 1949, ISBN 3-596-22003-3.

- Ernst Klee: *Das Personenlexikon zum Dritten Reich - Wer war was vor und nach 1945*. Fischer, Frankfurt a.M. 2003, ISBN 3-10-039309-0.

- François Bayle: *Croix gammée contre caducée. Les expériences humaines en Allemagne pendant la deuxième guerre mondiale*. Neustadt 1950.

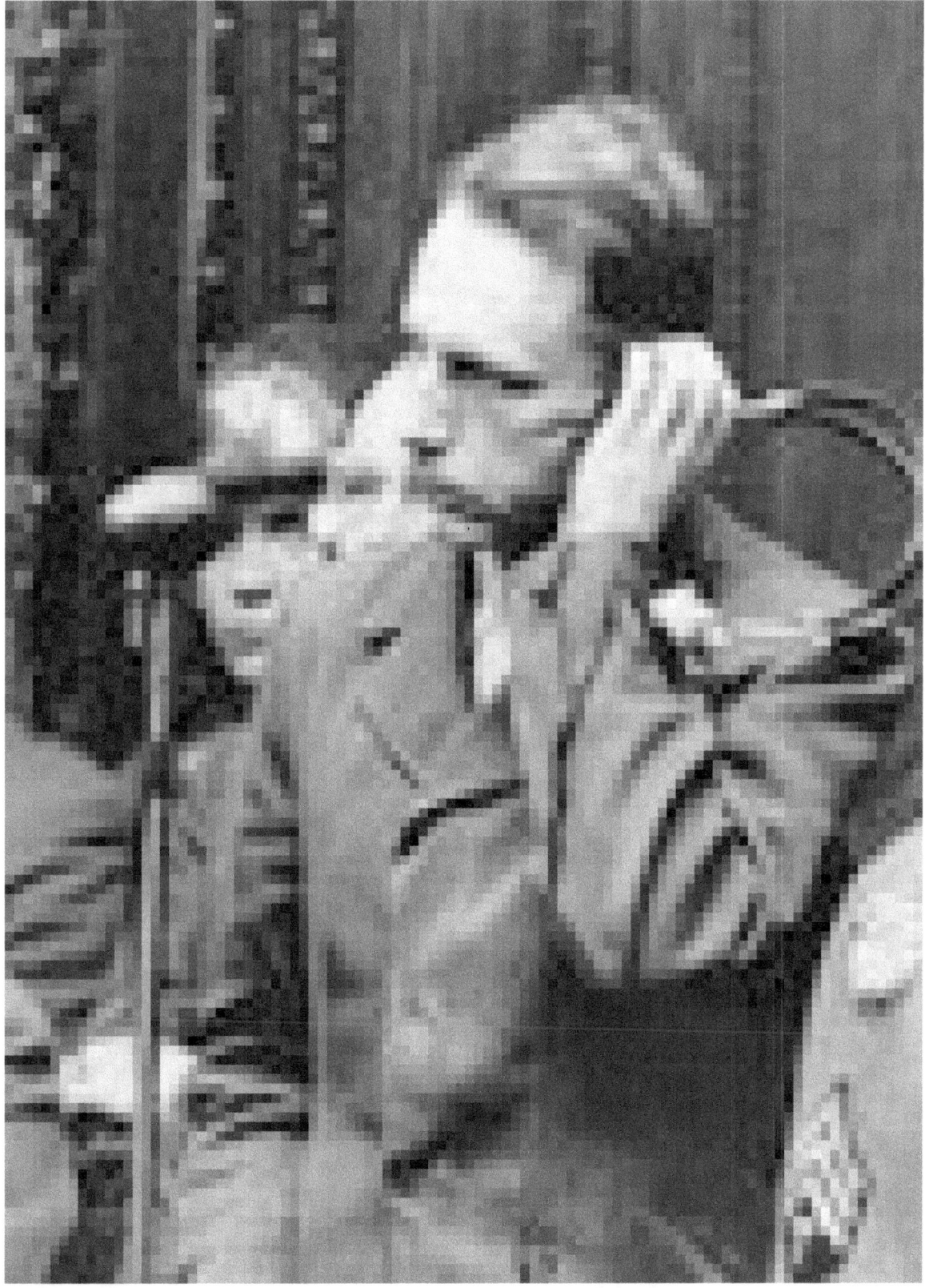

Wilhelm Beiglböck pleading "not guilty" at the Doctors' Trial.

Chapter 3

Block 10

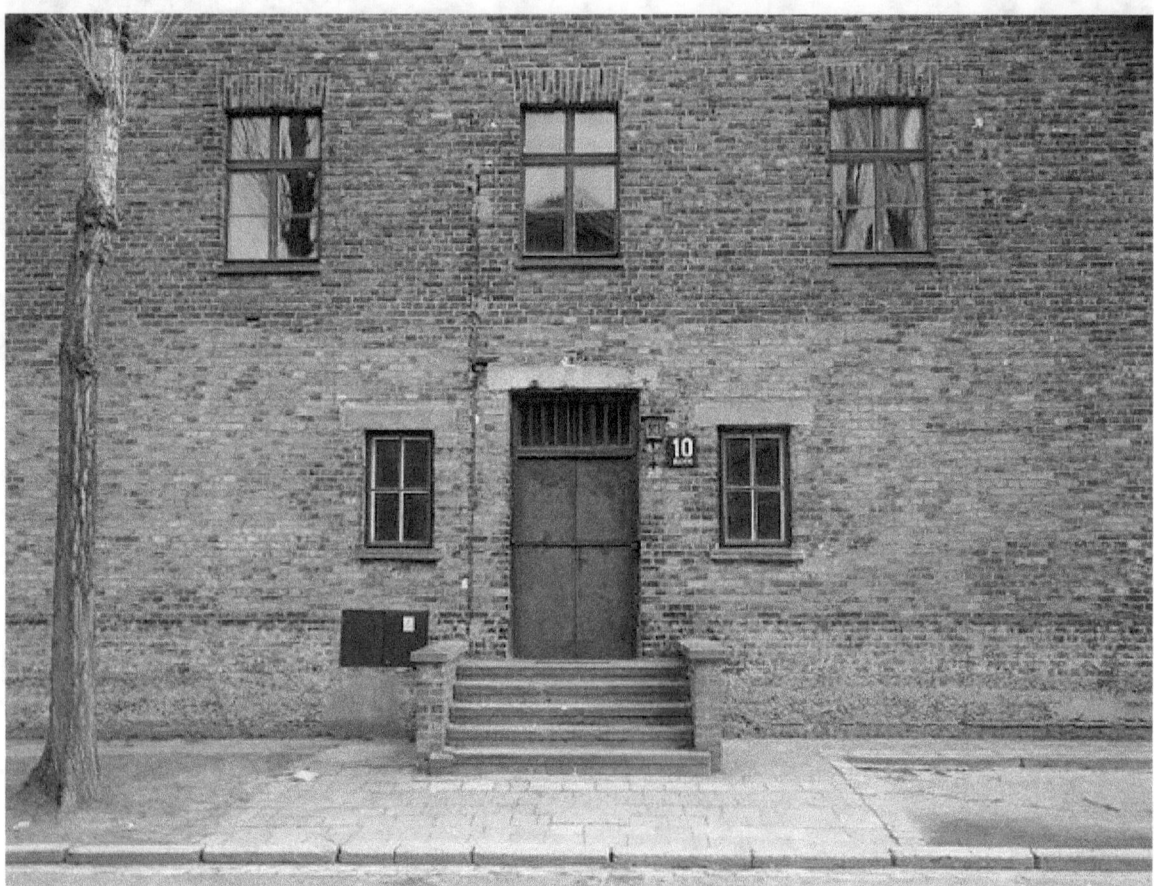

Block 10

Block 10 was a cellblock at the Auschwitz Concentration Camp where women and men were used as experimental subjects for German doctors. The experiments in Block 10 ranged from skin testing for reaction to relatively gentle substances to giving phenol injections to the heart for immediate dissection.

Although Block 10 was in the men's camps, the experiments conducted were mostly for women. To please the "elite" prisoners, the Germans would house prostitutes in Block 10. The main doctors who worked in Block 10 were Carl Clauberg, Horst Schumann, Eduard Wirths, Bruno Weber and August Hirt. Each of them had different methods in doing experiments on the inmates.

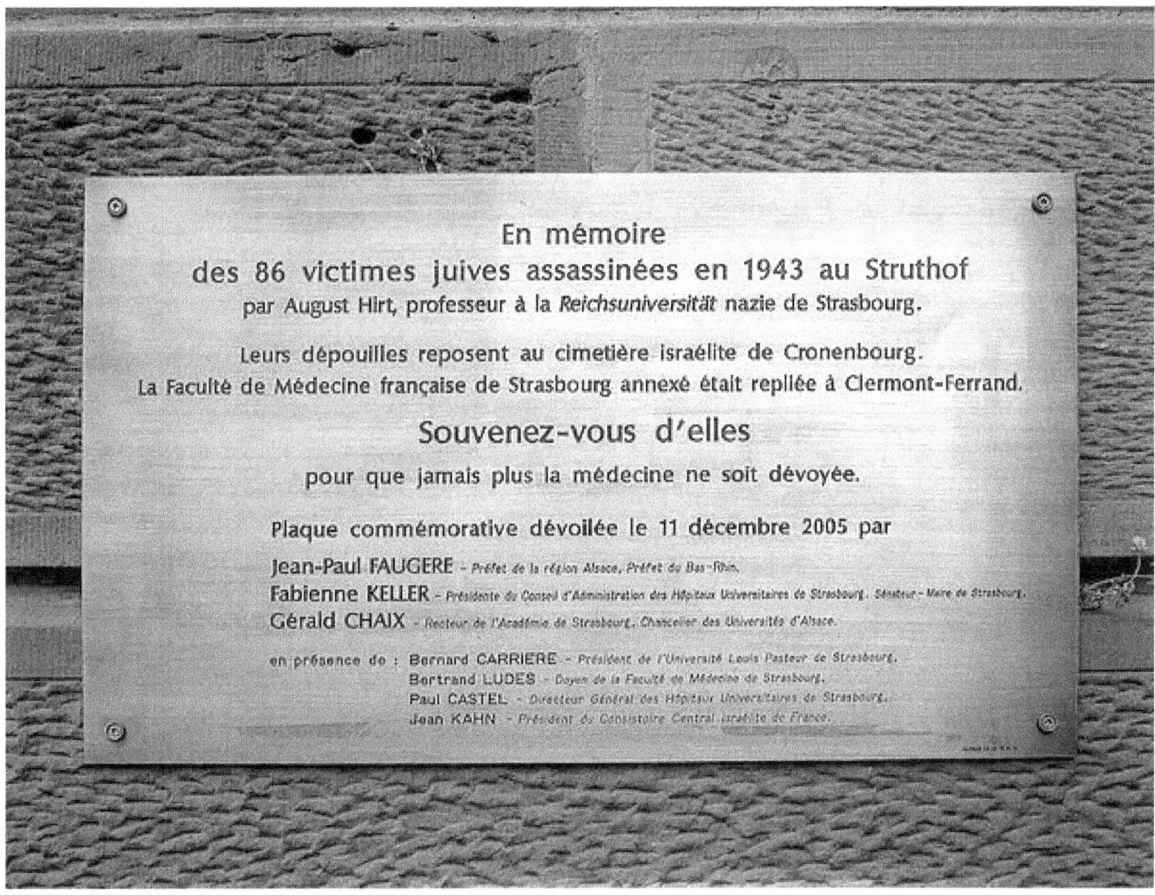

Memorial plaque at the Institute of Anatomy in Strasbourg. Translated, it reads, in part: "In memory of 86 Jews murdered in 1943 at Struthof by August Hirt, professor at the Nazi Reichsuniversität *in Strasbourg. Their remains rest in the Jewish cemetery in Cronenbourg....Remember them so that medicine shall never again be perverted."*

The victims at Auschwitz were also exported anywhere else experimental subjects were needed. For example, twenty Jewish children were transported to the Neuengamme concentration camp in Hamburg where they were injected with virulent tubercular serum and subjected to other experiments, and later murdered at the Bullenhuser Damm school.

3.1 The doctors

- Carl Clauberg — He focused on sterilization by injection. His method was to inject a caustic substance into the cervix in order to obstruct the fallopian tubes. His experimental subjects were married women between the ages of twenty and forty who had already had children.

- Horst Schumann — His experimental subjects were healthy men and women in their late teens or early twenties, on whom he attempted X-ray sterilization. Women were put between plates that pressed against abdomen and their back. He placed the men's penis and scrotum on a special plate. Radiation burns and intestinal damage were a frequent result.

3.2 References

- "Block 10". An Auschwitz Alphabet. Retrieved 2007-05-01.

- Ruth Jolanda Weinberger (2007-01-26). "The Deadly Origins of a Life-saving Procedure". *The Jewish Daily Forward*. Archived from the original on 2007-02-09. Retrieved 2007-05-01.

- Hans-Joachim Lang: *Die Frauen von Block 10. Medizinische Experimente in Auschwitz.* Hamburg 2011. ISBN 978-3-455-50222-0

Coordinates: 50°01′31″N 19°12′13″E / 50.0254°N 19.2035°E

Chapter 4

Franz von Bodmann

Franz Hermann Johann Maria Freiherr von Bodmann, sometimes written as **Bodman** (born 23 March 1908 in Zwiefaltendorf - died 25 May 1945 in Altenmarkt im Pongau) was a German SS-Obersturmführer who served as a camp physician in several Nazi concentration camps.

Von Bodmann joined the Nazi Party in May 1932 (membership number 1,098,482) and the SS itself in 1934 (member number 267,787). From October 1939 to June 1940 and from July 1941 to January 1942 he served with the 79th SS-Standarte in Ulm in the Second Bataillon as a physician.[1] It was 1941 that he was promoted to the rank of Obersturmführer.[2]

Von Bodmann was appointed camp physician at Auschwitz concentration camp in February 1942 and the following year held a similar position at Majdanek concentration camp.[1] He subsequently filled the same role at Natzweiler-Struthof concentration camp and from September 1943 at Vaivara concentration camp.[2] At some point he also worked at Neuengamme concentration camp although the exact dates are unknown.[2] Eyewitnesses claimed that at Auschwitz von Bodmann killed inmates personally by injecting Phenol into their veins and also stated that he carried out similar procedures at other camps.[3] Von Bodmann's departure from Auschwitz, where he had no superiors and as such acted largely as he pleased, was hastened when he contracted typhus not long after arriving.[4]

He left the camps in September 1944 when he was sent to work for SS-Wirtschafts-Verwaltungshauptamt and then to the Hauptamt Volksdeutsche Mittelstelle. His final assignment was as troop physician to the 5th SS Panzer Division Wiking.[1] He was taken as a prisoner of war and held in a military hospital where he killed himself just after the end of the Second World War.[2]

4.1 References

[1] Aleksander Lasik, 'Die Organisationsstruktur des KL Auschwitz', in: Aleksander Lasik, Franciszek Piper, Piotr Setkiewicz, Irena Strzelecka, *Auschwitz 1940-1945. Studien zur Geschichte des Konzentrations und Vernichtungslagers Auschwitz., Band I: Aufbau und Struktur des Lagers*, Staatliches Museum Auschwitz-Birkenau, Oświęcim 1999, p. 286

[2] Ernst Klee, *Das Personenlexikon zum Dritten Reich: Wer war was vor und nach 1945.*, Frankfurt am Main 2007, p. 57

[3] Ernst Klee, *Auschwitz, die NS-Medizin und ihre Opfer.*, Frankfurt am Main, 1997, p. 410

[4] Hermann Langbein, *People in Auschwitz*, UNC Press Books, 2004, p. 336

Chapter 5

Karl Brandt

For other people named Karl Brandt, see Karl Brandt (disambiguation).

Karl Brandt (January 8, 1904 – June 2, 1948) was a German physician and *Schutzstaffel* (SS) officer during the Third Reich. Trained in surgery, Brandt joined the Nazi Party in 1932 and became Adolf Hitler's escort physician in August 1934.[1] A member of Hitler's inner circle at the Berghof, he was selected by Philipp Bouhler, the head of Hitler's Chancellery, to administer the *Aktion T4* euthanasia program. Brandt was later appointed the Reich Commissioner of Sanitation and Health (*Bevollmächtiger für das Sanitäts und Gesundheitswesen*). Accused of involvement in human experimentation and other war crimes, Brandt was indicted in late 1946 and faced trial before a U.S. military tribunal along with 22 others in *United States of America v. Karl Brandt, et al*. He was convicted, sentenced to death, and later hanged on June 2, 1948.[2]

5.1 Early life

Brandt was born in Mulhouse in the then German Alsace-Lorraine territory (now in Haut-Rhin, France) into the family of a Prussian Army officer.[3] He became a medical doctor and surgeon in 1928, specializing in head and spinal injuries.[4] He joined the Nazi Party in January 1932, and first met Hitler in the summer of 1932.[5] He became a member of the SA in 1933 and a member of the SS on July 29, 1934; appointed the officer rank of *Untersturmführer*.[5] From the Summer of 1934 forward, he was Hitler's "Escort Physician". Karl Brandt married Anni Rehborn (born 1907), a champion swimmer, on March 17, 1934. They had one son, Karl Adolf Brandt (born October 4, 1935).

5.2 Career in the Third Reich

In the context of the 1933 Nazi law *Gesetz zur Verhütung erbkranken Nachwuchses* (Law for the Prevention of Hereditarily Diseased Offspring), he was one of the medical scientists who performed abortions in great numbers on women deemed genetically disordered, mentally or physically handicapped or racially deficient, or whose unborn fetuses were expected to develop such genetic "defects". These abortions had been legalized, as long as no healthy Aryan fetuses were aborted.[6]

On September 1, 1939, Brandt was appointed by Hitler co-head of the T-4 Euthanasia Program, with Philipp Bouhler.[7] Additional power was afforded Brandt when on July 28, 1942, he was appointed Commissioner of Sanitation and Health (*Bevollmächtiger für das Sanitäts und Gesundheitswesen*) by Hitler and was thereafter only bound by the Führer's instructions alone.[8] He received regular promotions in the SS; by April 1944, Brandt was a SS-*Gruppenführer* in the *Allgemeine-SS* and a SS-*Brigadeführer* in the Waffen-SS.[2] On April 16, 1945, he was arrested by the Gestapo for moving his family out of Berlin so they could surrender to American forces. He was condemned to death by a military court and then sent to Kiel.[5] Brandt was released from arrest by order of Karl Dönitz on May 2, 1945. He was later placed under arrest by the British on May 23, 1945.

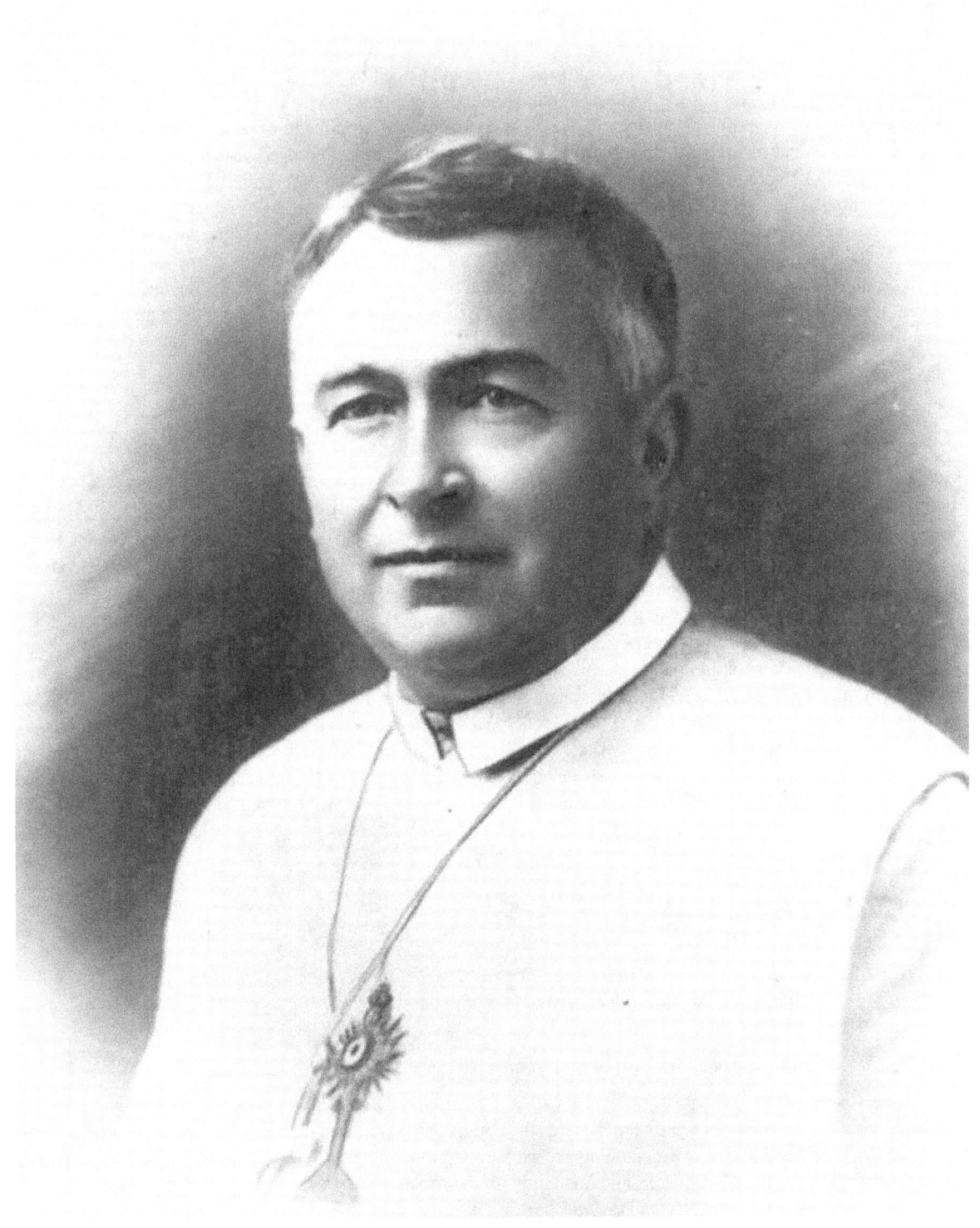

*Jan Maria Michał Kowalski **murdered** at Hartheim Euthanasia Centre.*

5.3 Brandt's medical ethics

See also: Action T4

Brandt's medical ethics, particularly regarding euthanasia, were influenced by Alfred Hoche, whose courses he attended. Like many other German doctors of the period, Brandt came to believe that the health of society as a whole should take precedence over that of its individual members. Because society was viewed as an organism that had to be cured, its weakest, most invalid and incurable members were only parts that should be removed. Such hapless creatures should therefore be granted a "merciful death" (*Gnadentod*).[9] In addition to these considerations, Brandt's explanation at his trial for his criminal actions – particularly ordering experimentation on human beings – was that "... Any personal code of ethics must give way to the total character of the war".[2] Historian Horst Freyhofer asserts that, in the absence of at least Brandt's "tacit" approval, it is highly unlikely that the grotesque and cruel medical experiments for which the Nazi doctors are infamous, could have been performed.[10] Brandt and Hitler discussed multiple killing techniques during the initial planning of the euthanasia program, during which Hitler asked Brandt, "which is the most humane way;" Brandt suggested the use of poisonous gas, whereupon the two agreed.[11]

5.4 Life in the inner circle

Karl Brandt and his wife Anni were members of Hitler's inner circle at Berchtesgaden where Hitler maintained his private residence known as the Berghof.[2] This very exclusive group functioned as Hitler's de facto family circle. It included Eva Braun, Albert Speer, his wife Margarete, Dr. Theodor Morell, Martin Bormann, Hitler's photographer Heinrich Hoffmann, Hitler's adjutants and his secretaries. Brandt and Hitler's chief architect Albert Speer were good friends as the two shared technocratic dispositions about their work. Brandt looked at killing "useless eaters" and the handicapped as a means to an end, namely since it was in the interest of public health. Similarly, Speer viewed the use of concentration camp labor for his defense and building projects in much the same way.[12] As members of this inner circle, the Brandts had a residence near the Berghof and spent extensive time there when Hitler was present. In his memoirs, Speer described the familial but numbing lifestyle of Hitler's intimate companions who were forced to stay up most of the night—night after night—listening to the Nazi leader's repetitive monologues or to an unvarying selection of music. Despite Brandt's personal closeness to Hitler, the dictator was furious when he learned shortly before the end of the war that the doctor had sent Anni and their son toward the American lines in hopes of evading capture by the Russians.[2] Only the intervention of Heinrich Himmler, Albert Speer, and the direct order of Admiral Doenitz after Brandt had been captured by the Gestapo and sent to Kiel in the war's closing days, saved him from execution.[2]

5.5 Trial and execution

Brandt was tried along with twenty-two others at the Palace of Justice in Nuremberg, Germany. The trial was officially titled *United States of America v. Karl Brandt et al.*, but is more commonly referred to as the "Doctors' Trial"; it began on December 9, 1946. He was charged with four counts:

1) Conspiracy to commit war crimes and crimes against humanity as described in counts 2 and 3;

2) War crimes: performing medical experiments, without the subjects' consent, on prisoners of war and civilians of occupied countries, in the course of which experiments the defendants committed murders, brutalities, cruelties, tortures, atrocities, and other inhuman acts. Also planning and performing the mass murder of prisoners of war and civilians of occupied countries, stigmatized as aged, insane, incurably ill, deformed, and so on, by gas, lethal injections, and diverse other means in nursing homes, hospitals, and asylums during the Euthanasia Program and participating in the mass murder of concentration camp inmates;

3) Crimes against humanity: committing crimes described under count 2 also on German nationals;

4) Membership in a criminal organization, the SS. The charges against him included special responsibility for, and participation in, Freezing, Malaria, LOST Gas, Sulfanilamide, Bone, Muscle and Nerve Regeneration and Bone Transplantation, Sea-Water, Epidemic Jaundice, Sterilization, and Typhus Experiments.[13]

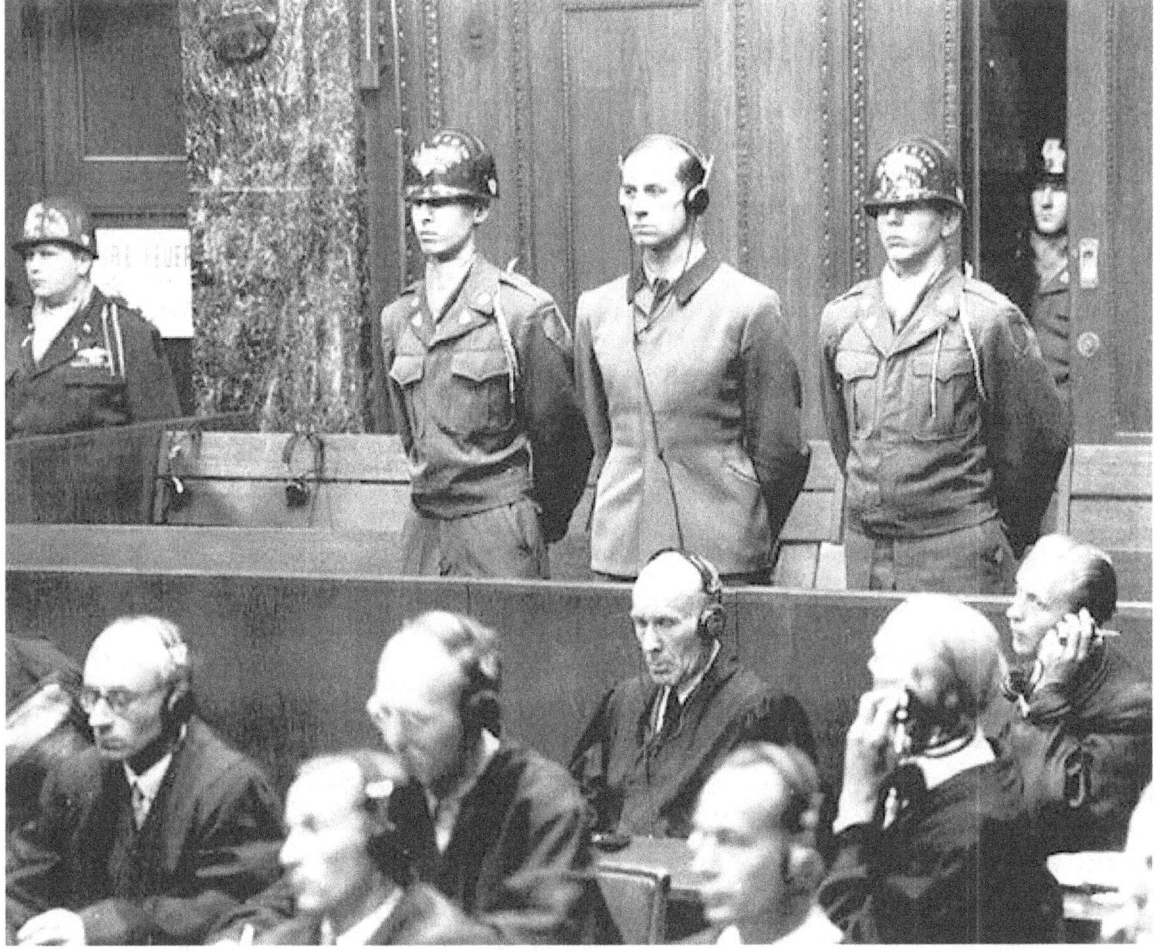

Brandt on trial, August 20, 1947

After a defense led by Robert Servatius, on August 19, 1947, Brandt was found guilty on counts 2-4 of the indictment. With six others, he was sentenced to death by hanging, and all were executed at Landsberg Prison on June 2, 1948.[2] Nine other defendants received prison terms of between fifteen years and life, while a further seven were found not guilty.[14]

While on the gallows, Brandt remarked: "It is no shame to stand upon the scaffold. This is nothing but political revenge. I have served my Fatherland as others before me ..." His speech was cut short when a black hood was placed over his head.[15]

5.6   See also

- Action 14f13

- Nazi human experimentation

- Nazi Germany

5.7   Notes

[1] Ben-Amos, Batsheva. "Karl Brandt: The Nazi Doctor. Medicine and Power in the Third Reich (review)". Retrieved 10 November 2014.

[2] Hamilton 1984, p. 138.

[3] Schmidt: Hitlers Arzt, Berlin 2009, ISBN 978-3-351-02671-4

[4] Lifton, Robert Jay (1986). *The Nazi Doctors: Medical Killing and the Psychology of Genocide*. United States: Basic Books. p. 114. ISBN 0-465-04905-2. Retrieved 2013-03-23.

[5] Joachimsthaler 1999, p. 296.

[6] 1935: Das Gesetz zur Änderung des Gesetzes zur Verhütung erbkranken Nachwuchses führt eine von der nationalsozialistischen Haltung zu Eugenik und Sterilisation motivierte Option auf Schwangerschaftsabbruch bei einer zu Sterilisierenden (Sechs-Monats-Fristenregelung) ein. Formale Bedingung für eine straffreie Abtreibung war unter anderem die „Einwilligung der Schwangeren"; in der Praxis dürften die Wünsche und Vorbehalte von als „minderwertig" definierten Frauen allerdings oft missachtet worden sein.

[7] Thompson, D.: *The Nazi Euthanasia Program*, Axis History Forum, March 14, 2004. URL last accessed April 24, 2006.

[8] Götz Aly, Peter Chroust, and Christian Pross, eds., *Cleansing the Fatherland: Nazi Medicine and Racial Hygiene* (Baltimore: Johns Hopkins University Press, 1994), p. 76.

[9] Lifton (1986). *The Nazi Doctors: Medical Killing and the Psychology of Genocide*, p. 64

[10] Horst Freyhofer, *Nuremberg Medical Trial* (New York: Peter Lang Publishing, 2004), 51.

[11] NARA, RG 238: Interrogation of Karl Brandt, 01 October 1945 p.m., p. 7. As found in *Origins of Nazi Genocide: From Euthanasia to the Final Solution* by Henry Friedlander (Chapel Hill: University of North Carolina Press, 1997), p. 86.

[12] Lifton, (1986) *The Nazi Doctors: Medical Killing and the Psychology of Genocide*, p. 115.

[13] National Archives and Records Administration, Records of the United States Nuremberg War Crimes Trials, 15 vols. See vol 1 and 2, *Karl Brandt: The Medical Case* (Washington DC: National Archives and Records Service, 1951-1952).

[14] See U.S. Library of Congress, Nuremberg Tribunal Indictments at: http://www.loc.gov/rr/frd/Military_Law/pdf/NT_Indictments.pdf

[15] Annas, George J. (1995). *The Nazi Doctors and the Nuremberg Code*. United States: Oxford University Press. p. 106. ISBN 0-19-507042-9. Retrieved 2015-03-03.

5.8 References

- Aly, Götz, Peter Chroust, and Christian Pross, eds. *Cleansing the Fatherland: Nazi Medicine and Racial Hygiene*. Baltimore: Johns Hopkins University Press, 1994.

- Burleigh, Michael, and Wolfgang Wippermann. *The Racial State: Germany 1933-1945*. Cambridge & New York: Cambridge University Press, 1991.

- Dawidowicz, Lucy S. *The War Against the Jews: 1933-1945*. New York: Bantam Books Inc., 1975.

- Ehrenreich, Eric. *The Nazi Ancestral Proof: Genealogy, Racial Science, and the Final Solution*. Bloomington: Indiana University Press, 2007.

- Freyhofer, Horst. *Nuremberg Medical Trial*. New York: Peter Lang Publishing, 2004.

- Friedlander, Henry. *Origins of Nazi Genocide: From Euthanasia to the Final Solution*. Chapel Hill: University of North Carolina Press, 1997.

- Fritz, Stephen G. *Ostkrieg: Hitler's War of Extermination in the East*. Lexington: The University Press of Kentucky, 2011.

- Hamilton, Charles (1984). *Leaders & Personalities of the Third Reich, Vol. 1*. R. James Bender Publishing. ISBN 0-912138-27-0.

- Hutton, Christopher. *Race and the Third Reich: Linguistics, Racial Anthropology and Genetics in the Dialectic of Volk*. Cambridge: Cambridge University Press, 2005.

- Joachimsthaler, Anton (1999) [1995]. *The Last Days of Hitler: The Legends, the Evidence, the Truth*. Trans. Helmut Bögler. London: Brockhampton Press. ISBN 978-1-86019-902-8.

- Koonz, Claudia. *The Nazi Conscience*. Cambridge, MA: Belknap Press of Harvard University Press, 2005.

- Lifton, Robert Jay. *The Nazi Doctors: Medical Killing and the Psychology of Genocide*. New York: Basic Books, 1986.

- Mayer, Arno. *Why Did the Heavens Not Darken?: The "Final Solution" in History*. London & New York: Verso Publishing, 2012.

- Proctor, Robert. *Racial Hygiene: Medicine under the Nazis*. Cambridge, MA: Harvard University Press, 1988.

- Schafft, Gretchen E. *From Racism to Genocide: Anthropology in the Third Reich*. Urbana and Chicago: University of Illinois Press, 2004.

- Schmidt, Ulf. *Karl Brandt: The Nazi Doctor: Medicine and Power in the Third Reich*. London, Hambledon Continuum, 2007.

- Skopp, Douglas R., *Shadows Walking, A Novel* (CreateSpace, Charlestown, South Carolina, 2010) ISBN 1439231990

- Spitz, Vivien. *Doctors from Hell: The Horrific Account of Nazi Experiments on Humans*. Boulder, CO: Sentient Publications, 2005.

Chapter 6

Bullenhuser Damm

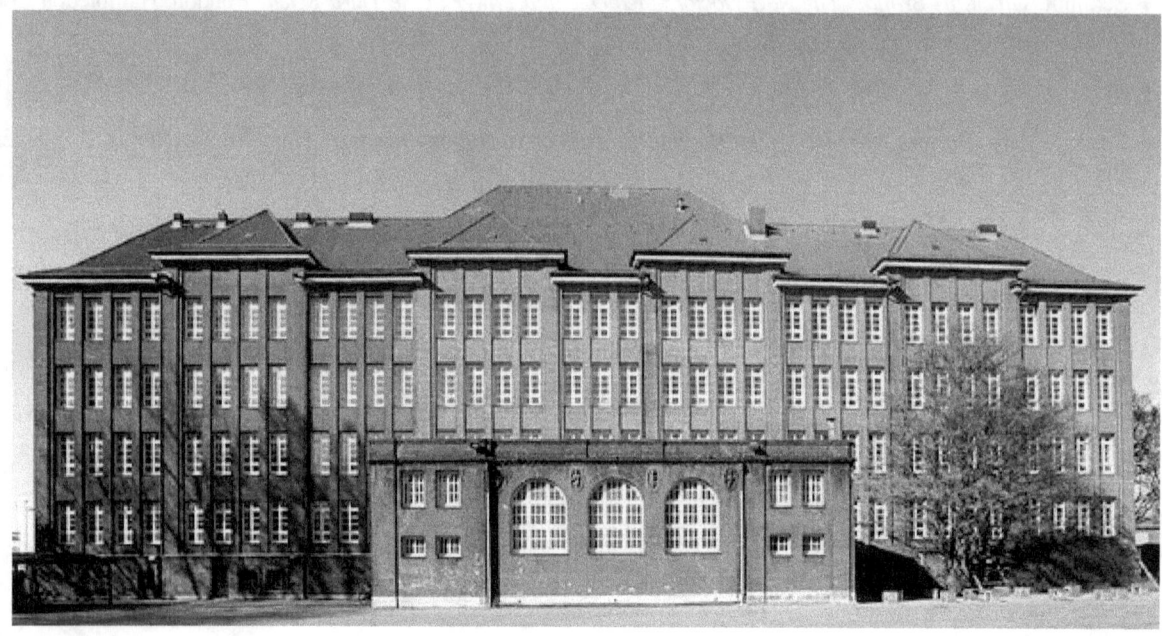

The school at Bullenhuser Damm

The **Bullenhuser Damm** School is located at 92–94 Bullenhuser Damm, a street in the Rothenburgsort section of Hamburg, Germany. During heavy air raids, many portions of Hamburg were destroyed including the Rothenburgsort section which received heavy damage.[1] The school was only slightly damaged. By 1943, the surrounding area was largely obliterated so the building was no longer needed as a school. In October 1944,[2] a subcamp of the Neuengamme concentration camp was established in the school to house prisoners used in clearing the rubble after air raids. The Bullenhauser Damm School was evacuated on April 11, 1945. Two SS men were left to guard the school: SS Unterscharführer Johann Frahm and SS Oberscharführer Ewald Jauch, and the janitor Wilhelm Wede.

On the night of April 20, 1945, 20 Jewish children who had been used in medical experiments at Neuengamme, their four adult Jewish caretakers and six Red Army prisoners of war (POWs) were killed in the basement of the school.[3] Later that evening, 24 Soviet POWs who had also been used in the experiments were brought to the school to be murdered. The names, ages and countries of origin were recorded by Hans Meyer, one of the thousands of Scandinavian prisoners released to the custody of Sweden in the closing months of the war. Neuengamme was used as a transit camp for these prisoners.[4]

21

6.1 Background

The SS physician Kurt Heissmeyer desired to obtain a professorship. In order to do so he needed to present original research. Although previously disproven, his hypothesis was that the injection of live tuberculosis bacilli into subjects would act as a vaccine. Another component of his experimentation was based on pseudoscientific Nazi racial theory that race played a factor in developing tuberculosis.

He attempted to prove his hypothesis by injecting live tuberculosis bacilli into the lungs and bloodstream of "Untermenschen" (subhumans), Jews and Slavs being considered by the Nazis to be racially inferior to Germans.

He was able to have the facilities made available and to test his subjects as a result of his personal connections: his uncle, SS general August Heissmeyer, and his close acquaintance, SS general Oswald Pohl.[5]

The medical experiments on tuberculosis infection were initially carried out on prisoners from the Soviet Union and other countries at the Neuengamme concentration camp. The experiments were then extended to Jews. For this he chose to use Jewish children. Twenty Jewish children (10 boys and 10 girls) from Auschwitz concentration camp were chosen by Josef Mengele and sent to Neuengamme. Mengele allegedly asked the children, "Who wants to go and see their mother?"

The children were accompanied to Neuengamme by four women prisoners. Two were Polish nurses and one was a Hungarian pharmacist, and they were killed upon arrival at Neuengamme. The fourth woman, Polish-born Jew Paula Trocki, was a doctor. She survived the war and later gave testimony in Jerusalem about what she had witnessed:

> The transport was accompanied by an SS guard. There were 20 children, one female medical doctor, three nurses. The transport was in a separate carriage that was coupled on a normal train. Presented in this manner it appeared to be an ordinary carriage. We had to take off the stars of David lest we attract any attention. To prevent people from approaching us they said it was a transport of people suffering from typhoid fever... The food was excellent; on that journey we were given chocolate and milk. After a two-day trip we arrived at Neuengamme at ten o'clock at night.
>
> — Paula Trocki, [6]

The children were injected with live tuberculosis bacilli, and they all became ill. Heissmeyer then had their axillary lymph nodes surgically removed from their armpits and sent to Dr Hans Klein at the Hohenlychen Hospital for study. All the children were photographed holding up one arm to show the surgical incision. Dr Klein was not prosecuted.

The collapsing western front and imminent approach of British troops prompted the perpetrators to murder the subjects of the experiment to cover up their crimes. The orders for the murders were issued from Berlin.

The children, their four adult caretakers and six Soviet prisoners were brought by truck to the Bullenhuser Damm School in the Hamburg suburb of Rothenburgsort. The school had been taken over by the SS to house prisoners from Neuengamme used to clear rubble from the surrounding area after Allied bombing raids. The SS evacuated the building around April 11, 1945 leaving a skeleton crew of two SS guards: Ewald Jauch and Johann Frahm and a janitor. They were accompanied by three SS guards (Wilhelm Dreimann, Adolf Speck, and Heinrich Wiehagen), as well as the driver, Hans Friedrich Petersen, and SS physician Alfred Trzebinski. The children as well as others were told they were being taken to Theresienstadt. Upon arriving at the school they were led into the basement. According to one of the SS men present, the children "sat down on the benches all around and were cheerful and happy that they had been for once allowed out of Neuengamme. The children were completely unsuspecting."

They were then made to undress and were then injected with morphine by Trzebinski. They were then led into an adjacent room and hanged from hooks set into the wall. The execution was overseen by SS Obersturmführer Arnold Strippel. The first child to be hanged was so light that the noose would not tighten. Frahm grabbed him in a bearhug and used his own weight to pull down and tighten the noose. The adults were hanged from overhead pipes; they were made to stand on a box, which was pulled away from under them. That same night, about 30 additional Soviet prisoners were also brought by lorry to the school to be executed; six escaped, three were shot trying to do so, and the rest were hanged in the basement.[7]

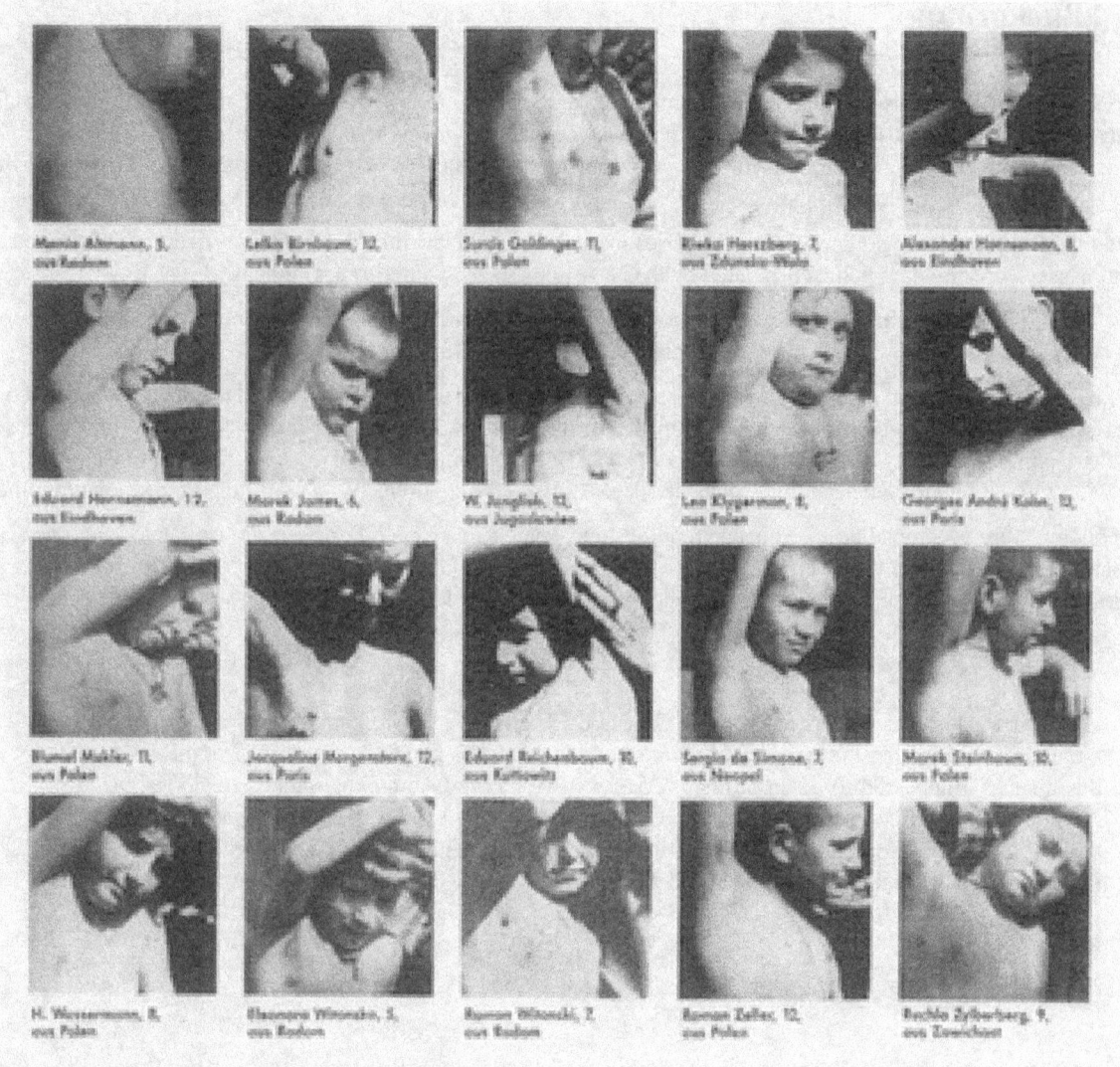

The children being forced to show the location of the scar where the axillary lymph nodes were excised.

6.2 Victims

- Marek James, a boy aged 6, from Radom, Poland; prisoner no. B 1159.

- H. Wassermann, a girl aged 8, from Poland.

- Roman Witonski, a boy aged 6, and his sister; prisoner number A-15160.

- Eleonora Witonska, a girl aged 5, from Radom, Poland; prisoner number A-15159. (Roman and Eleanora were deported to Auschwitz along with their mother, Rucza Witonska (prisoner number A-15158) from the ghetto in Radom, Poland. Their father, Seweryn Witonski, a pediatrician from Radom, was gunned down at an execution in the Szydlowiec cemetery. Ruzca worked in the laboratory of Josef Mengele. In November 1944, the children were separated from their mother when she was sent to the concentration camp in Gebhardsdorf in Lower Silesia. Roman and Eleonora were sent to the "Kinderheim" (orphanage) at Auschwitz. Rucza survived the war and tried to find her children. She later remarried. Rosa Grumelin has visited the memorial)[8]

- Roman Zeller, a boy aged 12, from Poland.

- Riwka Herszberg, a girl aged 7, from Zdunska Wola, Poland. (Her parents were Mania and Moishe Herszberg. They were kept in the family barracks for a period of time. Her mother survived the war.)

- Mania Altmann, a girl aged 5, from Radom, Poland.

- Surcis Goldinger, a girl aged 11, from Poland.

- Lelka Birnbaum, a girl aged 12, from Poland.

- Ruchla Zylberberg, a girl aged 8, from Zawichost, Poland. (Ruchla's sister, Esther, and her mother, Fajga (née Rosenblum), were gassed upon arrival in Auschwitz. Her father, Nison Zylberberg, survived the war in the Soviet Union, with his brother, Henry, and his sister, Felicja; he then emigrated to the United States. He died in Colorado on September 29, 2002 at the age of 86. He visited the memorial.)[9]

- Eduard Reichenbaum, a boy aged 10, from Katowice, Poland. (His brother Itzhak survived the war and emigrated to Haifa, Israel.)

- Blumel Mekler, a girl aged 11, from Sandomierz, Poland. (Her sister, Shifra, survived the war because, as she recalled, her mother told her to "run! Shifra! run!" as the round-up began. She was 8 at this time, and Blumel was 5. She was kept hidden by a Polish family. She emigrated to Tel Aviv, Israel and married. She has visited the memorial.)

- Eduard (Edo) Hornemann, a boy aged 12. (Born on January 1, 1933), he lived with his mother, Elisabeth, his father, Philip, and his brother, Alexander, at 29 Staringstraat in Eindhoven, the Netherlands. His parents worked at the Philips factory. Philip died on February 21, 1945 at Sachsenhausen, where he arrived after a stop at Dachau with the "death march". Elisabeth died of typhus in Auschwitz in October 1944.

- Alexander Hornemann, a boy aged 9. (b. May 31, 1936.)

- Georges André Kohn, a boy aged 12, from Paris, France. (b. April 23, 1932.)

- Jacqueline Morgenstern, a girl aged 12, from Paris. (b. May 26, 1932. A cousin, Henry Morgenstern, survived the war and has visited the memorial.)

- Sergio de Simone, a boy aged 7, from Naples, Italy; prisoner no. 179694. (b. November 29, 1937. Son of Italian Eduardo de Simone and his Yugoslav Jewish wife Gisella (née Perlow). Arrested March 21, 1944 in Fiume. First sent to San Sabba then on March 29, 1944 to Auschwitz. His mother survived the war and has visited the memorial.)

- Marek Steinbaum, a boy aged 10, from Radom, Poland. (His sister, Lola, survived the war and emigrated to the USA, living in San Francisco; she has visited the memorial.)

- W. Junglieb, a boy[10] aged 12, from Yugoslavia.

- Lea Klygermann, a girl aged 12, from Poland; prisoner no. A 16959.

The children were in the care of four male prisoners, two French professors and two Dutch prisoners, all of whom had been imprisoned because of their anti-German activities.

The two French professors were:

- Professor René Quenouille (b. December 6, 1887 in Lyon). He was a physician and radiologist at a hospital in Villeneuve-Saint-Georges, near Paris and a member of the French Resistance. He was arrested by the Gestapo, together with his wife, Yvonne, on March 3, 1943. Yvonne was released after three and a half months, but he was sentenced to death, although the sentence was later commuted to imprisonment.

- Professor Gabriel Florence (b. June 12, 1884). He was a biologist who taught at the University of Lyon. He fought in World War I and joined the French Resistance during World War II. He was arrested by the Gestapo on March 4, 1944.

The two Dutch prisoners were:

- Anton Holzel (b. May 7, 1909), who came from Deventer. He was a driver and a member of the Dutch Communist Party, who joined the Resistance after the German invasion. He became a waiter at the Novotel Den Haag, a hotel in The Hague, to facilitate the transfer of messages. He was arrested on September 11, 1941 and sent to Buchenwald. He was later transferred to Neuengamme.[11]

- Dirk Deutekom (b. December 12, 1895), who was a typographer. A member of the Dutch Resistance, he tried to hinder the deportation of Dutch Jews from the Netherlands. He was arrested in July, 1941 and sent to Buchenwald, where he was given a job in the infirmary, owing to his fluency in German. On June 6, 1944 he was transferred to the concentration camp at Neuengamme.

6.3   Criminal prosecutions

Some of those involved in the killings were tried by the British in the Curio Haus in Hamburg in 1946. Trzebinski, Neuengamme commandant Max Pauly, Dreimann, Speck, Jauch and Frahm were convicted and given the death sentence. They were hanged on October 8, 1946.

Two of those directly responsible for the children's suffering and murder, Kurt Heissmeyer and Arnold Strippel, escaped and remained at large. Strippel had served at other concentration camps before Neuengamme, including Buchenwald. He was recognized on the street in Frankfurt in 1948 by a former Buchenwald prisoner. He was tried for the murders of 21 Jewish inmates committed on November 9, 1939 as retribution for the failed assassination of Adolf Hitler at the Bürgerbräukeller in Munich by Georg Elser. Strippel was tried, convicted and sentenced to 21 life terms by a Frankfurt court in 1949.

In 1964, an investigation into his involvement with the Bullinghauser Damm School murders was begun by the Hamburg prosecutor's office. The statute of limitations had run out for manslaughter so he had to be charged with murder. Among the criteria for murder it had to be proven that the accused acted cruelly, insidiously or with motive. In 1967 the prosecutor, Helmut Münzberg, dropped the charges for lack of evidence, stating that Strippel had not acted cruelly as "the children had not been harmed beyond the extinction of their lives".

He was released from prison in 1969. After his release, he applied for a retrial, and in 1970 his original conviction was overturned and he was retried. At this retrial, he was convicted as being just an accessory to the Buchenwald murders and sentenced to six years' imprisonment. Because he had already served 20 years in prison, 14 years longer than this sentence, he was compensated with 121,477.92 Deutschmarks.

In 1979, partly as a result of articles written by Günther Schwarberg, Strippel's case was reopened. He was not reincarcerated, and in 1987 the case was abandoned by the Hamburg prosecutor's office, owing to Strippel's frailty.[12] Strippel died on May 1, 1994.

Kurt Heissmeyer returned to his home in Magdeburg in postwar East Germany and started a successful medical practice as a lung and tuberculosis specialist. He was eventually found out in 1959. In 1966, he was convicted and sentenced to life imprisonment. At his trial he stated, "I did not think that inmates of a camp had full value as human beings." When asked why he did not use guinea pigs he responded, "For me there was no basic difference between human beings and guinea pigs." He then corrected himself: "Jews and guinea pigs".[13] Heissmeyer died on August 29, 1967.

6.4   Memorial

The building at Bullenhuser Damm was used by the British as a transit camp for German POWs until 1947. It was then used by the Hydrograpichal Institute's meteorological service until 1949, when it again became a school, for 800 boys. In 1959, the organization representing Neuengamme survivors proposed to the Hamburg school board that a memorial plaque should be placed in the school. However, it was not until 1963 that the text for the plaque was approved. The text aroused controversy because it omitted mention of the Soviet victims and did not state that the children were Jewish or give any information about their personal identity. In 1980, information signs were placed in the basement of the school, and the Senate of Hamburg (government) declared the school to be a memorial site, renaming it Janusz Korczak School: Korczak was a Polish—Jewish pediatrician and author who died at Treblinka extermination camp with about 190 orphans.

A rose garden was established in 1985. Later, in the Schnelsen Quarter of the city several streets were named after the children who died at the school and a memorial tablet was installed. Much of the work of identifying the victims and of bringing the story to the public's attention was due to the efforts of Günther Schwarberg.[14]

In 2005, Wolfgang Peiner, Minister of Finance of Hamburg, published plans to sell the building. However, after several protests a spokesman denied these plans.

In 2011 a new exhibition (telling the story in German and English) was opened at the Memorial.

6.5   See also

- List of subcamps of Neuengamme

- Cap Arcona

6.6   References

[1] *Under the Bombs: The German Home Front, 1942–1945* By Earl R. Beck Publisher: The University Press of Kentucky (August 26, 1999) Language:English ISBN 0-8131-0977-9 ISBN 978-0-8131-0977-0

[2] http://bundesrecht.juris.de/begdv_6/anlage_6.html Official list (German)

[3] "Die Schule am Bullenhuser Damm" (in German). Retrieved 2008-04-20.

[4] *Bystanders to the Holocaust: a re-evaluation* By David Cesarani, Paul A. Levine page 246 Publisher: Routledge; illustrated edition (January 1, 2002) Language: English ISBN 0-7146-8243-8 ISBN 978-0-7146-8243-3

[5] Page 84–85: *Medicine and medical ethics in Nazi Germany: origins, practices, legacies* By Francis R. Nicosia, Publisher: Berghahn Books; illustrated edition (April 1, 2002) Language: English ISBN 1-57181-386-1 ISBN 978-1-57181-386-2

[6] Neumann, p. 141

[7] Neumann, Klaus (2000-12-22). *Shifting Memories: The Nazi Past in the New Germany (Social History, Popular Culture, and Politics in Germany)*. University of Michigan Press. ISBN 978-0-472-08710-5.

[8] Zwanzig Kinder erhängen dauert lange

[9] Shalom Funeral Service

[10] Die Schule am Bullenhuser Damm (The School in Bullenhuser Damm)

[11] *The Second World War: A Complete History* By Martin Gilbert Publisher: Holt Paperbacks; Revised edition (June 1, 2004) Language: English ISBN 0-8050-7623-9 ISBN 978-0-8050-7623-3

[12] *Shifting memories: the Nazi past in the new Germany* By Klaus Neumann: Page 143

[13] *Admitting the Holocaust: Collected Essays* By Lawrence L. Langer Publisher: Oxford University Press, USA (June 20, 1996) Language: English ISBN 0-19-510648-2 ISBN 978-0-19-510648-0

[14] Page 246: *Man, medicine, and the state: the human body as an object of government ...* By Wolfgang Uwe Publisher: Franz Steiner Verlag (December 1, 2006) Language: English ISBN 3-515-08794-X ISBN 978-3-515-08794-0

6.6.1   Bibliography

- Günther Schwarberg: *Meine zwanzig Kinder*. Steidl, Göttingen 1996, ISBN 3-88243-431-7 (German)

- Günther Schwarberg: *The murders at Bullenhuser Damm: the SS Doctor and the Children*. Bloomington: Indiana University Press, 1984. ISBN 978-0-253-15481-1

- Detlef Garbe, Günther Schwarberg: *Die Kinder vom Bullenhuser Damm.* Hamburg: Museum fuer Hamburgische Geschichte, 1995 (German)

- Gedenkstätte Bullenhuser Damm - Geschichte des Ortes, der Opfer und der Erinnerung. Hamburg, 2011 (German)

- The Bullenhuser Damm Memorial - The site, the victims and the history of commemoration. Hamburg, 2011

- »... dass du weißt, was hier passiert ist«: Medizinische Experimente im KZ Neuengamme und die Morde am Bullenhuser Damm. Bremen, 2012. ISBN 978-3-8378-2022-5 (German)

6.7   External links

- The 20 Children of Bullenhuser Damm (Italian)

- Georges-André Kohn at the Memorial to the Murdered Jews of Europe In Berlin

- Phillipe Kohn speaks about his brother's deportation and death

- Bullenhuser Damm (Dutch)

- Documentary on Sergio de Simone (Italian)

- Neuengamme Concentration Camp Memorial

- VR Movie: Rose Garden for the Children of Bullenhuser Damm

- Zeit Online The amazing career of the prosecutor Münzberg (German) - removed by Die Zeit from the on-line pages

Coordinates: 53°32′31″N 10°2′53″E / 53.54194°N 10.04806°E

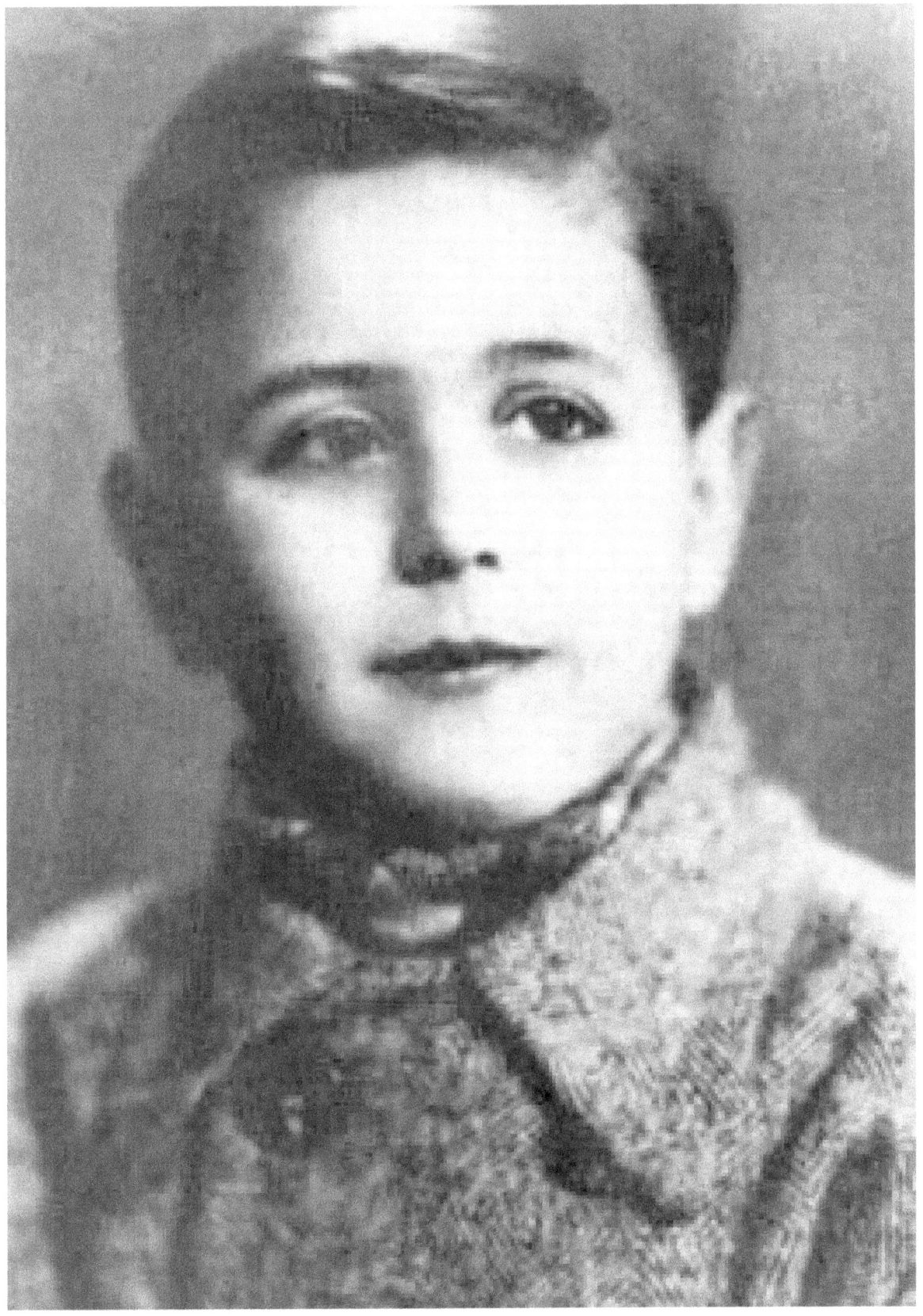

Sergio de Simone (b. Nov. 29, 1937 d. April 20, 1945) 7 yr. old Jewish Italian boy killed at the Bullenhauser Damm School

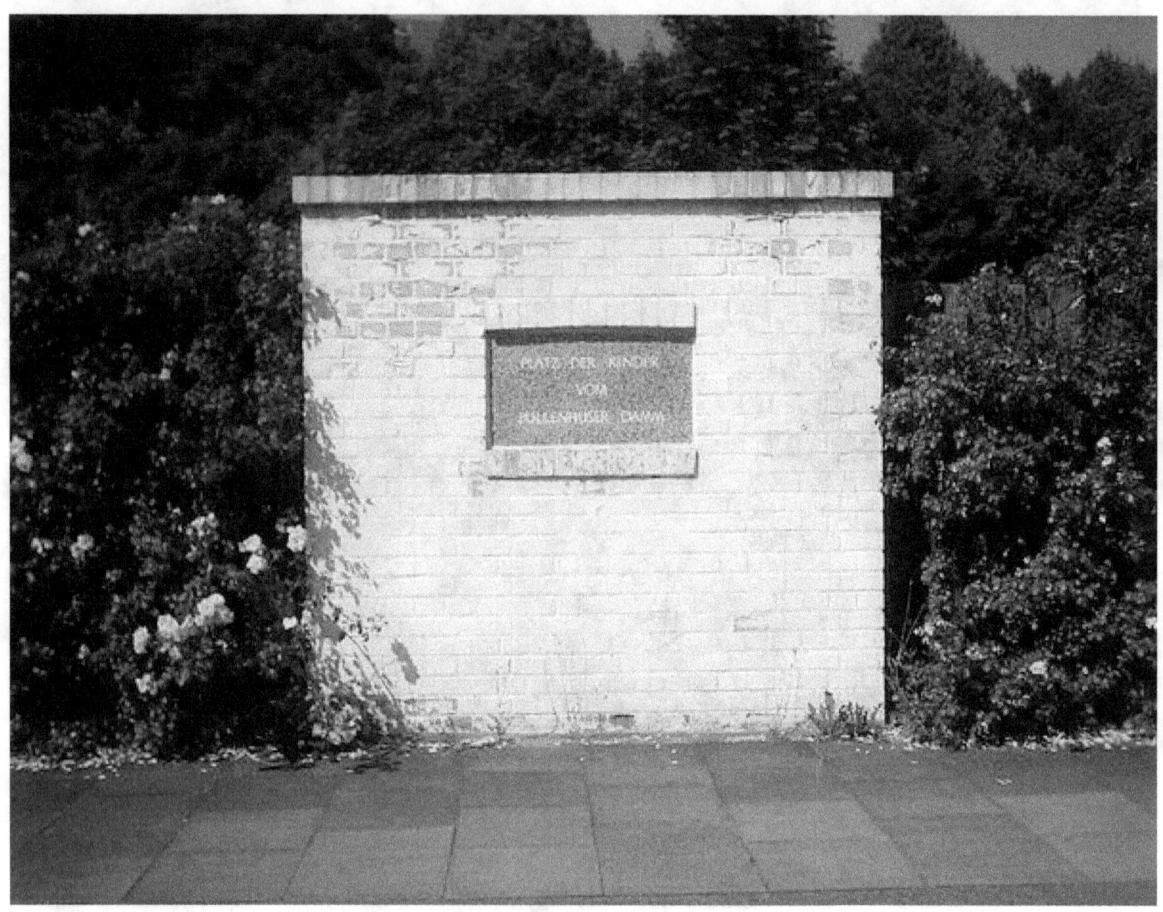

"Place of children from Bullenhuser Damm" in Hamburg, Germany.

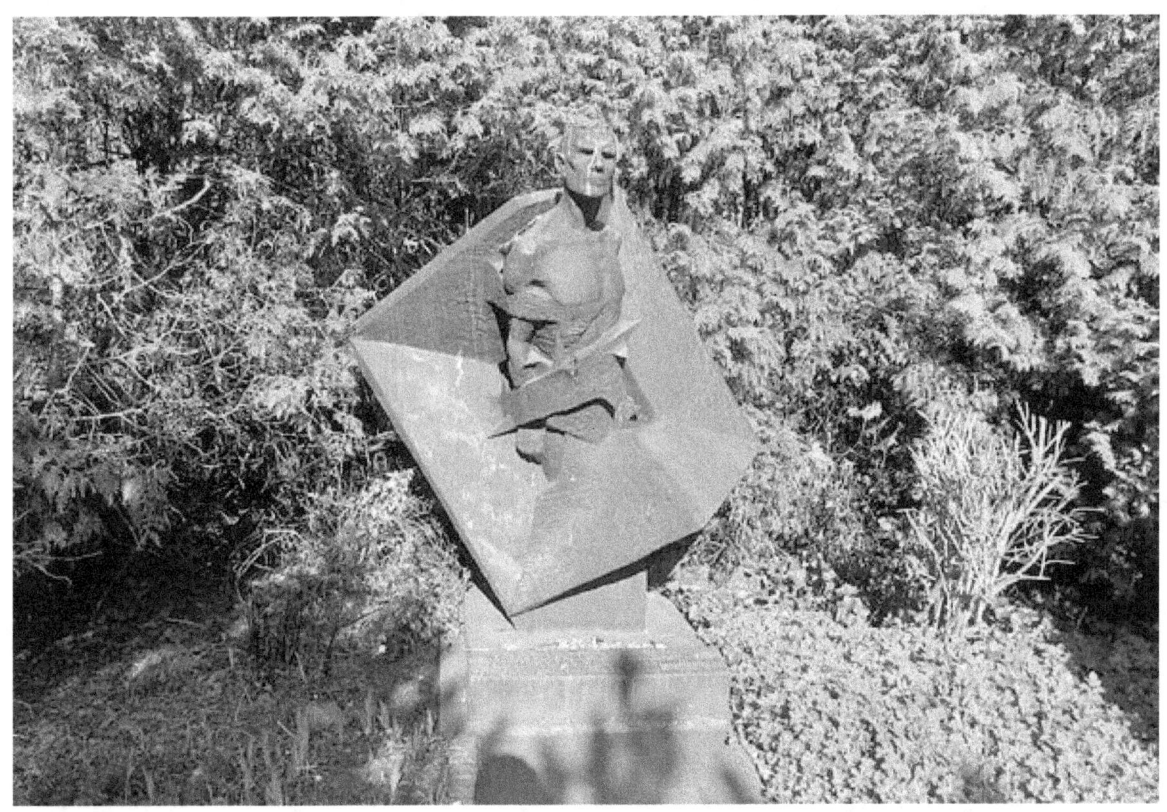

Memorial for the Russian prisoners

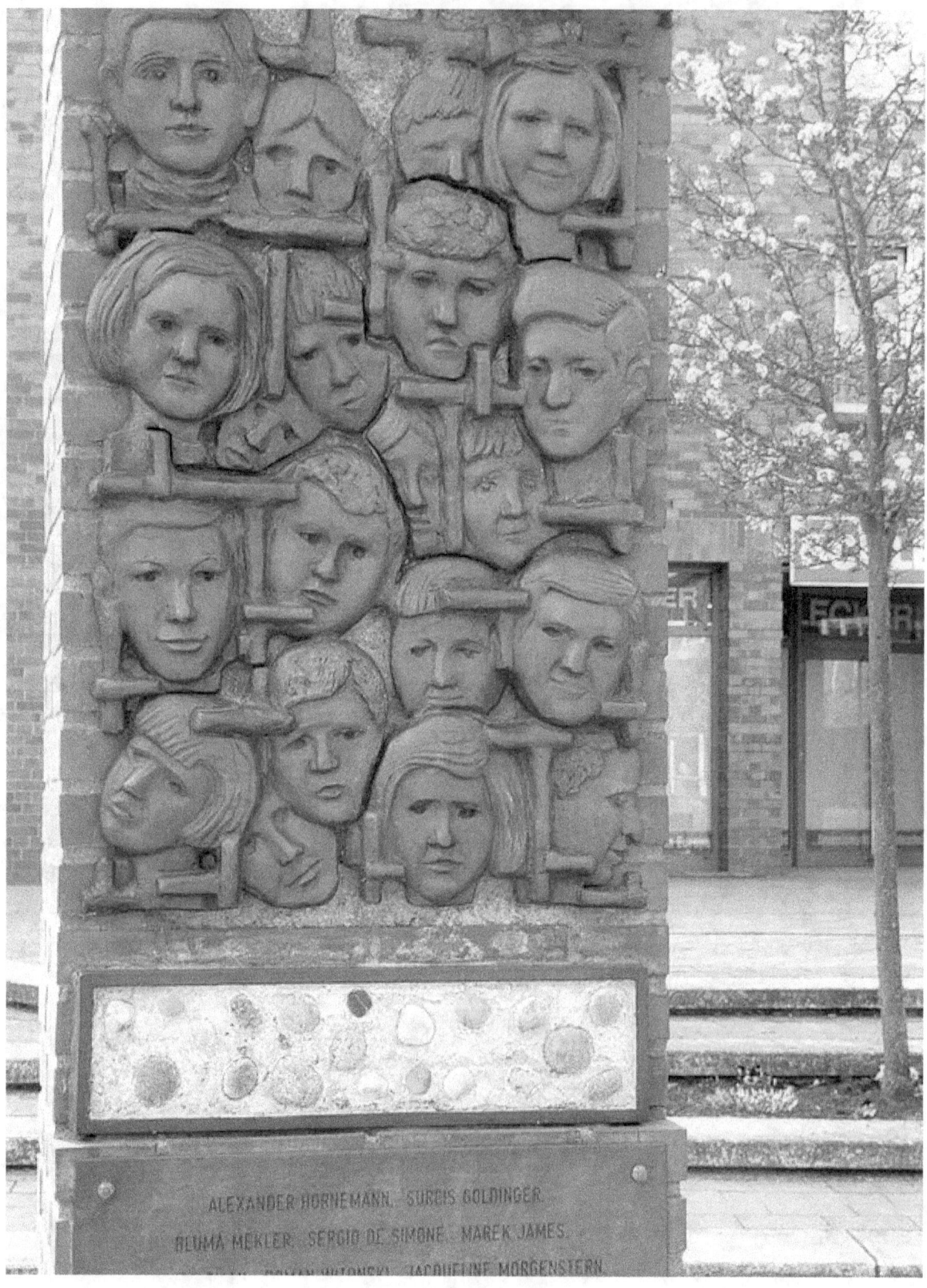

Memorial in Schnelsen

Chapter 7

Max Clara

Max Clara (1899–1966) was an Austrian anatomist. He was appointed as Chair of Anatomy at Leipzig University in 1935. Clara is known for having close ties with the Nazi Party, basing much of his controversial work on his studies of the bodies of executed prisoners. His main work, "Das Nervensystem des Menschen" (*The Nervous System of Humans*, alternatively *The Human Nervous System*)[1] was written in 1942 in Leipzig during the Third Reich's dictatorship.

In 1937, he discovered previously unknown cells found in human lungs, which were later eponymously named Clara cells.[2][3]

7.1   See also

- List of medical eponyms with Nazi associations

7.2   References

[1] Max Clara (1942). "Das Nervensystem des Menschen" [The Nervous System of Man] (in German). J.A. Barth. p. 772.

[2] Winkelmann, Andreas; Noack, Thorsten (2010). "The Clara cell - a "Third Reich eponym"?". *European Respiratory Journal Express* **36** (4): 722–727. doi:10.1183/09031936.00146609. PMID 20223917.

[3] Woywodt, A.; S. Lefrak; E. Matteson (October 1, 2010). "Tainted Eponyms in Medicine: the "Clara" Cell Joins the List". *European Respiratory Journal* **36** (4): 704–706. doi:10.1183/09031936.00046110. Retrieved 2010-11-02.

Chapter 8

Carl Clauberg

Carl Clauberg (28 September 1898 – 9 August 1957) was a German medical doctor who conducted medical experiments on human beings in Nazi concentration camps during World War II. He worked with Horst Schumann in X-ray sterilization experiments at Auschwitz concentration camp.

8.1 Biography

Carl Clauberg was born in 1898 in Wupperhof (now part of Leichlingen), Rhine Province, into a family of craftsmen. During the First World War he served as an infantryman. After the war he studied medicine and eventually reached the rank of chief doctor in the University gynaecological clinic in Kiel. He joined the Nazi party in 1933 and later on was appointed professor of gynaecology at the University of Königsberg. He carried out research on female fertility hormones (particularly progesterone) and their application as infertility treatments, obtaining a Habilitation for this work in 1937.[1] He received the rank of SS-Gruppenführer of the Reserve.

In 1942 he approached Heinrich Himmler (who knew of him through his treatment of the wife of a senior SS officer[1]) and asked him to give him an opportunity to sterilize women *en masse* for his experiments. Himmler agreed and Clauberg moved to Auschwitz concentration camp in December 1942. Part of the Block number 10 in the main camp became his laboratory. Clauberg looked for an easy and cheap way to sterilize women. He injected formaldehyde preparations into their uteruses - without anesthetics. His test subjects were Jewish and Tzigani women who suffered permanent damage and serious infections. Some of the subjects died because of the tests. Estimates of those who survived but were sterilized are around 700.

When the Red Army approached the camp, Clauberg moved to Ravensbrück concentration camp to continue his experiments on Romani women. Soviet troops captured him there in 1945.

After the war in 1948 Clauberg was put on trial in the Soviet Union and received 25 years. Seven years later he was released in the framework of a prisoners of war exchange between the Soviet Union and West Germany and returned to West Germany, where he was reinstated at his former clinic based on his prewar scientific output. Bizarre behavior, including openly boasting of his "achievements" in "developing a new sterilization technique at the Auschwitz concentration camp", destroyed any chance he might have had of staying unnoticed. After public outcry from groups of survivors, Clauberg was arrested in 1955 and was put on trial. He died of a heart attack before the trial could start.

8.2 Clauberg test

The Clauberg test is an obsolete bioassay to assess progestational activity based on the conversion of proliferative endometrium to secretory endometrium in immature rabbits.[2][3]

8.3   See also

- Block 10

8.4   References

[1] Robert Jay Lifton, "The Nazi doctors: Medical Killing and the Psychology of Genocide", Basic Books, 2000, ISBN 978-0465049059; pp. 271-278 of the online edition and references there, http://www.holocaust-history.org/lifton/LiftonT271.shtml

[2] Clauberg C. "Physiologie und Pathologie der Sexualhormone, im Besonderen des Hormons des Corpus luteum. I. Der biologische Test für das Luteumhormon (das spezielle Hormon des Corpus luteum) am infantilen Kaninchen.". *Zentralblatt für Gynänekologie , 1930, 54:2757-2770.*

[3] "Clauberg's method, alt. Clauberg's test". Whonameit?. Retrieved July 11, 2014.

8.5   Bibliography

- Ernst Klee: *Auschwitz, die NS-Medizin und ihre Opfer*. 3. Auflage. S. Fischer Verlag, Frankfurt am Main, 1997, ISBN 3-596-14906-1.

- Alexander Mitscherlich, *Fred Mielke: Medizin ohne Menschlichkeit: Dokumente des Nürnberger Ärzteprozesses*, 1. Aufl., Heidelberg: Fischer 1960. ISBN 3-596-22003-3, Taschenbuch wird 2008 in der 16. Auflage vertrieben.

- Jürgen Peter: *Der Nürnberger Ärzteprozeß im Spiegel seiner Aufarbeitung anhand der drei Dokumentensammlungen von Alexander Mitscherlich und Fred Mielke*. Münster 1994. 2. Auflage 1998.

- Till Bastian: *Furchtbare Ärzte. Medizinische Verbrechen im Dritten Reich*. Originalausgabe, 3. Auflage, Verlag C. H. Beck, München 2001, Becksche Reihe; Band 1113, ISBN 3-406-44800-3.

- R. J. Lifton, *The Nazi Doctors. Medical Killing and the Psychology of Genocide*. New York 1986), ISBN 3-608-93121-X.

- Hermann Langbein: *Menschen in Auschwitz*. Frankfurt am Main, Berlin Wien, Ullstein-Verlag, 1980, ISBN 3-548-33014-2.

- Hans-Joachim Lang: *Die Frauen von Block 10. Medizinische Experimente in Auschwitz*. Hamburg 2011. ISBN 978-3-455-50222-0.

8.6   External links

- Carl Clauberg at United States Holocaust Memorial Museum

- Carl Clauberg at Jewish Virtual Library

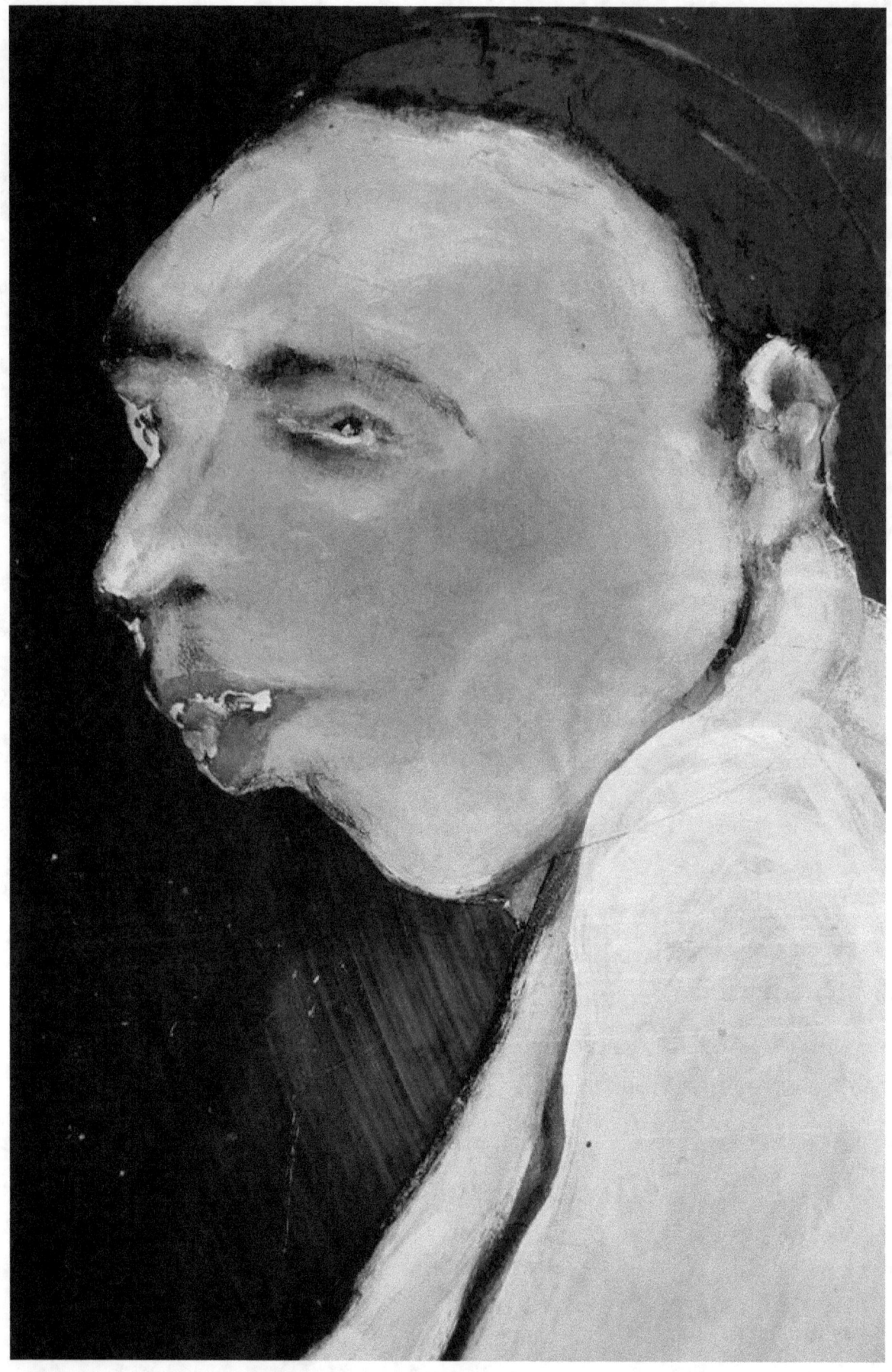

Dr. Carl Clauberg „The beast", *Image by the expressionist artist Stefan Krikl from his series* Doctors of Death, *1985*

Chapter 9

Club cell

Club cells, also known as **bronchiolar exocrine cells**,[1] and originally known as **Clara cells** (see nomenclature section), are dome-shaped cells with short microvilli, found in the small airways (bronchioles) of the lungs.[2]

Club cells are found in the ciliated simple epithelium. These cells may secrete glycosaminoglycans to protect the bronchiole lining. Bronchiolar cells gradually increase in number as the number of goblet cells decrease.

One of the main functions of club cells is to protect the bronchiolar epithelium. They do this by secreting a small variety of products, including club cell secretory protein uteroglobin, and a solution similar to the component of the lung surfactant. They are also responsible for detoxifying harmful substances inhaled into the lungs. Club cells accomplish this with cytochrome P450 enzymes found in their smooth endoplasmic reticulum. Club cells also act as a stem cell, multiplying and differentiating into ciliated cells to regenerate the bronchiolar epithelium.[3]

9.1 Mechanism

The respiratory bronchioles represent the transition from the conducting portion to the respiratory portion of the respiratory system. The narrow channels are usually less than 2 mm in diameter and they are lined by a simple cuboidal epithelium, consisting of ciliated cells and non-ciliated club cells, which are unique to bronchioles. In addition to being structurally diverse, club cells are also functionally variable. One major function they carry out is the synthesis and secretion of the material lining the bronchiolar lumen. This material includes glycosaminoglycans, proteins such as lysozymes, and conjugation of the secretory portion of IgA antibodies. These play an important defensive role, and they also contribute to the degradation of the mucus produced by the upper airways. The heterogeneous nature of the dense granules within the club cell's cytoplasm suggests that they may not all have a secretory function. Some of them may contain lysosomal enzymes, which carry out a digestive role, either in defense: Club cells engulf airborne toxins and break them down via their cytochrome P-450 enzymes (particularly CYP4B1, which is only present in the club cells) present in their smooth endoplasmic reticulum; or in the recycling of secretory products. Club cells are mitotically active. They divide and differentiate to form both ciliated and non-ciliated epithelial cells.

9.2 Role in disease

Club cells contain tryptase, which is believed to be responsible for cleaving the hemagglutinin surface protein of influenza A virus, thereby activating it and causing the symptoms of flu.[4] When the l7Rn6 protein is disrupted in mice, these mice display severe emphysema at birth as a result of disorganization of the Golgi apparatus and formation of aberrant vesicular structures within club cells.[5] Malignant club cells are also seen in bronchioalveolar carcinoma of the lung. Serum club cell proteins are used as a biomarker of lung permeability. Exposure to particulate air pollution may compromise the integrity of the lung epithelium and lead to rapid increase in epithelial barrier permeability,as reflected by increased serum club cell concentrations.[6]

9.3   Nomenclature

Club cells were previously called *Clara cells*, as they were first described by Max Clara (1899–1966), in 1937. Clara was an active member of the Nazi Party and used tissue taken from executed victims of the Third Reich for his research—including the work that led to his discovery of Clara cells.[7] In May 2012, the editorial boards of most of the major respiratory journals (including the journals of the American Thoracic Society, the European Respiratory Society and the American College of Chest Physicians) concluded that the continued use of Clara's eponym would be equivalent to honoring him; they therefore introduced a name-change policy, which went into effect beginning January 1, 2013.[8] The term "Clara" was used parenthetically after "club cell" for a 2-year period, after which "Clara cell" and "Clara cell secretory protein" were conclusively replaced with "club cell" and "club cell secretory protein", respectively.[9]

9.4   See also

- cGMP-dependent protein kinase

- List of medical eponyms with Nazi associations

- Skatole

9.5   References

[1] Peter J. Papadakos; Burkhard Lachmann (29 August 2007). *Mechanical Ventilation: Clinical Applications and Pathophysiology.* Elsevier Health Sciences. pp. 74–. ISBN 978-0-7216-0186-1. Retrieved 27 May 2011.

[2] Atkinson JJ, Adair-Kirk TL, Kelley DG, Demello D, Senior RM (2008). "Clara cell adhesion and migration to extracellular matrix". *Respir. Res.* **9** (1): 1. doi:10.1186/1465-9921-9-1. PMC 2249579. PMID 18179694.

[3] http://medical-dictionary.thefreedictionary.com/Clara+cell

[4] Taubenberger JK (August 1998). "Influenza virus hemagglutinin cleavage into HA1, HA2: No laughing matter". *Proc. Natl. Acad. Sci. U.S.A.* **95** (17): 9713–5. doi:10.1073/pnas.95.17.9713. PMC 33880. PMID 9707539.

[5] Fernández-Valdivia R, Zhang Y, Pai S, Metzker ML, Schumacher A (January 2006). "l7Rn6 Encodes a Novel Protein Required for Clara Cell Function in Mouse Lung Development". *Genetics* **172** (1): 389–99. doi:10.1534/genetics.105.048736. PMC 1456166. PMID 16157679.

[6] Provost EB, Chaumont A, Kicinski M, Cox B, Fierens F, Bernard A, Nawrot TS. "Serum levels of club cell secretory protein (Clara) and short- and long-term exposure to particulate air pollution in adolescents" Environ Int. 2014 Apr 4;68C:66-70. doi: 10.1016/j.envint.2014.03.011.

[7] Winkelmann, Andreas; Noack, Thorsten (2010). "The Clara cell - a "Third Reich eponym"?". *European Respiratory Journal* **36** (4): 722–7. doi:10.1183/09031936.00146609. PMID 20223917.

[8] Irwin, RS; Augustyn N; French CT; Rice J; Tedeschi V; Welch SJ (2013). "Spread the word about the journal in 2013: from citation manipulation to invalidation of patient-reported outcomes measures to renaming the Clara cell to new journal features". *Chest* **143**: 1–5. doi:10.1378/chest.12-2762. PMID 23276834.

[9] Akram, KM; Lomas NJ; Spiteri MA; Forsyth NR (2013). "Club cells inhibit alveolar epithelial wound repair via TRAIL-dependent apoptosis". *Eur Respir J* **41**: 683–694. doi:10.1183/09031936.00213411. PMID 22790912.

9.6   External links

- Histology image: 13805loa – Histology Learning System at Boston University

- *−415956935* at GPnotebook

- UIUC Histology Subject *1385*

- Histology at ucsf.edu

Chapter 10

Erwin Ding-Schuler

Erwin Oskar Ding-Schuler (September 19, 1912 — August 11, 1945) was a German surgeon and an officer in the Waffen-SS who attained the rank of Sturmbannführer (Major). He is notable for having performed experiments on inmates of the Buchenwald concentration camp.

Ding-Schuler joined the NSDAP in 1932 and the SS in 1936.[1] In 1937 he received his degree and passed his second state exam in medicine. An author of scientific publications, in 1939 he became camp physician at Buchenwald and head of the division for spotted fever and viral research of the Waffen-SS Hygiene Institute in Weimar-Buchenwald. Until 1945 he conducted extensive medical experiments (on some 1,000 inmates, many of whom lost their lives) in Experimental Station Block 46, using various poisons as well as infective agents for spotted fever, yellow fever, smallpox, typhus, and cholera.[2]

Erwin Ding-Schuler was arrested by U.S. troops on 25 April 1945 and committed suicide on 11 August 1945.[2][3][4][5]

10.1 See also

- Eugen Kogon

10.2 References

[1] Steiner, John Michael (1976). *Power Politics and Social Change in National Socialist Germany: A Process of Escalation into Mass Destruction*. Walter de Gruyter. p. 213. ISBN 0391005251.

[2] Zenter, Christian and Bedürftig, Friedemann (1991). Encyclopedia of the Third Reich, p. 199. New York: Macmillan. ISBN 0-02-897502-2

[3] Ernst Klee: *Das Personenlexikon zum Dritten Reich*. 2007, p. 111.

[4] Eugen Kogon: *Der SS-Staat. Das System der deutschen Konzentrationslager*. 1974, p. 320.

[5] Eugen Kogon, *The Theory and Practice of Hell* (1998) p. 265.

- Williamson, Gordon (2006). *The SS: Hitler's Instrument of Terror*. New York: Barnes & Noble Publishing. p. 304. ISBN 978-0-7607-8168-5.

Chapter 11

Doctors of Infamy

Doctors of Infamy: The Story of the Nazi Medical Crimes (1949) is a book by Alexander Mitscherlich and Fred Mielke which begins with a statement on the intention of its publication and includes a documentation of the Doctors' Trial in Nuremberg that was held from 9 December 1946 until 20 August 1947.[1]

In Germany, the first edition appeared in 1947. It was the interim report of the umbrella organization of doctors' associations in Western Germany who had sent out a commission of six observers to the Nuremberg trials. This commission was headed by young Mitscherlich because none of the established colleagues would have taken on this task in their own name.[2] This edition oappeared before the trial was closed and met with an action for injunction by certain doctors. As a result of the trial, some parts of the study were eliminated in the subsequent enlarged edition of 1949 which was the final report on the part of the doctors' associations. From 1960 onwards the book was made available in German in a paperback edition. For the 1977 reprint of this edition, Mitscherlich wrote a new preface. The most recent edition is the 18th impression of 2012.

11.1   Editions

- Alexander Mitscherlich and Fred Mielke, *Doctors of infamy. The story of the Nazi medical crimes*, translated from German by Heinz Norden. With statements of 3 American authorities identified with the Nuremberg medical trial and a note on medical ethics by Albert Deutsch, xxxix, 172 pages, Ill. with 16 pages of photographs; 8. Henry Schuman, New York 1949

Previous editions in German

- Alexander Mitscherlich, Fred Mielke, *Das Diktat der Menschenverachtung. Der Nürnberger Ärzteprozeß und seine Quellen*, 175 pages, Lambert Schneider, Heidelberg 1947

- Alexander Mitscherlich, Fred Mielke (Eds.), *Wissenschaft ohne Menschlichkeit. Medizinische und Eugenische Irrwege unter Diktatur, Bürokratie und Krieg*, Lambert Schneider, Heidelberg 1949

1960 paperback edition in German

- Alexander Mitscherlich, Fred Mielke (Eds.), *Medizin ohne Menschlichkeit. Dokumente des Nürnberger Ärzteprozesses* Fischer Taschenbuchverlag, Frankfurt 1960, ISBN 3-596-22003-3; in 1977, Alexander Mitscherlich contributed a new preface (alone, since his colleague Fred Mielke had died in 1959); most recent edition: 18th impression, Fischer Taschenbuchverlag, Frankfurt am Main 2012, ISBN 978-3-596-22003-8

11.2 Literature

- (About the English edition, in German) Julius Brandel, „Das Diktat der Menschenverachtung. Deutsche Aerzte versuchen ein amerikanisches Buch gegen Nazi-Aerzte zu verhindern", in: *Aufbau*, Volume 15, 18 February 1949, No. 7, page 19, columns a–c.

11.3 References

[1] The book also includes the Nuremberg Code (1947) on pages xxiii-xxv which was drafted by Leo Alexander.

[2] »Medizin ohne Menschlichkeit«. Vor 60 Jahren begann der Nürnberger Ärzteprozess, in: *Antifaschistisches Infoblatt*, 73, 4.2006:46–49.

Chapter 12

List of medical eponyms with Nazi associations

This article lists **medical eponyms** which have been associated with Nazi human experimentation or Nazi politics. While normally eponyms used in medicine serve to honor the memory of the physician or researcher who first documented a disease or pioneered a procedure, the propriety of such names resulting from unethical research practices is controversial. In some cases terms closely related to doctors in the Nazi era have fallen out of favor or there are active lobbying efforts to remove the original name from use. In other cases their use in the medical literature is sometimes presented with a caveat or footnote.

The declining use of the Nazi-era eponyms has itself been tracked in the literature.[1] Since 2007, the *Israel Medical Association Journal*[2] and *European Neurology*[3] have each published articles cataloging eponyms honoring Nazis and their collaborators. While the most direct Nazi experimenters (such as Josef Mengele) were never honored, others who were members of the Nazi party or whose research relied upon the Nazi program—such as conducting research on the remains of Nazi execution victims—have been honored.

Some physicians have used the Nazi associations as an argument to discontinue the use of eponyms in medical naming conventions altogether,[4] while others have argued that such Nazi-associated eponyms should be retained as "a means of conveying immortal dishonor."[5] Both the *Israel Medical Association Journal* and *European Neurology* articles advocated that eponyms honoring victims of the Nazis be retained, while eponyms honoring Nazi collaborators or benefactors be replaced.

12.1   List of eponyms

12.2   References

[1] Wu, Dave A.; Kenneth A. Katz (October 2005). "Declining Use of the Eponym "Reiter's syndrome" in the Medical Literature, 1998-2003". *Journal of the American Association of Dermatology* **53** (4): 720. doi:10.1016/j.jaad.2005.06.048.

[2] Strous, Rael D.; Morris C. Edelman (March 2007). "Eponyms and the Nazi Era: Time to Remember and Time For Change" (PDF). *Israel Medical Association Journal* **9** (3): 207–214. Retrieved 2010-10-28.

[3] Kondziella, Daniel (2009). "Thirty Neurological Eponyms Associated with the Nazi Era". *European Neurology* **62** (1): 56–64. doi:10.1159/000215880. Retrieved 2010-10-28.

[4] Woywodt, Alexander; Eric Matteson (2007). "Should Eponyms be Abandoned? Yes". *British Medical Journal* **335** (7617): 424. doi:10.1136/bmj.39308.342639.AD. PMC 1962844. PMID 17762033. Retrieved 2010-10-28.

[5] Leach, John Paul (April 24, 2003). "Correspondence: Hallervorden and History". *The New England Journal of Medicine* **348**: 1725–1726. doi:10.1056/NEJM200304243481721. Retrieved 2010-10-31.

[6] Woywodt, A.; S. Lefrak; E. Matteson (October 1, 2010). "Tainted Eponyms in Medicine: the "Clara" Cell Joins the List". *European Respiratory Journal* **36** (4): 704–706. doi:10.1183/09031936.00046110. Retrieved 2010-10-31.

[7] Winkelmann, A.; T. Noack (October 1, 2010). "The Clara Cell: a "Third Reich eponym"?". *European Respiratory Journal* **36** (4): 722–727. doi:10.1183/09031936.00146609. PMID 20223917. Retrieved 2010-11-01.

[8] Woywodt, A.; E. L. Matteson (2006-08-03). "Wegener's Granulomatosis—Probing the Untold Past of the Man Behind the Eponym" (PDF). *Rheumatology* **45** (10): 1303–1306. doi:10.1093/rheumatology/kel258. PMID 16887845. Retrieved 2010-10-28.

This list is incomplete; you can help by expanding it.

12.3 External Links

- Eponyms and the Nazi Era: Time to Remember and Time for Change R.D. Strous and M.C. Edelman

Chapter 13

Feeder of lice

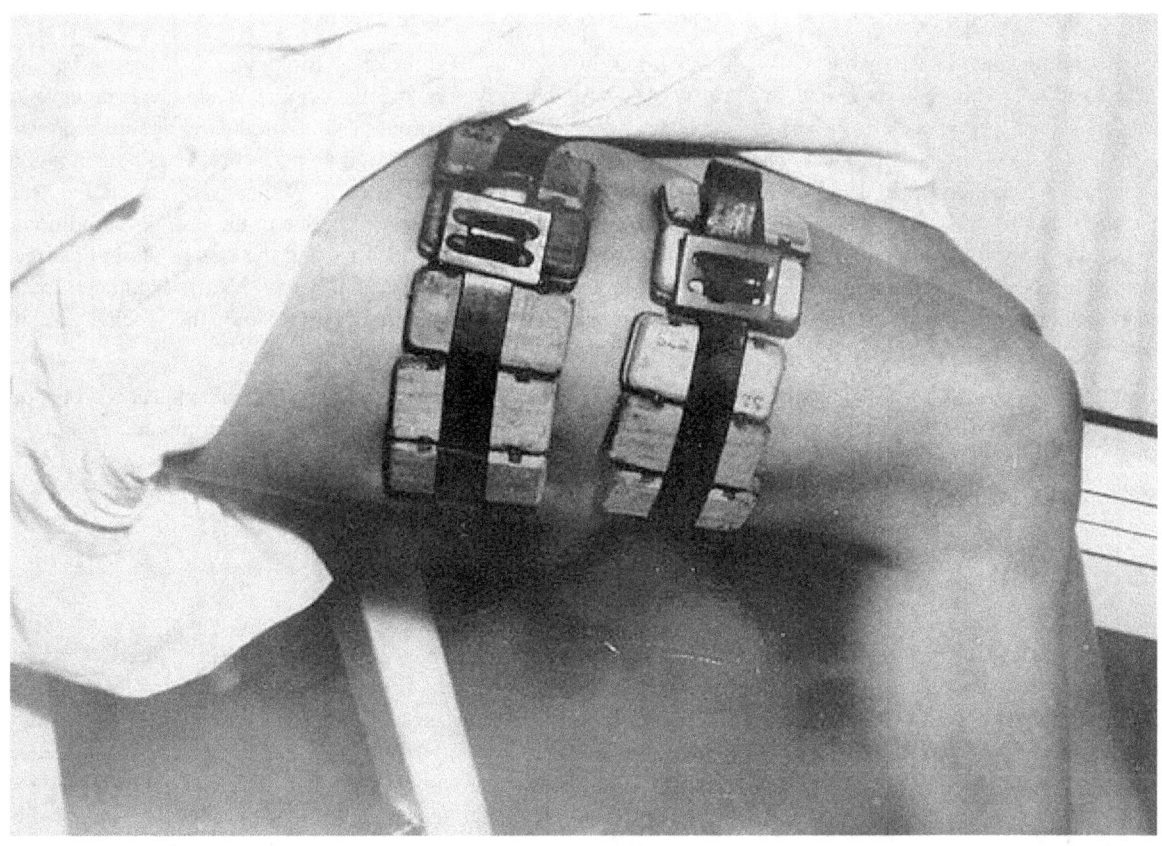

Cages with typhus carrying lice strapped onto a person's thigh. During World War II, feeding the lice with human subjects' blood was the only way to produce a viable typhus vaccine.

A **feeder of lice** was a job in interwar and Nazi-occupied Poland, in the city of Lwów at the *Institute for Study of Typhus and Virology* of Rudolf Weigl (Polish: *Instytut Badań nad Tyfusem Plamistym i Wirusami prof. Rudolfa Weigla*) in Lwów (Lviv, Ukraine). It involved serving as a source of blood for lice, a typhus vector, which could then be used to develop vaccines against the disease.

Initially begun in 1920 by Weigl, during the Nazi occupation of the city it became the primary means of support and protection for many of the city's Polish intellectuals, including the mathematician Stefan Banach and the poet Zbigniew Herbert. While the profession carried a significant risk of infection, thanks to Weigl's patronage the feeders of lice obtained additional food rations, were protected from being shipped to slave labor in Germany or German concentration camps, and were allowed additional mobility around the occupied city.

Typhus research involving human subjects, who were purposely infected with the disease, was also carried out in various Nazi concentration camps, in particular at Buchenwald and Sachsenhausen and to a lesser extent at Auschwitz.

13.1 Background

French bacteriologist Charles Nicolle showed in 1909 that lice (*Pediculus humanus corporis*) were the primary means by which the typhus bacteria (*Rickettsia prowazekii*) were spread.[1] In his experiments Nicolle infected a chimpanzee with typhus, retrieved the lice from it, and placed them on a healthy chimpanzee who developed the disease shortly thereafter.[2] Further work established that it was lice excrement rather than bites which spread the disease.[2] Nicolle received a Nobel Prize in Physiology and Medicine for his work on typhus in 1928.[2]

During World War I, beginning in 1914, Rudolf Weigl, a Polish parasitologist of Austrian background was drafted into the Austrian army and given the task of studying typhus and its causes.[1][3] Weigl worked at a military hospital in Przemyśl, where he supervised the newly established Laboratory for the Study of Spotted Typhus.[3]

After Poland regained its independence Weigl was hired, in 1920, as a Professor of Biology in the Medical Faculty at the Jan Kazimierz University in Lwów, at the *Institute for Study of Typhus and Virology*.[3] While there, he developed a vaccine against typhus made from grown lice which were then crushed into a paste. Initially the lice were grown on the blood of guinea pigs but the effectiveness of the vaccine depended on the blood being as similar to human blood as possible. As a consequence, by 1933, Weigl began using human volunteers as feeders. While the volunteers fed healthy lice, there was still the danger of accidental exposure to some of the typhus-carrying lice in the institute. Additionally, once the lice were infected with typhus, they required additional feeding, which carried the risk of the human feeder becoming infected with the disease. Weigl protected the donors by vaccinating them beforehand, and although some of them (including Weigl himself) developed the disease, none died. However, the production of the vaccine was still a potentially dangerous activity, and it was still difficult to produce the vaccine on a large scale.[1][4]

At the time Weigl's vaccine was the only one in existence which could be employed in practical applications outside of controlled settings. The first widespread use of his vaccine was carried out in China by Belgian missionaries between 1936 and 1943.[1][3]

13.2 Procedure

The development of the typhus vaccine involved several stages. First, the lice larvae had to be bred and then fed on human blood. Once they matured, they were removed from the feeders, held down in a clamp machine especially designed by Weigl, and anally injected with the strain of the typhus bacteria. At that point the infected louse had to be fed human blood for about five more days. This stage of the production process carried the greatest risk to the human feeder of contracting the disease. Weigl and his staff tried to prevent the danger by heavily vaccinating the feeders before hand. Once the louse was sufficiently infected, it was removed from the human feeder, killed in a solution of phenol, and then dissected. The contents of the louse abdomen (its feces) was removed and then ground up into a paste. The paste was then made into the typhus vaccine.[3]

The feeding was done through the use of specially-constructed small wooden boxes, 4 cm by 7 cm, developed by Weigl. The boxes were sealed with paraffin on the top which prevented the lice from escaping, and the underside consisted of a screen made of a fabric sieve, adopted by Weigl from sieves that were used by local peasants to separate wheat husks from the seeds. A typical box contained 400 to 800 lice larvae which would mature as the feeding took place. The sieve bottom allowed the lice to stick out their heads and feed on the human flesh. A standard feeding period took thirty to forty-five minutes, and was repeated with the same lice colony for twelve days. Usually, an individual feeder would accommodate from 7 to 11 boxes (of 400 to 800 lice each) on his or her leg, per feeding session. Typically men would place the boxes on their calves, to minimize the discomfort of the bites, while women feeders placed them on their thighs, so that the bite marks could be covered up by a skirt. A nurse had to watch over the feeding process as the lice would feed beyond the point of being gorged on the blood and could burst if left on the human flesh for too long.[3]

Other dangers that employment at the institute involved, in addition to the contraction of typhus, concerned allergic reactions to the vaccine or asthma attacks because of the louse feces dust.[3]

13.3   World War II

13.3.1   First Soviet occupation

After the invasion of Poland by Nazi Germany and the Soviet Union in 1939, Lwów initially came under Soviet occupation. During this period Weigl's institute continued to function, although Poles, particularly those escaping from the German-controlled areas, were banned from being employed there. The Soviet authorities deported ethnic Poles from the seized territories, sending them to Kazakhstan, Siberia and other areas deep within the Soviet Union. Nevertheless, despite the official prohibition on employment, Weigl used his prestige and influence (during this time Nikita Khrushchev visited the institute) to secure the release of several Polish would-be deportees and in some cases managed to obtain permission for those who had already been exiled to return.[3] These individuals were then given work in the institute as either nurses, interpreters (Weigl himself did not speak Russian)[3] or as some of the first lice feeders; people who were given the job as a means of protecting them from persecution by the Soviet authorities.[3]

The vaccine produced by the institute during this time was earmarked for the Red Army, aside from a small quantity which was used in the civilian sector.[5]

13.3.2   Nazi occupation

In June 1941, after the Nazi attack on the Soviet Union, Lwów was taken over by the Germans. Weigl's institute, now renamed *Institut für Fleckfieber und Virusforschung des OKH*, was kept open because, much like the Soviets before them, the Germans were interested in the applications of the typhus vaccine among their front line soldiers. The Institute was made directly subordinate to the German military, which, as it turned out, ended up giving its workers significant protection against the Gestapo. The Nazis converted a building of the former Queen Jadwiga Grammar School into Weigl's new laboratory and ordered that the production of the vaccine be stepped up, with the whole output being shipped to the German armed forces.[5]

Role of institute under Nazi occupation

In light of the *Sonderaktion Krakau*, a German operation in which many distinguished professors from Jagiellonian University in Kraków were arrested and sent to German concentration camps, the danger that a similar fate would befall Lwów intellectuals was very real. As a result, in July 1941, Weigl began hiring prominent Polish intellectuals of the city for his institute, many of whom had lost work as a result of the closure of all Polish institutions of higher learning by the Nazis. In fact, soon after, the Nazis carried out a massacre of Lwów professors.[6] Weigl managed to convince the occupation authorities to give him full discretion as to whom he hired for his experiments, even as he himself refused to sign the so-called Volksliste which would have identified him as an ethnic German (since he was of Austrian background) with access to privileges and opportunities unavailable to Poles. Similarly, he refused an offer to move to Berlin, direct a dedicated institute and become a Reichsdeutscher.[3] The group of scholars hired by Weigl were often brought in by Wacław Szybalski, an oncologist, who was also put in charge of supervising the lice feeding.[5]

Association with the institute offered a measure of protection. Weigl was able to continue his research, and even hire more people, some as research assistants, others as lice feeders, often among those threatened by Nazi authorities with deportation, or even resistance members.[1][3] The feeders of lice who were employed at the institute were issued a special version of the Kennkarte, the *"Ausweis"*, which noted both that they might be infected with typhus and that they worked for an institution of the German military, the *"Oberkommando des Heeres"* (Office of the Commander-in-Chief of the German Army). As a result, the workers of the institute, unlike other Poles in the city, could move freely about and, if stopped by the police or the Gestapo, were quickly released.[3]

Lwów academics and intellectuals as feeders

In autumn of 1941, the famous mathematician Stefan Banach began working at the institute as a lice feeder,[6] as did his son, Stefan Jr.[5] Banach continued to work at the institute feeding lice until March 1944, and managed to survive the war as a result, unlike many other Polish mathematicians who were killed by the Nazis (although he died of lung cancer shortly after the war's conclusion). Banach's employment at the institute also gave protection to his wife, Łucja (it was she who purchased the notebook that eventually became the famous Scottish Book), who was in particular danger because of her Jewish background.[5][7] The poet Zbigniew Herbert also spent the occupation as a lice feeder in Weigl's institute.[8] According to Alfred Jahn, a geographer and future rector of the University of Wrocław, "Almost the entire University of Lwów worked at Weigl's". Two other future rectors of the University of Wrocław, Kazimierz Szarski and Stanisław Kulczyński, also survived the war as feeders of lice.[9]

With numerous academics gathering in one place under the pretense of lice feeding and research, underground education and research often took place. The actual feeding time took only about an hour a day, which left the remainder of the day free for conspiratorial activity and scientific discourse.[3]

Anti-Nazi resistance fighters as feeders

Additionally, Weigl began employing members of the Polish anti-Nazi resistance, the Home Army, in his institute, which provided them with sufficient cover to carry out their underground activities. Aleksander Szczęścikiewicz and Zygmunt Kleszczyński, two leaders of the underground scout movement, the Grey Ranks (*Szare Szeregi*), also worked at the institute. Due to his special position, Weigl was allowed to have a radio at the institute – otherwise ownership of a radio by Poles was punishable by death – which was used by him and members of the Polish resistance to gather up-to-date news of the war otherwise censored by German propaganda.[3]

Attempts to save Jews via employment in the institute

When the Germans began the systematic murder of the Lwów Jews, Weigl tried to save as many as he could by hiring them as well. Among others, work at the institute saved the life of the bacteriologist Henryk Meisel. Weigl also tried to protect the bacteriologist Filip Eisenberg, from Jagiellonian University, by offering him a position. Unfortunately, Eisenberg believed that he could survive the war by hiding in Kraków, turned down Weigl's offer, and in 1943 was caught by the Nazis and sent to the Belzec extermination camp where he was murdered. In the end, about 4000 people (feeders, technicians and nurses) passed through Weigl's institute, of whom about 500 are known by name.[9]

Smuggling of the vaccine

While all of the vaccines produced by the institute during this time were supposed to go to the German army, some portion was smuggled out by the employees associated with the Polish resistance and shipped to partisan units of the Home Army, as well as underground movements in the Lwów and Warsaw ghettos, and even to sick individuals in the Auschwitz and Majdanek concentration camps.[3][9] According to the famous Polish-Jewish pianist and diarist, Władysław Szpilman (the protagonist of the 2002 movie *The Pianist*), because of his vaccine, Weigl became "as famous as Hitler in the Warsaw ghetto", with "Weigl as a symbol of Goodness and Hitler as a symbol of Evil".[3]

13.3.3   Soviet re-capture of the city

After the Red Army, along with the Home Army (Operation Tempest) recaptured Lwów in July 1944, Weigl's institute was disbanded and moved to central Poland, along with most other Polish inhabitants of Lwów.[3] Weigl would continue his research in Kraków at Jagiellonian University.[1]

13.4   Lice feeding around the world

Human lice feeders were also used in America in the 1940s. The *Wilmington Morning Star* reported that the U.S. government's researchers paid around 60 lice feeders $60 a month, rising to $120 due to the lack of people willing to participate. Humans were used because lice failed to thrive on animals, until it was discovered that some could live on an "Easter bunny" called Samson. Samson and his descendants were used to conduct hundreds of experiments.[10]

13.5   Notable feeders

- Jerzy Albrycht

- Stefan Banach (mathematician, founder of Functional Analysis)

- Feliks Barański (mathematician)

- Jerzy Broszkiewicz (author, essayist)

- Józef Chałasiński (sociologist)

- Leszek Elektorowicz (poet, essayist)

- Zbigniew Herbert (poet)

- Adam Hollanek (science fiction author)

- Artur Hutnikiewicz (historian of Polish literature)

- Alfred Jahn (geographer, polar explorer)

- Bronisław Knaster (mathematician)

- Seweryn Krzemieniewski (biologist)

- Jan Noskiewicz (zoologist)

- Lesław Ogielski (veterinarian, medical researcher)

- Władysław Orlicz (mathematician)

- Stanisław Skrowaczewski (classical conductor)

- Stefania Skwarczyńska (historian of literature)

- Kazimierz Smulikowski (geologist)

- Wacław Szybalski (oncologist)

- Mirosław Żuławski (writer, screen writer) – who wrote about his work as a lice feeder in his screenplay *Trzecia część nocy* (*The Third Part of the Night*)

[6][11]

13.6   Legacy

Weigl continued his research on typhus after the war. After his death, his studies were picked up by his friends, students, and his second wife, Anna-Herzig Weigl.[3]

Rudolf Weigl was posthumously awarded the medal of Righteous among the Nations by the Yad Vashem in 2003.[12] His contributions to saving lives during the Nazi occupation of Poland have been compared to those of Oskar Schindler.[3][13]

13.7 References

[1] "Stefan Krynski - Rudolf Weigl (1883-1957)". Lwow.home.pl. 1957-08-11. Retrieved 2012-02-17.

[2] Irwin W. Sherman; American Society for Microbiology (2006). *The power of plagues.* Wiley-Blackwell. p. 122. ISBN 978-1-55581-356-7. Retrieved 19 February 2012.

[3] "Waclaw Szybalski: The genius of Rudolf Stefan Weigl (1883-1957), a Lvovian microbe hunter and breeder - In Memoriam". Lwow.home.pl. Retrieved 2012-02-17.

[4] Baumslag, Naomi (2005). *Murderous medicine: Nazi doctors, human experimentation, and Typhus.* Greenwood Publishing Group. p. 133. ISBN 0-275-98312-9.

[5] Jakimowicz, Emilia; Mironowicz, Adam, eds. (2011). *Stefan Banach. Remarkable Life, Brilliant Mathematics.* Gdansk: Gdansk University Press. pp. 17, 21. ISBN 978-83-7326-827-2.

[6] Kałuża, Roman (1996). *Through a reporter's eyes: The life of Stefan Banach.* Ann Konstant. Birkhäuser. ISBN 0-8176-3772-9.

[7] Pietsch, Albrecht (2007). *History of Banach spaces and linear operators.* Birkhäuser. p. 638. ISBN 0-8176-4367-2.

[8] Łukasiewicz, Jacek (2001). *Herbert. A to Polska właśnie.* Wydawnictwo Slaskie. p. 20. ISBN 83-7023-889-0.

[9] "Rudolf Stefan Weigl. Profesor Rudolf Weigl był Polakiem z wyboru.". Lwow.com.pl. Retrieved 2012-02-17.

[10] *Wilmington Morning Star*, 5 July 1949

[11] "Dlaczego Stefan Banach?". *www.lwow.com.* Moj Lwow. Retrieved February 29, 2012.

[12] Righteous Among the Nations Honored by Yad Vashem By 1 January 2011. Poland, YAD VASHEM

[13] Pennington, Thomas Hugh (2003). *When food kills: BSE, E. coli, and disaster science.* Oxford University Press. p. 190. ISBN 0-19-852517-6.

13.8 External links

- List of 507 individuals employed by Weigl's institute during Nazi occupation

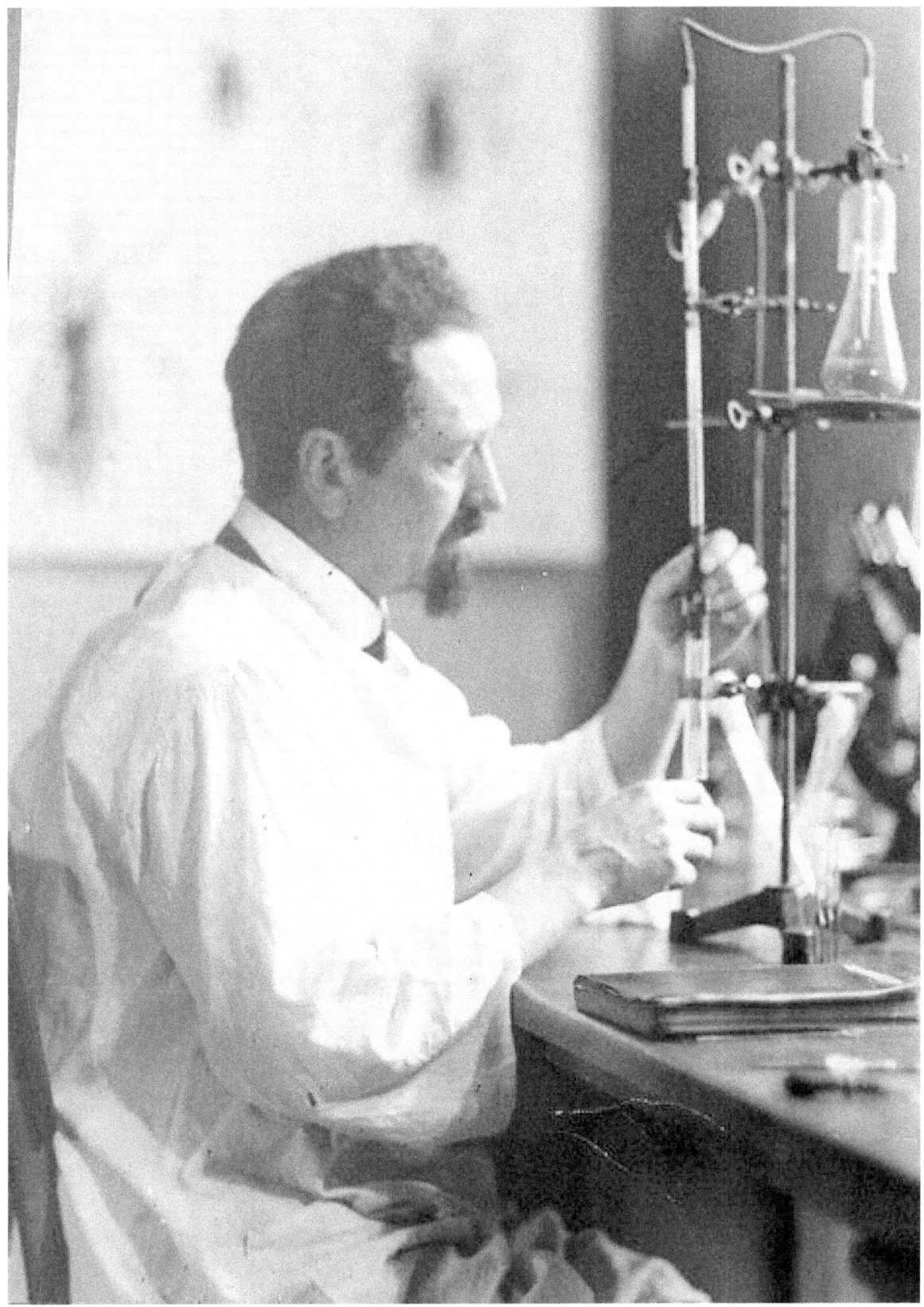

Rudolf Weigl, the developer of first viable typhus vaccine in his laboratory in Lwów

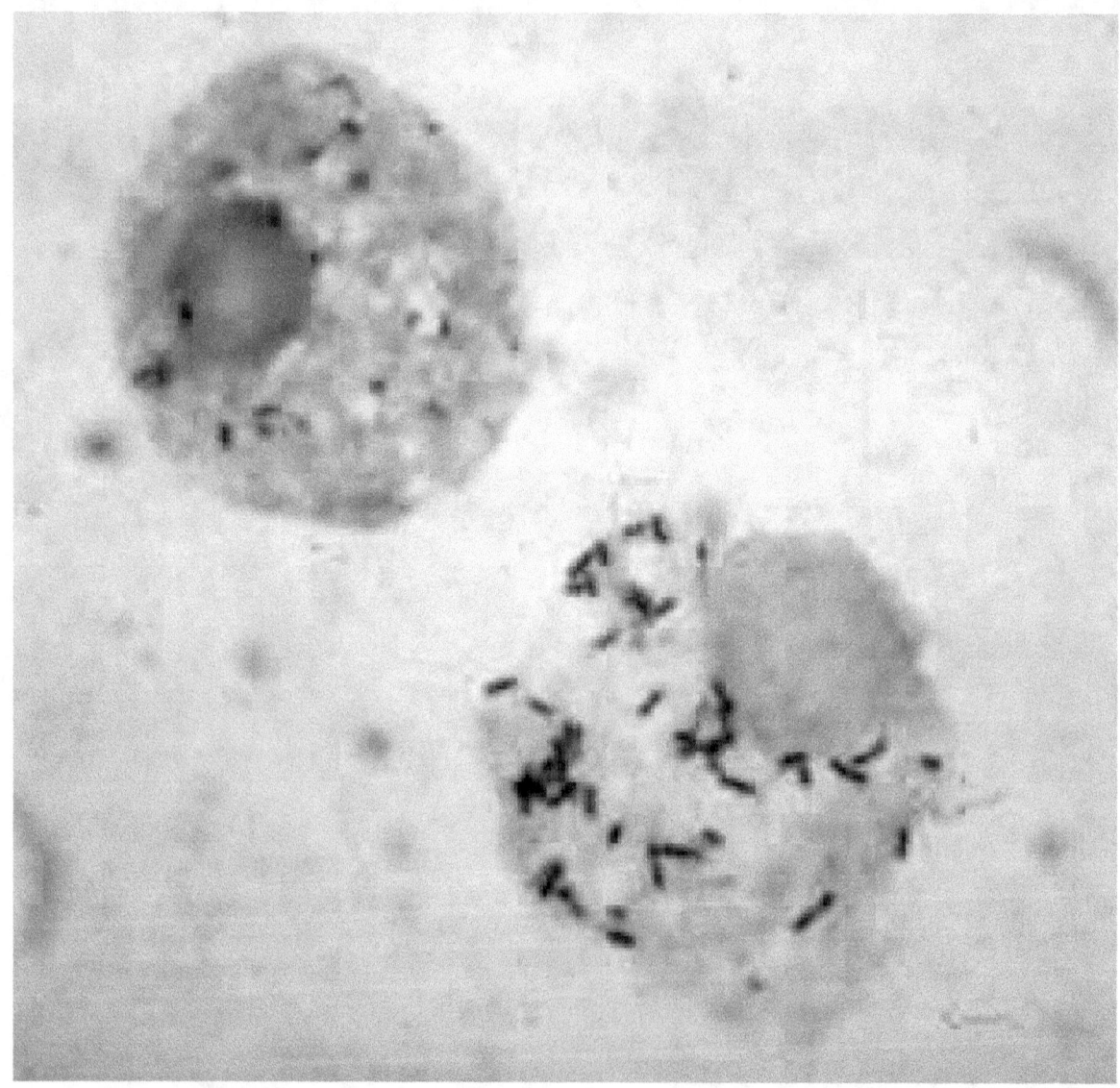

Rickettsia – *typhus-causing bacteria*

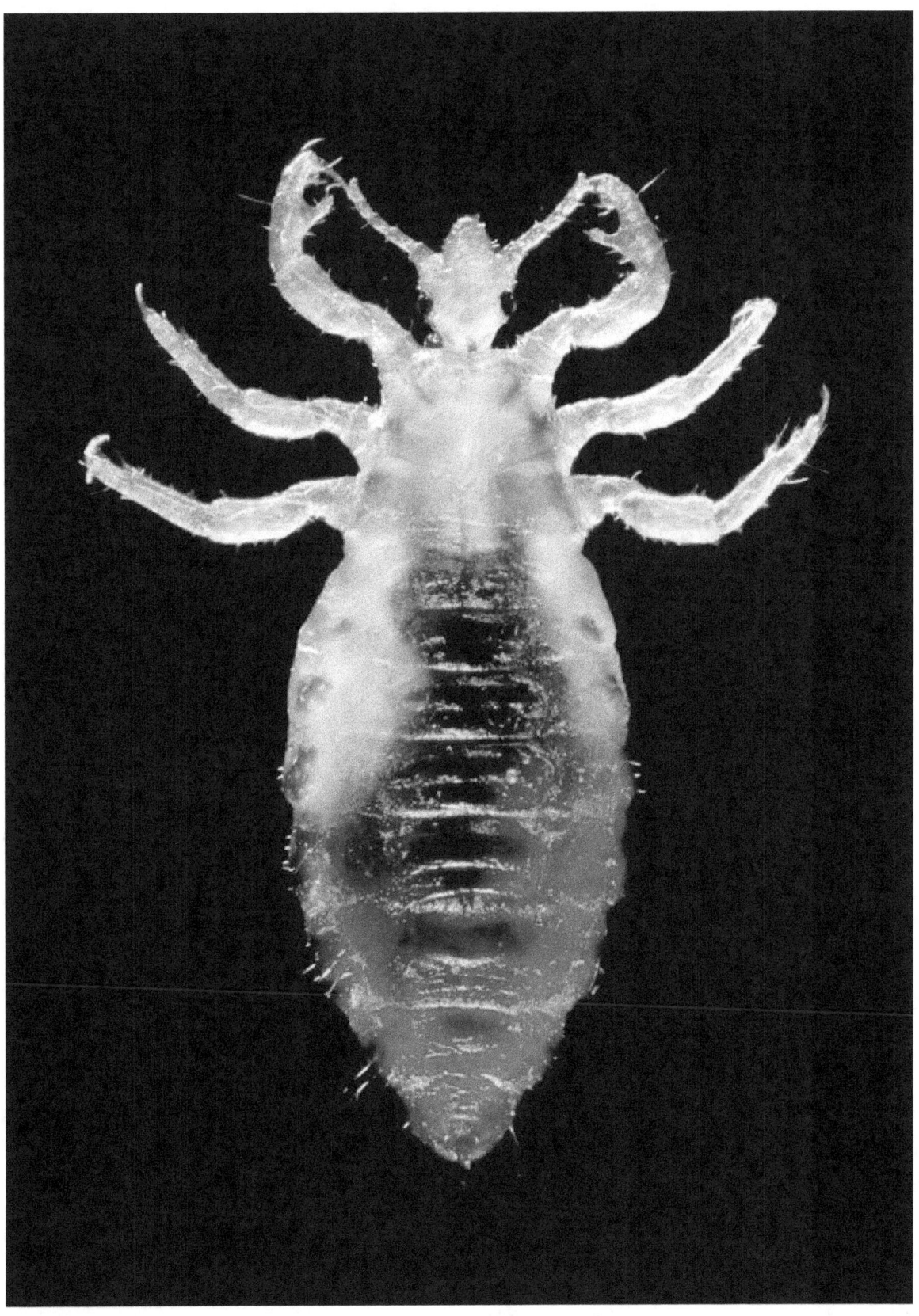

Typhus-spreading body louse

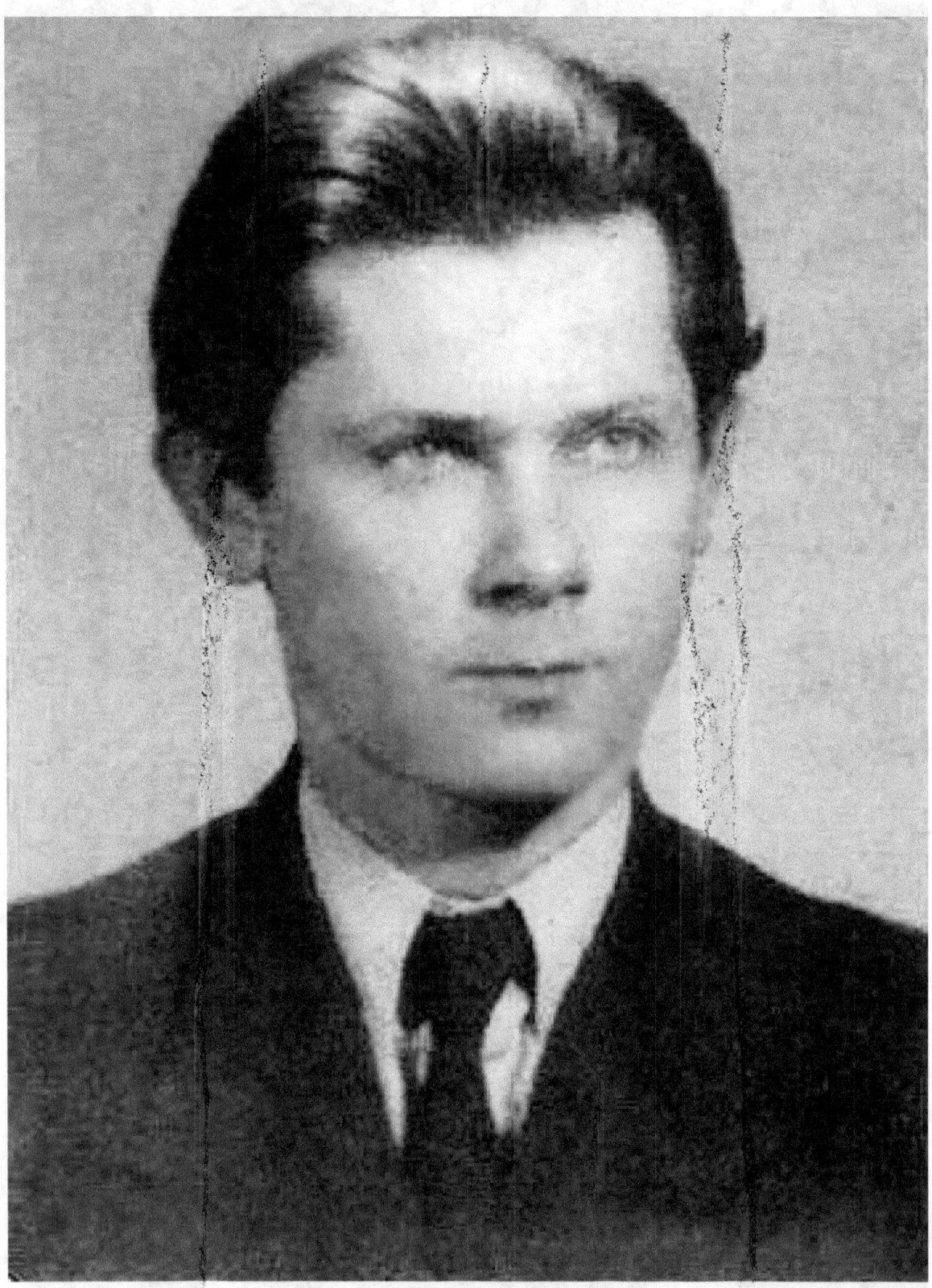

Poet Zbigniew Herbert, one of the feeders in German-occupied Lwów

Chapter 14

Fritz Fischer (medical doctor)

Fritz Ernst Fischer (5 October 1912 – 2003) was a German medical doctor who, under the Nazi regime, participated in medical experiments conducted on inmates of the Ravensbrück concentration camp.

Fischer was born in Berlin. He studied medicine first at Bonn, later at Berlin and Leipzig, and finally graduated in Hamburg in 1938. He joined the SS in 1934 (ultimately reaching the rank of *Sturmbannführer* [major]) and became a member of the NSDAP in June 1937. On 1 November 1939, he was assigned to the Waffen-SS of the SS-Department of the Hohenlychen Sanatorium as a physician and SS Second Lieutenant.

In 1940, he became troop physician of the SS Division *Leibstandarte Adolf Hitler*. After having been wounded he was posted back to Hohenlychen and worked in the camp hospital of the Ravensbrück concentration camp as a surgical assistant to Karl Gebhardt. He participated in the surgical experiments carried out on concentration camp inmates there.

After World War II, he was tried in the Doctors' Trial in Nuremberg, convicted of war crimes and crimes against humanity, and was condemned to life imprisonment. His sentence was reduced to 15 years in 1951 and he was released in March 1954. Fischer subsequently regained his license to practice medicine and started a new career at the chemical company Boehringer in Ingelheim, where he stayed until his retirement.

Based on available records, when he died in 2003 he was the last known living of those indicted at the Doctor's Trial.

14.1 References

- Schäfer, S.: *Zum Selbstverständnis von Frauen im Konzentrationslager: das Lager Ravensbrück*, p. 130f. PhD thesis 2002, TU Berlin. (PDF file, 741 kB). In German.

- Schmidt, U.: *Lebensläufe: Biographien und Motive der Angeklagte aus der Perspektive des medizinischen Sachverständigen, Dr. Leo Alexander, 1945-1947*, in Dörner, K., Ebbinghaus, A. (ed.): *Vernichten und Heilen: Der Nürnberger Ärzteprozess und seine Folgen*; Aufbau-Verlag, Berlin 2001; ISBN 3-351-02514-9; pp. 374–404.

- Waltrich, H.: *Zur Geschichte der Heilanstalten vom Roten Kreuz in Hohenlychen, part 2*, Ökostadt-Nachrichten 28 (1999).

14.2 Further reading

- Klier, F.: *Die Kaninchen von Ravensbrück. Medizinische Versuche an Frauen in der NS-Zeit.*; Droemer Verlag, Munich 1994, ISBN 3-426-77162-4.

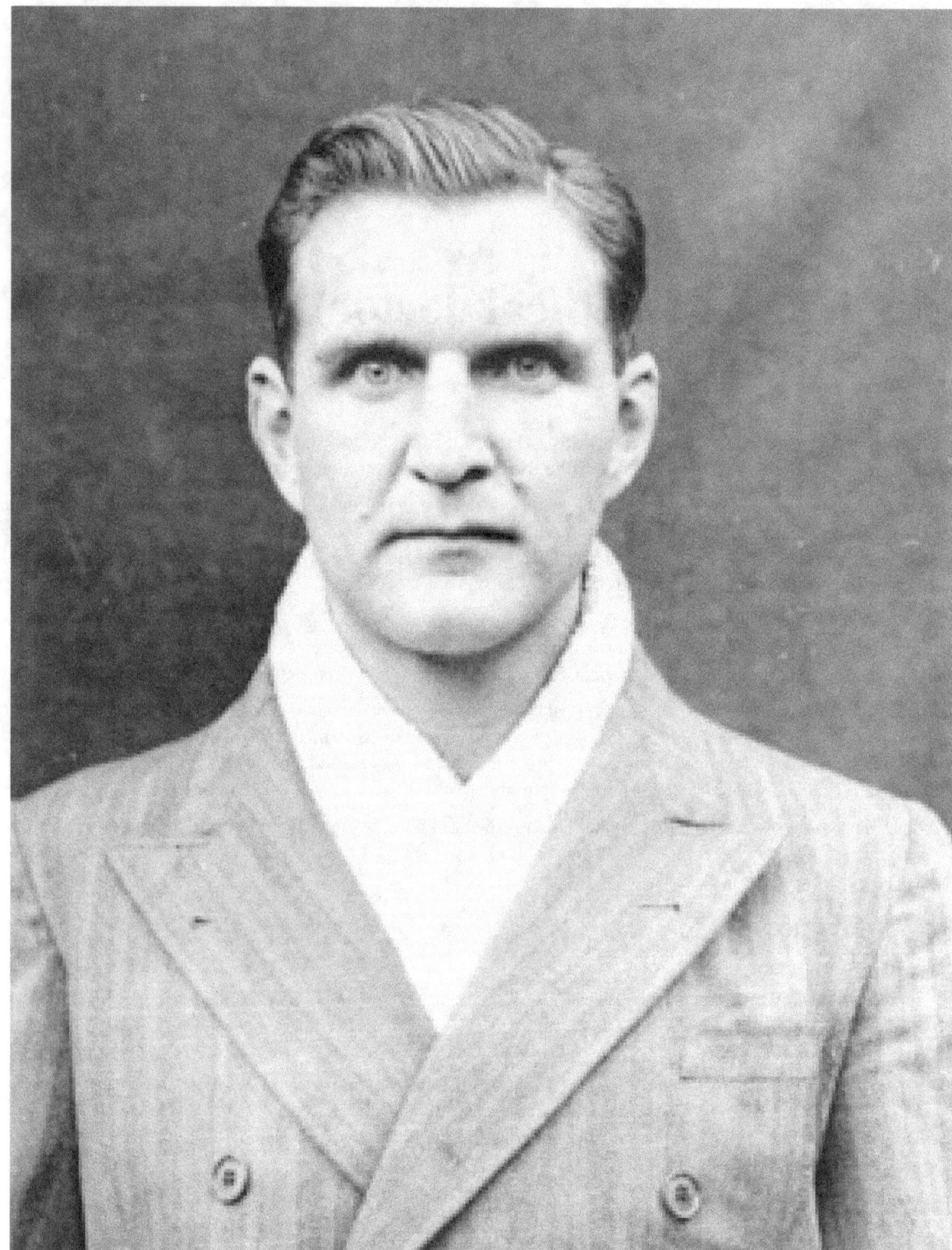

Fritz Fischer as a defendant in the Doctors' Trial.

14.3 External links

- Affidavit of Fritz Ernst Fischer

Chapter 15

Forgiving Dr. Mengele

Forgiving Dr. Mengele is a documentary film about **Eva Mozes Kor**, a victim of the Holocaust, and Dr. Josef Mengele and his staff, who experimented on her and her twin sister Miriam Mozes, as well as approximately 1,400 other twin pairs.

The documentary was directed by Bob Hercules and Cheri Pugh, who also served as producers. They followed Eva for over four years, chronicling her story and her journey to Israel.

Forgiving Dr. Mengele premiered at the Gene Siskel Film Center in Chicago, Illinois, on February 24, 2006. It was scheduled to play for a week, and then travel to other cities in the US. The film is distributed by First Run Features, which handles independent films and documentaries.

15.1 Biographical information on Eva

Eva Mozes Kor and her sister Miriam were born on Jan. 30, 1934 in northern Transylvania Portz, Romania. In 1944, Nazis transported her immediate family to Auschwitz-Birkenau. Because Eva and Miriam were twins, Dr. Mengele selected them to remain alive for experiments.

After a 70-hour ride without food or water, Eva and Miriam, along with their mother, arrived at the selection platform. Eva gripped her mother's hand and looked around: her father and her two older sisters were nowhere in sight. She never saw them again. Soon the twin girls were ripped from their mother, whom they also never saw again.

Eva later recalled how she and her family arrived at the Auschwitz railhead:

> 'When the doors to our cattle car opened, I heard SS soldiers yelling, "Schnell! Schnell!" (Quick!), and ordering everybody out. My mother grabbed Miriam and me by the hand. She was always trying to protect us because we were the youngest. Everything was moving very fast, and as I looked around, I noticed my father and my two older sisters were gone. As I clutched my mother's hand, an SS man hurried by shouting, "Twins! Twins!" He stopped to look at us. Miriam and I looked very much alike. "Are they twins?" he asked my mother. "Is that good?" she replied. He nodded yes. "They are twins," she said ...

> Once the SS guard knew we were twins, Miriam and I were taken away from our mother, without any warning or explanation. Our screams fell on deaf ears. I remember looking back and seeing my mother's arms stretched out in despair as we were led away by a soldier. That was the last time I saw her..."

Eva and Miriam remained in Auschwitz for nine months, enduring experimentation such as being injected with potentially lethal strains of bacteria (and not given treatment). After World War II, they went to Romania and then immigrated to Israel. Eva served in the Israeli Army for ten years. After meeting a tourist who was a Holocaust survivor living in the United States, the two were married, and she moved to the US. In Terre Haute, Indiana, they raised a family and she became a successful realtor and created the C.A.N.D.L.E.S. Museum (Children of Auschwitz Nazi Deadly Lab Experiment Survivors). The museum is dedicated to education about the Holocaust and operates under the mission to "eliminate hatred and prejudice from our world." Her husband, Michael, is a pharmacist, and her son, Alex, is active in the museum and education. He has made trips to Auschwitz on his mother's behalf and has documented these experiences.

15.2 External links

- *Forgiving Dr. Mengele* at the Internet Movie Database
- "A Holocaust Survivor's Path To Peace: Forgiving Josef Mengele" - article in *Der Spiegel*.

Chapter 16

Karl Gebhardt

Karl Franz Gebhardt (23 November 1897 in Haag in Oberbayern – 2 June 1948 in Landsberg Prison, Landsberg am Lech) was a German medical doctor. He served as Medical Superintendent of the Hohenlychen Sanatorium, Consulting Surgeon of the *Waffen-SS*, Chief Surgeon in the Staff of the Reich Physician SS and Police, and personal physician to Heinrich Himmler.[1]

Gebhardt was the main coordinator of a series of surgical experiments performed on inmates of the concentration camps at Ravensbrück and Auschwitz. These experiments were an attempt to defend his approach to the surgical management of grossly contaminated traumatic wounds, against the then-new innovations of antibiotic treatment of injuries acquired on the battlefield.[1]

During the Subsequent Nuremberg Trials, Gebhardt stood trial in the Doctors' Trial (American Military Tribunal No. I). He was convicted of war crimes and crimes against humanity and condemned to death on 20 August 1947. He was hanged on 2 June 1948, in Landsberg Prison in Bavaria.[1]

16.1   Career before World War II

In his student days Gebhardt had been a supporter of the national counter-revolutionary movement and was active among other things in the Volunteer Corps "the Upland Alliance." Gebhardt studied medicine in Munich beginning in 1919.[1] In 1924, after two years as an unpaid assistant physician he received a post as an intern at the Surgical Clinic of the University of Munich.[2] Gebhardt trained under the tutelage of Ferdinand Sauerbruch and later under Erich Lexer, finally gaining his habilitation in 1932.[1] Gebhardt had a distinguished career prior to World War II, contributing a great deal to the development of the field of sports medicine. He wrote articles on physical medicine and rehabilitation, a textbook on sports rehabilitation[3] and he disseminated his ideas in Germany and throughout the rest of Europe.[4]

Gebhardt's Nazi career began with him joining the *Nationalsozialistische Deutsche Arbeiterpartei* (NSDAP, more commonly known as the Nazi Party) on 1 May 1933. In 1935, he moved to Berlin, where he was appointed associate professor. That year, Gebhardt joined the *Schutzstaffel* (SS) and was also appointed Medical Superintendent of Hohenlychen Sanatorium in the Uckermark,[1] which he changed from a sanatorium for tuberculosis patients into an orthopedic clinic. At Hohenlychen Sanatorium, Gebhardt started the first sports medicine clinic in Germany and developed sports programs for amputees and other disabled people. Gebhardt was also appointed to the *Deutsche Hochschule für Leibesübungen* (German College for Physical Education) in 1935, where he became the first professor of sports medicine in Berlin.[4]

In 1936 he distinguished himself in his post as a head of the Medical Department of the *Akademie für Sport und Leibeserziehung* (Academy for Exercise and Physical Training) as senior physician of the 1936 Summer Olympics. Hohenlychen Sanatorium became the sports sanatorium for the Third Reich and served as the central hospital for the athletes who participated in the 1936 Summer Olympics. In 1937 he became chair holder for orthopedic surgery at the University of Berlin. In 1938, Gebhardt was appointed as Heinrich Himmler's personal physician.[4]

16.2 World War II

Gebhardt served as Chief Surgeon of the Staff of the *Reich* during World War II, and under his direction the Hohenlychen Sanatorium became a military hospital for the *Waffen-SS*.[4]

On 27 May 1942, Himmler ordered Gebhardt dispatched to Prague in order to attend to Reinhard Heydrich, who was wounded by an anti-tank grenade during Operation Anthropoid earlier that day.[5] Heydrich was SS-*Obergruppenführer* and *General der Polizei*, and the acting *Reichsprotektor* of the Protectorate of Bohemia and Moravia. When Heydrich developed a fever after surgery for his extensive wounds, Theodor Morell, personal physician to Adolf Hitler, suggested to Gebhardt that he should treat Heydrich with sulfonamide (an early antibiotic). Gebhardt refused Morell's advice, expecting Heydrich to recover without antibiotic therapy. Heydrich died of sepsis on 4 June 1942, eight days after the attack.[6] Gebhardt's refusal to prescribe sulfonamide contributed to Heydrich's death and had many unfortunate implications for concentration camp prisoners, upon whom he later conducted medical experiments.[7][8]

In early 1944, Gebhardt treated Albert Speer for fatigue and a swollen knee. He nearly killed Speer until he was replaced by another doctor, Dr. Friedrich Koch, who intervened on Speer's behalf. Gebhardt eventually rose to the rank of *Gruppenführer* in the *Allgemeine SS* and a *Generalleutnant* in the *Waffen-SS*.

By 22 April 1945, the day before the Red Army entered the outskirts of Berlin, Joseph Goebbels brought his wife and children into the *Vorbunker* to stay. German dictator Adolf Hitler and a few loyal personnel were present in the adjoining *Führerbunker* to direct the final defence of Berlin.[9] Gebhardt, in his capacity as leader of the German Red Cross, approached Goebbels about taking the children out of the city with him, but he was dismissed by Goebbels.[10]

16.3 Medical experiments in concentration camps

During the war, Gebhardt conducted medical and surgical experiments on prisoners in the concentration camps at Ravensbrück (which was close to Hohenlychen Sanatorium) and Auschwitz. At Ravensbruck he had initially faced opposition from camp commandant Fritz Suhren, who feared future legal problems given the status of most camp inmates as political prisoners, but the SS leadership backed Gebhardt and Suhren was forced to cooperate.[11]

Gebhardt was blamed for the death of Reinhard Heydrich, which some believed could have been prevented had Heydrich been treated with sulfonamide. Himmler suggested to Gebhardt that he should conduct experiments proving that sulfonamide was useless in the treatment of gangrene and sepsis. In order to vindicate his decision to not administer sulfa drugs in treating Heydrich's wounds, he carried out a series of experiments on Ravensbrück concentration camp prisoners, breaking their legs and infecting them with various organisms in order to prove the worthlessness of the drugs in treating gas gangrene. He also attempted to transplant the limbs from camp victims to German soldiers wounded on the Russian front. The Ravensbrück experiments were slanted in Gebhardt's favor; women in the sulfonamide-treated experimental group received little or no nursing care, while those in the untreated control group received better care. Not surprisingly, those in the control group were more likely to survive the experiments.[7][8]

16.4 Trial and execution

During the Subsequent Nuremberg Trials, Gebhardt stood trial in the Doctors' Trial (9 December 1946–20 August 1947), along with 22 other doctors. He was found guilty of war crimes and crimes against humanity and sentenced to death on 20 August 1947. He was hanged on 2 June 1948, in Landsberg Prison in Bavaria.[1]

Two of Gebhardt's assistants were also tried and convicted at Nuremberg. Fritz Fischer worked in the hospital of the Ravensbrück concentration camp as a surgical assistant to Gebhardt, and participated in the surgical experiments carried out on the inmates.[12] He was initially condemned to life imprisonment, but his sentence was reduced to 15 years in 1951 and he was released in March 1954. Fischer subsequently regained his medical license and resumed his career at the chemical company Boehringer Ingelheim, where he remained employed until his retirement. He died in 2003 at the age of 90.

Herta Oberheuser was another of Gebhardt's assistants at the Ravensbrück concentration camp. She was the only female

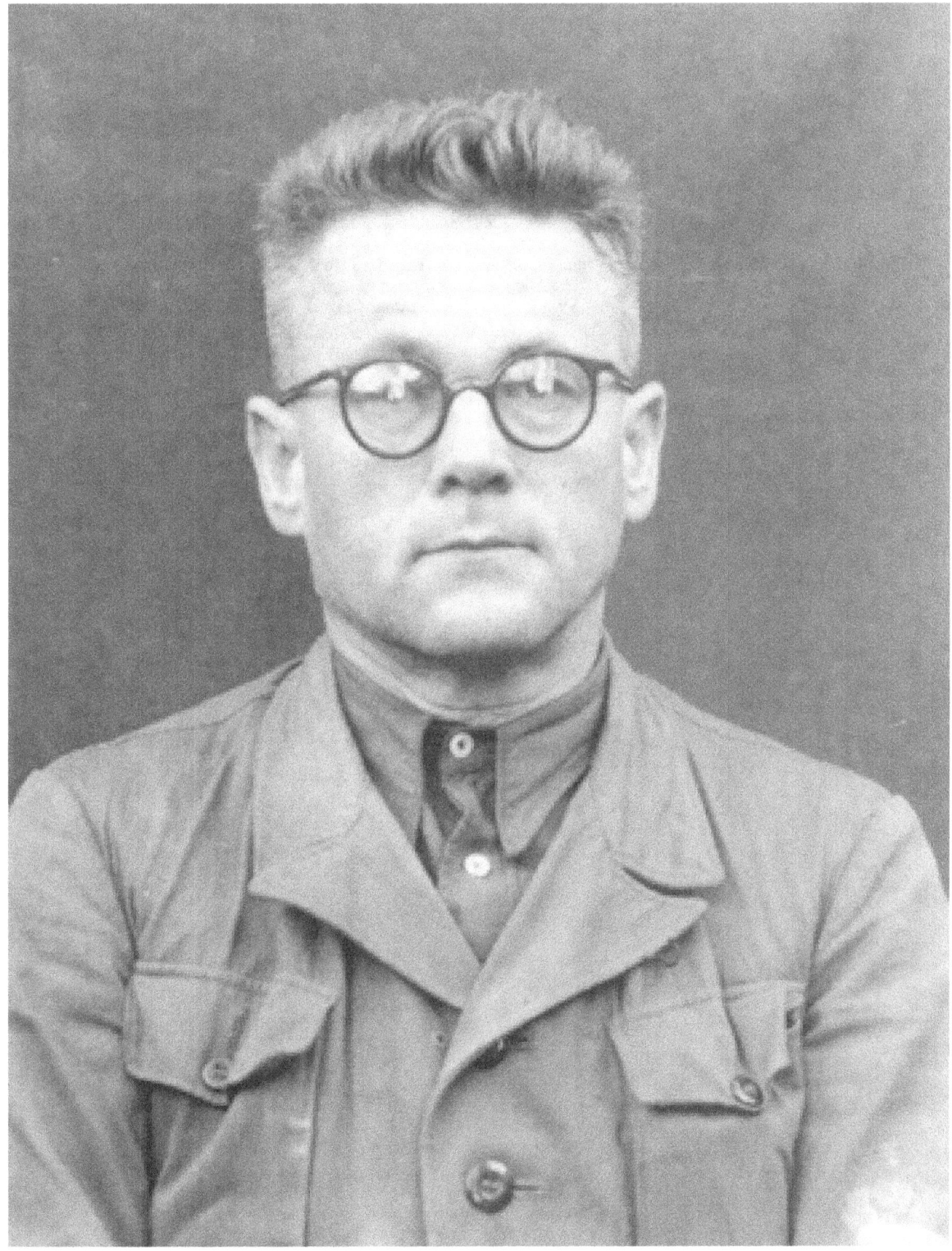

Photograph of Karl Gebhardt as a defendant in the Doctors' Trial at Nuremberg. Courtesy of the United States Holocaust Memorial Museum.

defendant in the Doctors' Trial, where she was sentenced to 20 years in prison. She was released in April 1952 and became a family doctor in Stocksee, Germany. She lost her position in 1956 after a Ravensbrück survivor recognized her, and her medical license was revoked in 1958.[13] She died on 24 January 1978 at the age of 66.

16.5 References

[1] Dörner, K, ed. (2001). *The Nuremberg Medical Trial 1946/47:guide to the microfiche edition.* Munich: K.G. Saur Verlag GmbH. p. 91. ISBN 3598321546.

[2] "Chirurgische krankengymnastik (book review)". *British Journal of Surgery* **20** (80): 708. 1933. doi:10.1002/bjs.1800208042.

[3] Gebhardt, K (1931). *Chirurgische krankengymnastik* (in German). Leipzig: Johann Ambrosius Barth. pp. 1–42.

[4] Silver, JR (2011). "Karl Gebhardt (1897–1948): a lost man" (PDF). *Journal of the Royal College of Physicians of Edinburgh* **41** (4): 366–71. doi:10.4997/JRCPE.2011.417. PMID 22184577.

[5] Moorehead, C (2011). *A Train in Winter.* London: Chatto & Windus. pp. 252–3. ISBN 978-0-7011-8281-6.

[6] Williams, Max (2003). *Reinhard Heydrich: The Biography.* 2—Enigma. Church Stretton: Ulric Publishing. p. 165. ISBN 978-0-9537577-6-3.

[7] Time Inc. (1947-02-24). "Human laboratory animals". *Life* (New York City: Time Inc.) **22** (8): 81–4. Retrieved 2012-06-10.

[8] "Nuremberg Trials 60th Anniversary Euthanasia, Medical Experiments, and Sterilization". *The Anti-Defamation League Dimensions Online* **19** (Fall). 2006.

[9] Beevor, A (2002). *Berlin: The Downfall 1945.* Viking Press/Penguin Books. pp. 380, 381. ISBN 0-670-88695-5.

[10] Tony Le Tissier (1999). *Race for the Reichstag: The 1945 Battle for Berlin*, Routledge, p. 62

[11] Heberer P, Matthäus J (2008). *Atrocities on Trial: Historical Perspectives on the Politics of Prosecuting War Crimes*, University of Nebraska Press, p. 136

[12] Affidavit of Fritz Ernst Fischer

[13] Herta Oberheuser

- Bio-sketch

Chapter 17

Karl Genzken

Karl August Genzken (born June 8, 1885 in Preetz, Holstein – October 10, 1957 in Hamburg, Germany) was a Nazi physician who conducted human experiments on prisoners of several concentration camps. He was a *Gruppenführer* (Major General) of the Waffen-SS and the Chief of the Medical Office of the Waffen-SS. Genzken was tried as a war criminal in the Doctors' Trial at Nuremberg.

17.1   Military career

Genzken had joined the NSDAP on July 7, 1926 (party member No. 39,913). He joined the SS on November 5, 1933 (No. 207,954).

In 1934, he was reactivated as a reserve officer in the Naval Medical Service. After that, he transferred to the SS Operational Main Office then was promoted from an assistant medical director to the medical superintendent of the SS Hospital in Berlin, and appointed Chief of the Medical Office of the Waffen-SS in 1942. He rose to the rank of Major General in the Waffen-SS.

Genzken was involved in a series of human experiments that were carried out on prisoners of several concentration camps. Genzken was accused and convicted of involvement in the typhus experiments conducted from December 1941 - February 1945, which were conducted for the benefit of the German armed forces to test the effectiveness of vaccines against typhus, smallpox, cholera, and other diseases. The experiments were conducted at Buchenwald and Natzweiler. Genzken was also accused of involvement in sulfanilamide experiments, poison experiments, and incendiary bomb experiments but was not convicted on these counts.

17.2   Trial and conviction

Genzken was found guilty of war crimes, crimes against humanity, and membership in an illegal organization by the American Military Tribunal No. I. He was condemned in August 1947 to life imprisonment by the tribunal. His sentence was later reduced to 20 years and he was released in April 1954.

17.3   See also

- Concentration Camps Inspectorate

- Doctors' Trial

- Nazi human experimentation

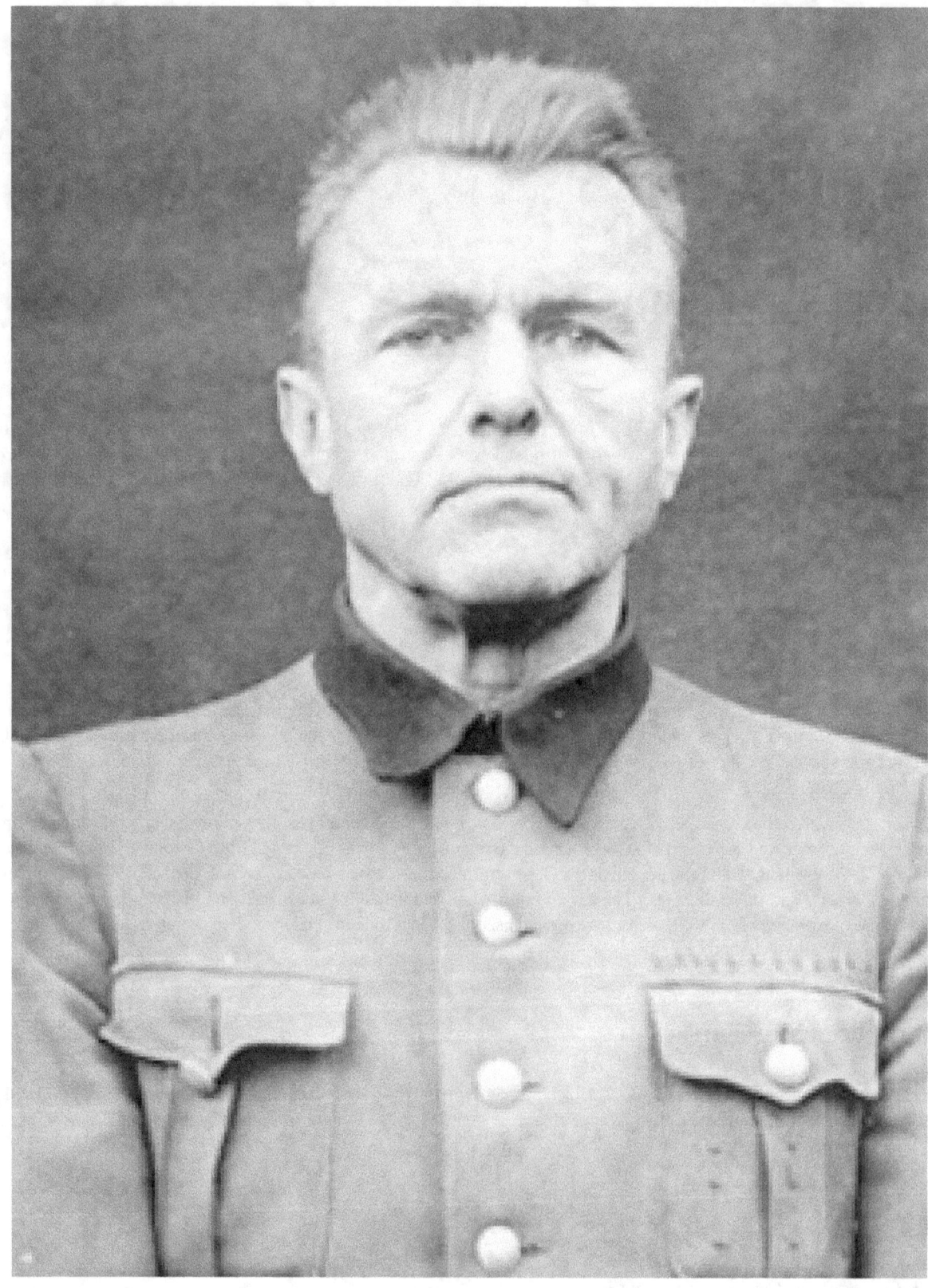

Karl August Genzken as a defendant in the Doctors' Trial at Nuremberg.

- Ex-Nazis

17.4 References

McHaney, James M.; Alexander G. Hardy; Arnost Horlick-Hochwald; Esther Jane Johnson (June 16, 1947). "Closing Brief for the United States of America Against Karl Genzken". Harvard Law School Library. Retrieved 2007-12-18.

- OCLC's Authority records for 20070228

Chapter 18

Julius Hallervorden

Julius Hallervorden (October 21, 1882 – May 29, 1965) was a German physician and neuroscientist. In 1938, he became the head of the Neuropathology Department of the Kaiser Wilhelm Institute for Brain Research. He was a member of the Nazi Party, and admitted to knowingly performing much of his research on the brains of executed prisoners. Along with Hugo Spatz, he is credited with the discovery of Hallervorden-Spatz syndrome (now, in light of revelations of his Nazi past, more commonly referred to as Pantothenate kinase-associated neurodegeneration).[1][2]

18.1 See also

- List of medical eponyms with Nazi associations

18.2 References

[1] Strous, Rael D.; Morris C. Edelman (March 2007). "Eponyms and the Nazi Era: Time to Remember and Time For Change" (PDF). *Israel Medical Association Journal* **9** (3): 207–214. Retrieved 2010-11-01.

[2] Shevell, Michael; Jüergen Peiffer (August 2001). "Julius Hallervorden's wartime activities: implications for science under dictatorship". *Pediatr Neurol* **25** (2): 162–165. PMID 11551747.

Chapter 19

Siegfried Handloser

Siegfried Adolf Handloser (25 March 1885 – 3 July 1954) was a Doctor, Prof. Dr. med., Generaloberstabsarzt (thee stars, OF-8) of the German Armed Forces Medical Services, Chief of the German Armed Forces Medical Services. He was one of the accused in the Doctors' Trial in Nuremberg—after the main Nuremberg Trials.

Born in Konstanz he had been a member of the German Army Medical Service since the First World War. In 1938, Handloser was promoted to the position of Army Group physician of the Army Group Command 3. In October, 1939, he was named honorary professor.

He had held the position of Chief of the Medical Services of the Armed Forces during World War II. It was the most important medical position in the entire German Armed Forces and the Waffen-SS.

Yet despite his full knowledge, he had done nothing to stop medical experiments conducted on concentration camp prisoners; this was sufficient to implicate him in the several medical cases dealt with during the Doctors' Trial.

He was convicted by the American Military Tribunal No. I in August, 1947, and sentenced to life imprisonment. This was later reduced to 20 years and, in 1954, he was released. Shortly afterwards, Handloser died of cancer in Munich at the age of 69.

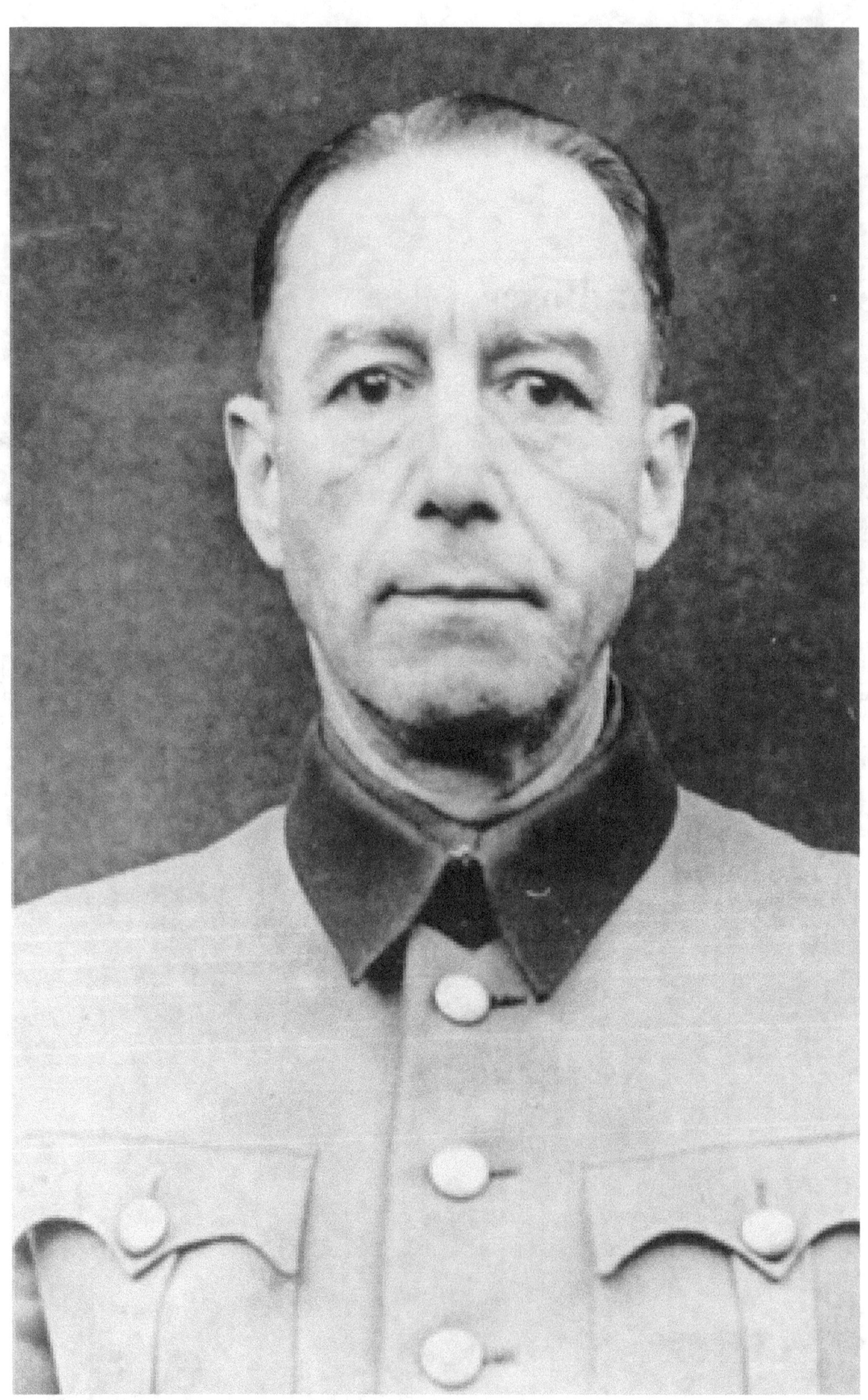

Mug shot of Siegfried Handloser ca 1946

Chapter 20

Aribert Heim

Aribert Ferdinand Heim (28 June 1914 – 10 August 1992)[1] was an Austrian SS doctor, also known as Dr. Death. During World War II he served at the Mauthausen-Gusen concentration camp in Mauthausen, killing and torturing inmates by various methods, such as direct injections of toxic compounds into the hearts of his victims.[2]

After the war, Heim lived for many years in Cairo, Egypt, under the alias of Tarek Farid Hussein, and died there on 10 August 1992 according to testimony by his son and lawyer. This information, though set forth by a German court, has been challenged.[3][4] In 2009, a BBC documentary stated that German police had found no evidence of Heim's death on their recent visit to Cairo;[5] nevertheless, three years later, a court in Baden-Baden confirmed again that Heim had died in 1992, based on new evidence provided by his family and lawyer.[1]

20.1   Life

Heim was born in Bad Radkersburg, Austria-Hungary. He was the son of a policeman and a housewife. He studied medicine in Graz, and received his diploma in Vienna. Heim joined the SS after the Anschluss. He volunteered for the Waffen-SS in the spring of 1940, rising to the rank of Hauptsturmführer (Captain).

20.1.1   Mauthausen concentration camp

Aribert Heim worked in Mauthausen as a doctor starting in October 1941 at the age of 26, and he only worked there for six weeks.[6] The prisoners at Mauthausen called Heim "Dr. Death", or the "Butcher of Mauthausen" for his cruelty.[7] He was known there for performing operations without anaesthesia. For about two months (October to December 1941), Heim was stationed at the Ebensee concentration camp near Linz (Austria), where he carried out experiments on Jews and others similar to those performed at Auschwitz by Josef Mengele. According to Holocaust survivors, Jewish prisoners were poisoned with various injections directly into the heart, including petrol, phenol, available poisons or even water, to induce death.[8]

He is reported to have removed organs from living prisoners without anesthesia, killing hundreds.[9] A prisoner by the name of Karl Lotter also worked in the Mauthausen hospital at the time Aribert Heim was there.[10] Mr. Lotter testified that in 1941, he witnessed Aribert Heim butcher a prisoner who came to him with an inflamed foot.[10] Mr. Lotter provided more gruesome details about how Aribert butchered the 18-year-old prisoner.[10] Mr. Lotter stated that Aribert gave the prisoner anesthetic and then proceeded to cut him open, castrate him, and take out one of his kidneys.[10] The prisoner died, and his head was cut off, boiled and stripped of its flesh.[10] Aribert Heim then allegedly used this young man's skull as a paperweight on his desk.[10] In a sworn statement that was given eight years after the incident Lotter stated that Heim, "needed the head because of its perfect teeth".[10]

Other survivors of the Holocaust talk of Aribert removing tattooed flesh from prisoners and using the skin to make seat coverings, which he gave to the command-ant of the camp.[6]

20.1.2 Later service

From February 1942, Heim served in the 6th SS Mountain Division Nord in northern Finland, especially in Oulu's hospitals as an SS doctor. His service continued until at least October 1942.[11][12]

On 15 March 1945 Heim was captured by US soldiers and sent to a camp for prisoners of war. He was released and worked as a gynecologist at Baden-Baden until his disappearance in 1962; he had telephoned his home and was told that the police were waiting for him. Having been questioned on previous occasions, he surmised the reason (an international warrant for his arrest had been in place since that date) and went into hiding.[9] According to his son Rüdiger Heim, he drove through France and Spain onward to Morocco, moving finally to Egypt via Libya.[13] After Alois Brunner (Adolf Eichmann's top assistant), Heim had been the second most wanted Nazi officer.

20.2 Sightings and investigations

In the years following his disappearance, Heim was the target of a rapidly escalating manhunt and ever-increasing rewards for his capture. Following his escape there were reported sightings in Latin America, Spain and Africa, as well as formal investigations aimed at bringing him to justice, some of which took place even after he had apparently died in Egypt. The German government offered €150,000 for information leading to his arrest, while the Simon Wiesenthal Center launched Operation Last Chance, a project to assist governments in the location and arrest of suspected Nazi war criminals who are still alive.[14] Tax records prove that, as late as 2001, Heim's lawyer asked the German authorities to refund capital gains taxes levied on him because he was living abroad.[14]

Heim reportedly hid out in South America, Spain and the Balkans, but only his presence in Spain has ever been confirmed.[13] He was alleged to have moved to Spain after fleeing Paysandú, Uruguay, when he was located by the Israeli Mossad. Efraim Zuroff, of the Wiesenthal Center, initiated an active search for his whereabouts,[14] and in late 2005, Spanish police incorrectly determined that he was located in Palafrugell.[15] According to *El Mundo*, Heim had been helped by associates of Otto Skorzeny, who had organised one of the biggest ODESSA bases in Franco's Spain.[16] Press reports in mid-October 2005 suggested that Heim's arrest by Spanish police was "imminent". Within a few days, however, newer reports suggested that he had successfully evaded capture and had moved either to another part of Spain or else to Denmark.[17][18][19][20]

Fredrik Jensen, a Norwegian and a former SS Obersturmführer, was put under police investigation in June 2007, and charged with assisting Heim in his escape. The accusation was denied by Jensen.[21]

In July 2007, the Austrian Justice Ministry declared that it would pay €50,000 for information leading to his arrest and extradition to Austria.[22]

On 6 July 2008 Dr. Efraim Zuroff, the Wiesenthal Center's chief Nazi-hunter, headed to South America as part of a public campaign to capture the most wanted Nazi in the world and bring him to justice,[14] claiming that Heim was alive and hiding in Patagonia, either in Chile or in Argentina. He elaborated on 15 July 2008 that he was sure Heim was alive and the groundwork had been laid to capture him within weeks.[8][23][24][25][26][27][28]

In 2008, Heim was named as one of the ten most wanted Nazi war criminals by the Simon Wiesenthal Center.[9][29]

20.3 Later years and death

In 2006, a German newspaper reported that he had a daughter, Waltraud, living on the outskirts of Puerto Montt, Chile who said he died in 1993.[30] However, when she tried to recover a million-dollar inheritance from an account in his name, she was unable to provide a death certificate.[31][32][33]

In August 2008, Heim's son Rüdiger asked that his father be declared legally dead, in order to take hold of his assets; he intended to donate them to projects working to document the atrocities committed in the camps.[34]

After years of apparently false sightings, the circumstances surrounding Heim's escape, life in hiding and death were jointly reported by the German broadcaster ZDF and the New York Times in February 2009. They reported that he lived under a false name, Tarek Farid Hussein, in Egypt and that he died of intestinal cancer in Cairo in 1992.[35]

In an interview at the family's villa in Baden-Baden his son Rüdiger admitted publicly for the first time that he was with his father in Egypt at the time of his death. Heim says it was during the Olympics, and that he died the day after the games ended. According to Efraim Zuroff, Rüdiger Heim had - until the publishing of the ZDF research results - constantly denied having any knowledge of the whereabouts of Aribert Heim.[14]

On 18 March 2009, the Simon Wiesenthal Center filed a criminal complaint due to suspicion of false testimony.[36]

In 2012, a regional court in Baden-Baden confirmed that Heim died under the assumed identity of Tarek Hussein Farid in Egypt in 1992, based on evidence that his family and lawyer had presented.[1]

20.4 Family

Aribert Heim has an ex-wife, Freida Heim, and two sons with Freida. Their names are Albert Christian Heim and Rudiger Holf Heim. He also has an illegitimate daughter in Chile named Waltraud. Aribert's one-time lover, Gertrud Boser, is Waltraud's mother.[5] After World War II, Aribert Heim escaped to Baden-Baden with his family where he opened a successful gynecology practice until he received word from a friend that he was wanted in suspicion of crimes he allegedly committed while working at Mauthausen.[37] Currently, Freida and her sons reside in Baden-Baden Germany in the home that Aribert Heim shared with his family before he went into hiding.[5]

20.5 References

[1] "German court confirms Nazi 'Doctor Death' died in 1992". BBC. 2012-09-21. Retrieved 2012-09-21.

[2] "The life and crimes of 'Dr Death'". *BBC News*. 5 February 2009.

[3] From the Briefcase of Dr. Aribert Heim, New York Times, February 4, 2009.

[4] "Nazi camp doctor 'died in 1992'". *BBC News*. 4 February 2009.

[5] "The Hunt for Dr Death". *The Last Nazis*. Episode 1. 12 September 2009. BBC Two. Retrieved 10 March 2014.

[6] Carroll, Rory, Goni, Uki. "G2: The Hunt for Doctor Death: As an SS Medic, Aribert Heim Carried Out Horrific Experiments on Concentration Camp Prisoners. He Escaped and is Thought to be Hiding in Argentina - but the Net may Finally be Closing. Rory Carroll and Uki Goni on the Search for the Last of the Nazis.". *ProQuest*. The Guardian: 4. Retrieved 26 October 2015.

[7] Dsl with Wires (September 21, 2012). "Search for 'Dr Death' Ends: Nazi War Criminal Aribert Heim Declared Dead". Der Spiegel Online. Retrieved 21 July 2013.

[8] "Nazi doctor 'is alive in Chile'". BBC. 2008-07-08. Retrieved 2008-07-08.

[9] "Most Wanted Nazis", Bridget Johnson, About.com

[10] Harris, Ed. "Butcher of Mauthausen' is the most Wanted Nazi". *ProQuest*. Evening Standard. Retrieved 27 October 2015.

[11] (Finnish) ETSITTY NATSIRIKOLLINEN TOIMI LÄÄKÄRINÄ MYÖS SUOMESSA *A-Piste*. 30 November 2007.

[12] (German) "Es geht mir gut" *Der Spiegel. 9 July 2008.*

[13] "Meistgesuchter Nazi-Verbrecher seit 1992 tot". ZDF. Retrieved 4 February 2009.

[14] Zuroff, Efraim (2009). "Dr. Heim, the most wanted Nazi in the world". *Operation Last Chance: One Man's Quest to Bring Nazi Criminals to Justice*. Palgrave Macmillan. pp. 185–207. ISBN 0-230-61730-1.

[15] Nazi war criminal escapes Costa Brava police search, *The Guardian*, 17 October 2005

[16] (Spanish) A la caza del último nazi, *El Mundo*, 30 October 2005

[17] Germany expresses 'utmost interest' in seeing Nazi face justice, *Ireland Online*, 17 October 2005.

[18] Nazi 'Dr. Death' tracked to Spain, *Ottawa Sun / AP*, 16 October 2005.

[19] German courts seek Nazi fugitive thought to be in Chile, *The Santiago Times*, 26 April 2006.

[20] Warrant of Apprehension Austrian Justice Ministry, July 2007.

[21] Accused of hiding "Doctor Death", *Aftenposten*, 23 August 2007

[22] Report: Net closing in on top Nazi criminal Aribert Heim, *Haaretz*, 28 July 2007

[23] Nazi hunter looking for 'Dr. Death' in S. America | International | Jerusalem Post

[24] "SS doctor 'still alive in Chile'". BBC News. 2008-07-15. Retrieved 2008-07-15.

[25] "Nazi hunters search Chile for 'Dr. Death'".

[26] Concentration camp doctor Aribert Heim is the most-wanted Nazi war criminal Telegraph.co.uk 30 April 2008

[27] Nazi doctor 'is alive in Chile' BBC NEWS 9 July 2008

[28] The Hunt for Nazi War Criminal Aribert Heim, aka "Dr. Death" Investigation Discovery 10 July 2008

[29] "Fugitive Hunt", *Dateline World Jewry*, World Jewish Congress, July/August 2008

[30] Nazi hunter: 'Give up, Dr. Death' - World news - Americas - msnbc.com

[31] http://news.bbc.co.uk/1/hi/world/7871121.stm>

[32] (German) Geheimorganisation angeblich auf Nazi Jagd, ORF, accessed 2007-10-14

[33] (Spanish) Un tribunal alemán pide a la justicia chilena datos sobre el paradero del 'carnicero de Mathausen', *El Pais*, 28 April 2006

[34] "Son of Nazi wants him declared dead".

[35] "Nazi 'Dr. Death' hunt leads to Cairo." *CNN*. Retrieved on February 5, 2009.

[36] Mekhennet, Souad; Kulish, Nicholas (5 February 2009). "Uncovering Lost Path of the Most Wanted Nazi". *The New York Times*.

[37] Myers, Kevin. "Why I Wish Nazi-Hunters Well in Search for Death Camp Fiend". *Proquest*. The Guardian. Retrieved 12 November 2015.

20.6 Further reading

- N.Y. Times (2009) From the Briefcase of Dr. Aribert Heim: The Personal Archives of the Most Wanted Nazi War Criminal, New York Times, retrieved 4 February 2009 (dozens of Aribert Heim's personal documents have been scanned and are available for viewing on the N.Y. Times' multimedia website)

- Nicholas Kulish and Souad Mekhennet, Being the Son of a Nazi, *The Atlantic*, March 22, 2014 (article about Heim's later years by the authors of *The Eternal Nazi*

Chapter 21

Hans Heinze

Hans Heinze, sometimes referred to as ***Euthanasie-Heinze*** ("Euthanasia Heinze"; 18 October 1895 – 4 February 1983) was a Nazi German psychiatrist and eugenicist. In 1997/1998 his rehabilitation as a consequence of the request submitted by a German historian as a means of obtaining research material caused controversy.

21.1   Life

After service as a medical orderly during World War I Heinze trained as a psychiatrist at Leipzig, where he worked from 1924 in child psychiatry. He was later appointed director of the child psychiatry department of the University Clinic in Berlin, and also, in 1934, director of the *Landesheilanstalt* in Potsdam, holding the two posts simultaneously. On 2 October 1939 he was appointed Dozent for neurology and psychiatry in the medical faculty of Berlin University, where on 6 April 1943 he became a professor.

In November 1938 Heinze took over the direction of the *Landes-Pflegeanstalt Brandenburg an der Havel* mental institution, commonly now referred to as the Brandenburg Euthanasia Centre,[1] with about 2,500 patients, 1,000 of them children. Here he supervised the murder by injection, starvation and poisoning of thousands of children whose brains he then supplied to Nazi researchers.[2] He also trained physicians for the T4 Euthanasia Programme.

After the war Heinze remained in post at Brandenburg-Görden. The Russians were interested in some of his work and offered him the direction of an institution in the Crimea, but when he turned this down, tried him for war crimes, convicting him on 14 March 1946. He was imprisoned for seven years, mostly in the Soviet Special Camp No. 7 at Sachsenhausen, where he worked as the camp doctor.[3][4]

He was released on 14 March 1952 and declined offers of senior medical posts in the Volkspolizei and at the University of Jena in order to return to his family in West Germany. He took up the directorship of the department of child and adolescent psychiatry in the hospital of Wunstorf in Lower Saxony, where he remained until his retirement, and where he died in 1983.[5]

21.2   German judicial investigation

In 1962 the legal authorities of Lower Saxony opened a preliminary investigation into Heinze, but the proceedings were halted after Heinze, represented by the lawyer Kurt Giese (formerly a senior lawyer in the Private Chancellery of the Führer) was declared psychologically unfit for the process.[5]

21.3 Rehabilitation

In 1997 Dr Klaus-Dieter Müller, a German historian seeking research material, approached the Russian military authorities for their files on Heinze, which he was only able to obtain by entering a request for Heinze's rehabilitation (a recognition by the Russian authorities of Heinze's innocence of the crimes for which he had been imprisoned). As a result of Müller's request the Russian military legal service reviewed Heinze's case and in 1998 declared him rehabilitated. This caused considerable discussion in Germany of the extent to which historians should take responsibility for the consequences of their researches.[6][7]

21.4 Publications

- *Veränderungen des Liquor cerebrospinalis und ihre Bedeutung für die Auffassung vom Wesen des Ischias*, Leipzig 1923

- *Kindliche Charaktere und ihre Abartigkeiten*, Paul Schröder with explanatory case studies by Hans Heinze, Breslau 1931

- *Zur Phänomenologie des Gemüts*, Berlin 1932

- *Die Entstehung und Funktion des intervillösen Raumes*, Halle 1933

- *Rasse und Erbe: Ein Wegweiser auf dem Gebiet der Rassenkunde, Vererbungslehre und Erbgesundheitspflege für den Gebrauch an Volks- und Mittelschulen*, Halle 1934

- *"Zirkuläres Irresein (manisch-depressives): Psychopathologische Persönlichkeiten"*, Handbuch der Erbkrankheiten ("Handbook of Hereditary Illnesses"), ed. Arthur Julius Gütt,Vol. 4, revised by Hans Heinze et al., Thieme, Leipzig 1942[8]

- *Ein Geschwisterpaar mit Myoklonusepilepsie*, Bonn 1955

21.5 Notes and references

[1] not the same buildings that are now Brandenburg-Görden Prison

[2] "The Rise of hatred & violence in Germany - Freedom Magazine". *Freedom Magazine*. 1995. p. 58. Retrieved April 27, 2014.

[3]

[4] p. 17, Ernst Klee: „Was sie taten – Was sie wurden", p. 136

[5] Ernst Klee: „Was sie taten – Was sie wurden", pp. 137/138

[6] „Verfolgung unterm Sowjetstern in der SBZ/DDRF", XV. Bautzen-Forum der Friedrich-Ebert-Stiftung, Büro Leipzig, 13 and 14 May 2004, ISBN 3-89892-296-0 (PDF; 695 kB)

[7] Warum ein Nazi-Massenmörder rehabilitiert wurde. *Spiegel Online, 24 August 2004]*

[8] The Deutsche Nationalbibliothek lists this 6-volume handbook of Nazi euthanasia medicine only at Leipzig, in the former DDR. In the former BRD the copies at Frankfurt/Main were apparently disposed of; in any event they are not now to be found in the OPAC.

21.6 See also

- Euthanasia

21.7   External links

- Archived version; original version link is dead: List of FBI Files on Nazi War Crimes page 2

21.8   Bibliography

- Götz Aly (ed.): *Aktion T4. 1939–1945. Die „Euthanasie"-Zentrale in der Tiergartenstraße 4.* 2nd expanded edition. Edition Hentrich, Berlin 1989, ISBN 3-926175-66-4 (*Reihe deutsche Vergangenheit. Stätten der Geschichte Berlins* 26), (exhibition catalogue)

- Henry Friedlander: *Der Weg zum NS-Genozid. Von der Euthanasie zur Endlösung.* Berlin, Berlin-Verlag 1997, ISBN 3-8270-0265-6

- Ernst Klee, ed. (1985) (in German), *Dokumente zur „Euthanasie"*, Frankfurt am Main: Fischer, ISBN 3-596-24327-0

- Ernst Klee: *„Euthanasie" im NS-Staat. Die „Vernichtung lebensunwerten Lebens".* 11th edition. Fischer-Taschenbuch-Verlag, Frankfurt am Main 2004, ISBN 3-596-24326-2 (*Fischer-Taschenbücher. 4326 Die Zeit des Nationalsozialismus*)

- Ernst Klee: *Hans Heinze.* In: Ernst Klee: *Das Personenlexikon zum Dritten Reich. Wer war was vor und nach 1945.* (updated edition). Fischer-Taschenbuch-Verlag, Frankfurt am Main 2005, ISBN 3-596-16048-0, p. 43 (*Fischer* 16048)

- Ernst Klee: *Was sie taten – was sie wurden. Ärzte, Juristen und andere Beteiligte am Kranken- oder Judenmord.* 12th edition. Fischer-Taschenbuch-Verlag, Frankfurt am Main 2004, ISBN 3-596-24364-5 (*Fischer-Taschenbücher. 4364 Die Zeit des Nationalsozialismus*)

- Ernst Klee: *Verschonte Medizinverbrecher. Die Professoren Heinze und Hallervorden.* In: *Dachauer Hefte.* 13, 1997, ISSN 0257-9472, pp. 143–152

- Alexander Mitscherlich, Fred Mielke (ed.): *Medizin ohne Menschlichkeit. Dokumente des Nürnberger Ärzteprozesse* (new edition). Fischer-Taschenbuch-Verlag, Frankfurt am Main 1987, ISBN 3-596-22003-3 (*Fischer-Taschenbücher* 2003)

- Spiegel Online, 24 August 2004@ *Warum ein Nazi-Massenmörder rehabilitiert wurde*

- Manfred Müller-Küppers: Die Geschichte der Kinder- und Jugendpsychiatrie unter besonderer Berücksichtigung der Zeit des Nationalsozialismus in: *Forum der Kinder- und Jugendpsychiatrie und Psychotherapie* Heft 2, 2001

- Hans-Walter Schmuhl: "Hirnforschung und Krankenmord. Das Kaiser-Wilhelm-Institut für Hirnforschung 1937 - 1945 (PDF; 243 kB)" Series: Ergebnisse, 1. Stand 2000

- dsb.: Medizin in der NS-Zeit: Hirnforschung und Krankenmord in: *Deutsches Ärzteblatt* 2001; Year 98. A 1240–1245, Heft 19

Chapter 22

Kurt Heissmeyer

Kurt Heissmeyer (December 26, 1905 – August 29, 1967) was a Nazi SS physician[1] involved in medical experimentation on concentration camp inmates including children.

22.1 Medical experiments

In order to obtain a professorship, Heissmeyer needed to present original research.

Although previously disproven, his hypothesis was that the injection of live tuberculosis bacilli into subjects would act as a vaccine. Another component of his experimentation was based on pseudoscientific Nazi racial theory that race played a factor in developing tuberculosis.

He attempted to prove his hypothesis by injecting live tuberculosis bacilli into the lungs and bloodstream of "Untermenschen" (subhumans), Jews and Slavs being considered by the Nazis to be racially inferior to Germans.

He was able to have the facilities made available and to test his subjects as a result of personal connections: his uncle, SS general August Heissmeyer,[2][3][4] and his close acquaintance, SS general Oswald Pohl.[5]

His experiment was conducted on 20 Jewish children at Neuengamme concentration camp. The children, along with their four adult caretakers, were murdered by being hanged in the basement of Bullenhuser Damm School in Hamburg.

After the war, Heissmeyer escaped detection and returned to his home in Magdeburg in postwar East Germany and started a successful medical practice as a lung and tuberculosis specialist. He was eventually found out in 1959. In 1966, he was convicted and sentenced to life imprisonment. At his trial he stated, "I did not think that inmates of a camp had full value as human beings." When asked why he didn't use guinea pigs he responded, "For me there was no basic difference between human beings and guinea pigs." He then corrected himself: "Jews and guinea pigs".[6] Heissmeyer died on 29 August 1967.

22.2 See also

- Bullenhuser Damm

22.3 References

[1] Medicine and medical ethics in Nazi Germany: origins, practices, legacies By Francis R. Nicosia, Jonathan Huener p.84

[2] The Nazi Doctors by Robert Jay Lifton: Medical Killing and the Psychology of Genocide Publisher: Basic Books (August 2000) Language: English ISBN 0-465-04905-2 ISBN 978-0-465-04905-9

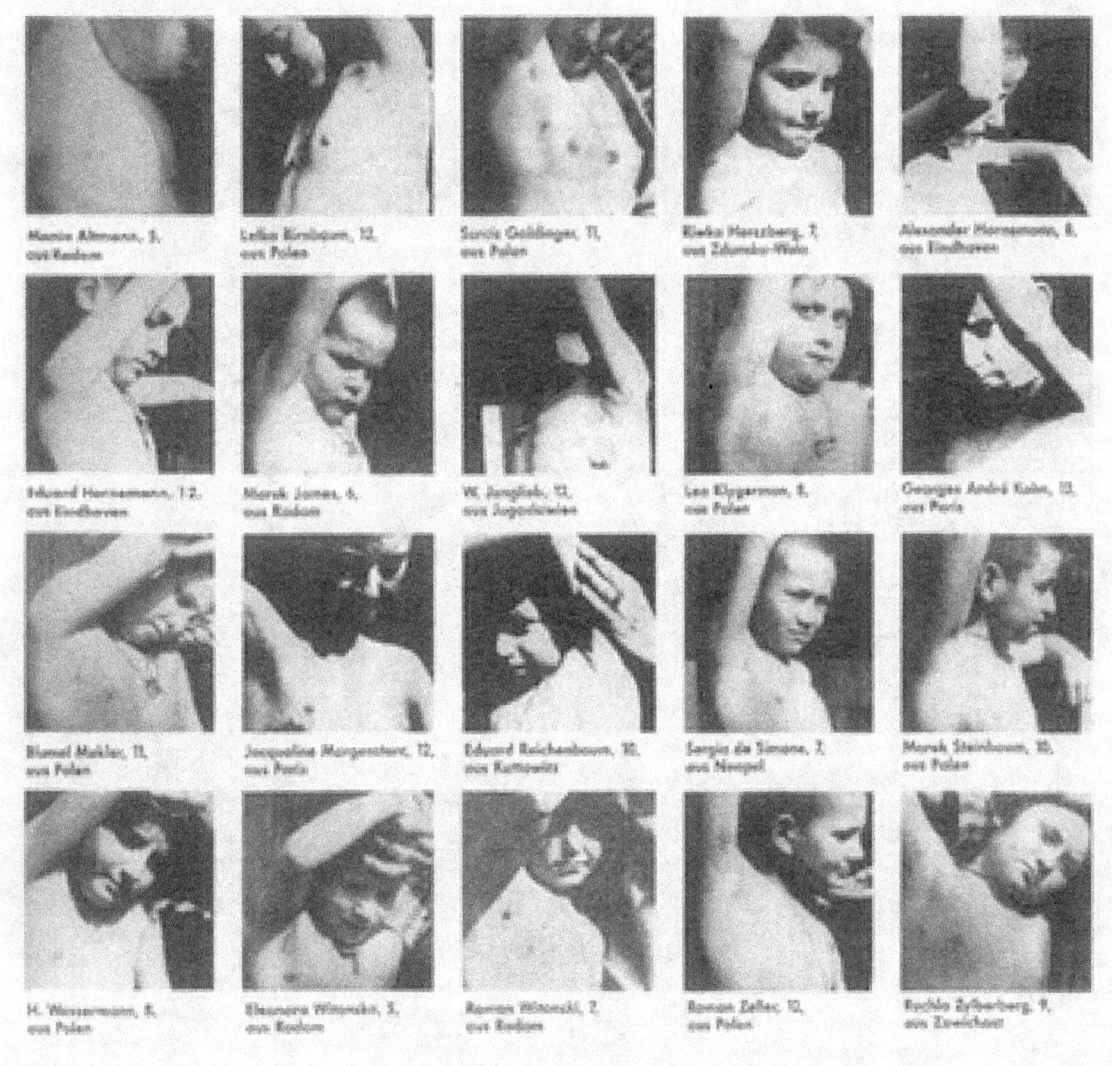

The children being forced to show the location of the scar where the axillary lymph nodes were excised.

[3] The Murders at Bullenhuser Damm: The SS Doctor and the Children by Gunther Schwarberg Publisher: Indiana Univ Pr; First Edition (April 1984) Language: English ISBN 0-253-15481-2 ISBN 978-0-253-15481-1

[4] Doctors Under Hitler By Michael H. Kater Publisher: The University of North Carolina Press (February 2, 2000) Language: English ISBN 0-8078-4858-1 ISBN 978-0-8078-4858-6

[5] Page 84–85:Medicine and medical ethics in Nazi Germany: origins, practices, legacies By Francis R. Nicosia,Publisher: Berghahn Books; illustrated edition (April 1, 2002) Language: English ISBN 1-57181-386-1 ISBN 978-1-57181-386-2

[6] Admitting the Holocaust: Collected Essays By Lawrence L. Langer Publisher: Oxford University Press, USA (June 20, 1996) Language: English ISBN 0-19-510648-2 ISBN 978-0-19-510648-0

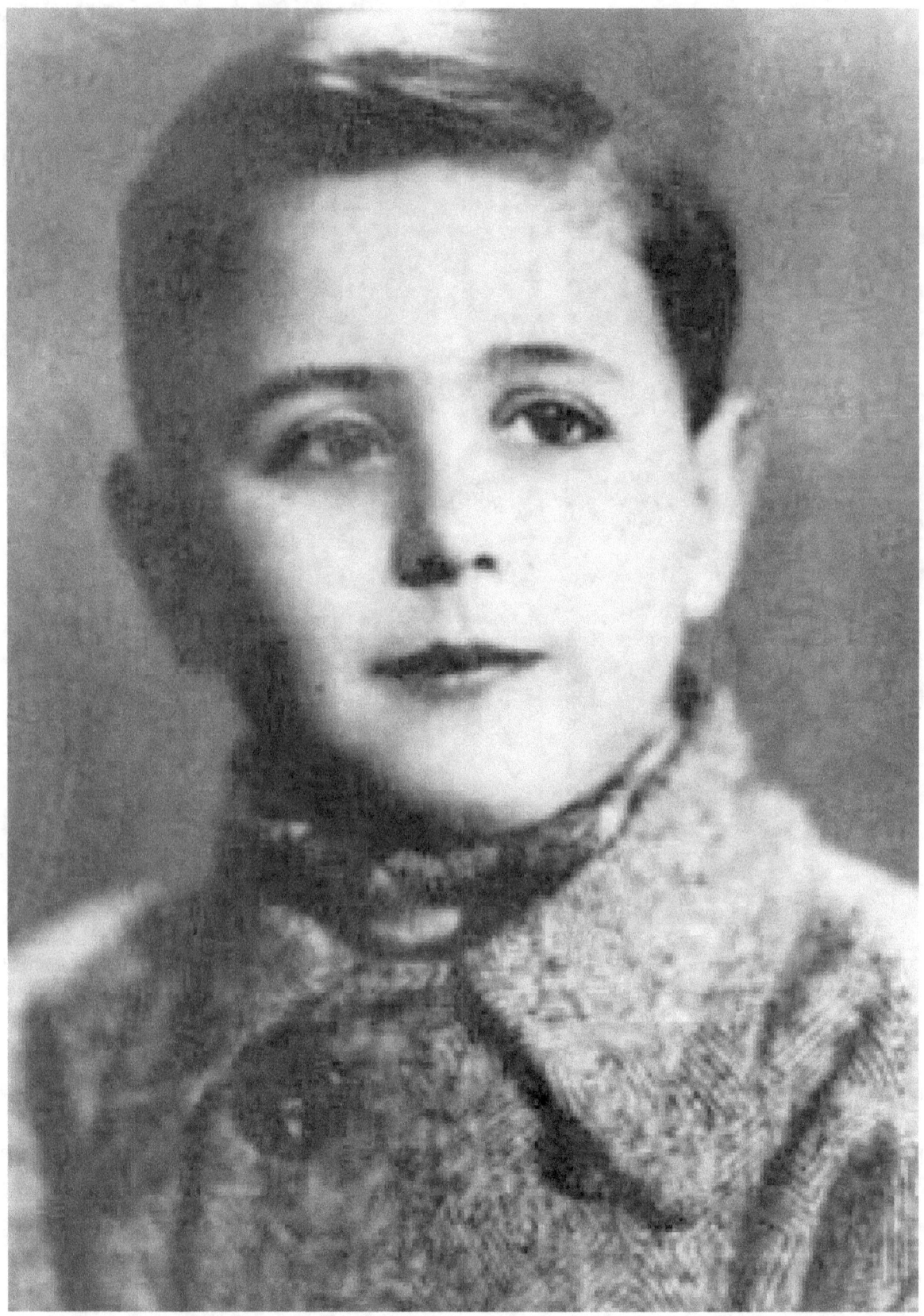

Sergio de Simone (b. Nov. 29, 1937 d. April 20, 1945) 7 yr. old Jewish Italian boy killed at the Bullenhuser Damm School

Chapter 23

Erich Hippke

Erich Hippke (7 March 1888 in Prökuls – 10 June 1969 in Bonn) was a German Air Force General Surgeon.[1]

23.1 Life

In the time of the Nazi Germany, from 1937 to December 1943, Hippke was the Chief Medical Officer of Luftwaffe. He was also a member of the Board of Trustees of the Kaiser Wilhelm Institute for Brain Research. Hippke was the true source of the ideas for the so-called "freezing experiments" on behalf of the Luftwaffe, conducted at Dachau concentration camp by Sigmund Rascher.[2]

He was succeeded by Oskar Schröder on May 15, 1944.[3]

He was arrested only in December 1946. By that time he was a general practitioner working in Hamburg, Germany. He avoided the Doctors' Trial and left Nuremberg without charge.[4] He was never charged with a crime but American investigators of the Nazi medical atrocities later concluded that he was actually the source of the idea for those deadly experiments on humans.[5][6]

23.2 See also

- Erhard Milch

- Dachau concentration camp

- Nazi human experimentation

- Dachau Trials

- Hans Schwerte

- Siegfried Knemeyer

23.3 References

[1] Heller, Kevin (2011). Oxford University Press, ed. *The Nuremberg Military Tribunals and the Origins of International Criminal Law*. ISBN 978-0199554317.

[2] Moreno, Jonathan D. (2000). *Undue Risk: Secret State Experiments on Humans*. Routledge. pp. 7–17. ISBN 978-0415928359.

[3] Mackowski, Maura Phillips (2005). Texas A&M University Press, ed. *Testing the Limits: Aviation Medicine and the Origins of Manned Space Flight pg.95*. ISBN 1585444391.

[4] Klee, Ernst (2008). *The people lexicon to the Third Reich: Who was what before and after 1945*. Koblenz: Ed. Kramer. ISBN 9783981148343.

[5] Heller, Kevin (2011). Oxford University Press, ed. *The Nuremberg Military Tribunals and the Origins of International Criminal Law*. ISBN 978-0199554317.

[6] *Hippkes letter to Wolff of 6 March 1943*. In at *Nuremberg Trials Project*. (Nürnberger Document NO-262).

Chapter 24

August Hirt

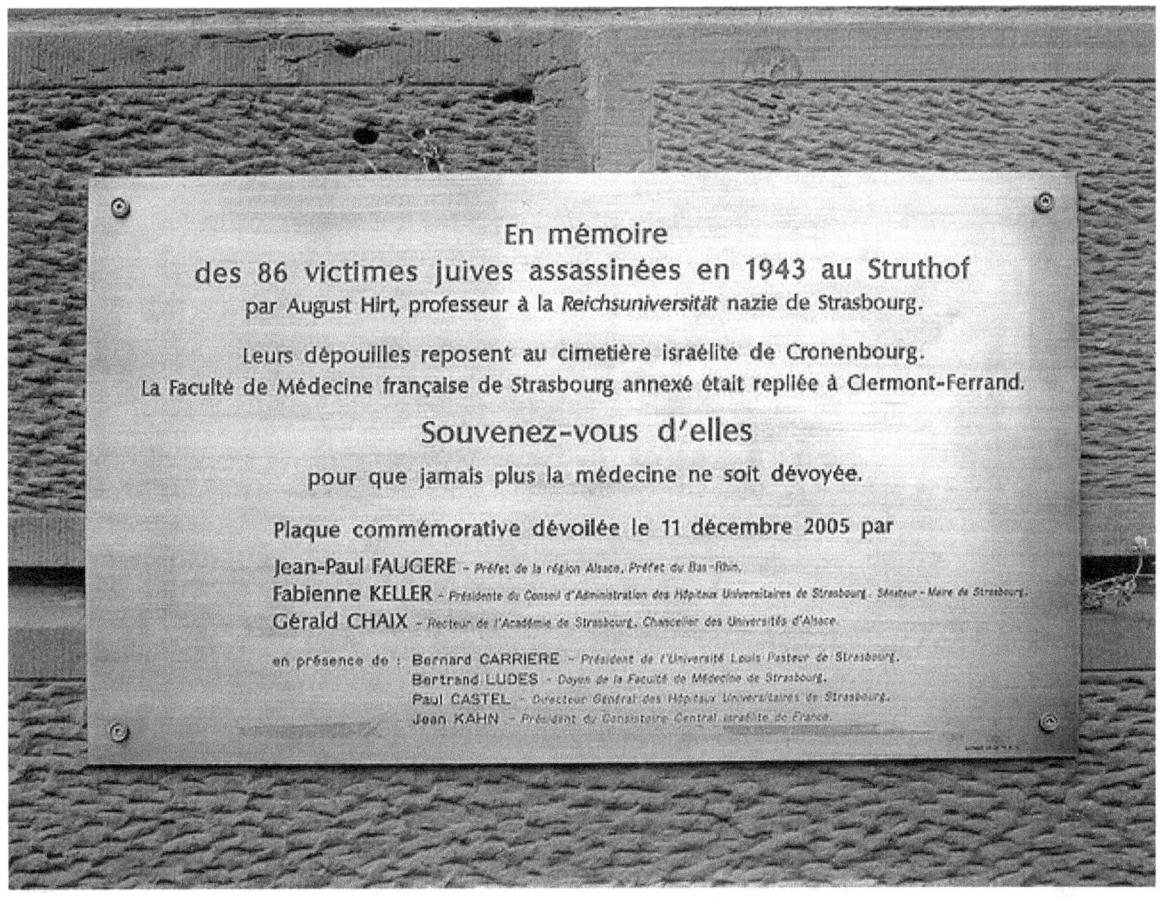

Memorial of the 86 Jewish victims murdered in 1943 at Struthof by August Hirt. Located at Institut of Anatomie of Strasbourg.

August Hirt (April 28, 1898 – June 2, 1945) was an anatomist with Swiss and German nationality who served as a chairman at the Reich University in Strasbourg during World War II. He performed experiments with mustard gas on inmates at the Natzweiler-Struthof concentration camp and played a role in the murders of 86 people at Auschwitz. The skeletons of his victims became specimens at the l'Institut anatomique de Strasbourg. He was an SS-Hauptsturmführer (captain)

24.1 Early life

Hirt was the son of a Swiss business man. In 1914, he volunteered, while still a high school student, to fight in World War I on the German side. In October 1916, he was wounded in the upper jaw by a bullet. He received the Iron Cross and returned to Mannheim in 1917. He went on to study medicine at the University of Heidelberg. In 1921, he took German citizenship. In 1922, Hirt obtained his doctorate in Literature with "Der Grenzstrang des Sympathicus bei einigen Sauriern". He then worked at the Anatomical Institute in Heidelberg and in 1925 he was authorized to teach thanks to a thesis on nerve cells.

in September 1932 Hirt joined the Militant League for German Culture. On 1 April 1933 he joined the SS (SS-Nr. 100 414), and was promoted to Hauptsturmführer (captain) on 1 July 1937, but he was only a member of the Nazi Party from 1 May 1937, when he enrolled in the universities of the Reich (Mitgliedsnr. 4012784). From 1 March 1942, he was a member of the personal staff of the RuSHA, the organisation in charge of "racial and ideological purity" of the members of the SS. He attained the rank of Sturmbannführer (commandant) in 1944.

From 1 April 1936 Hirt was associate director fo the Institut d'anatomie de University of Greifswald. On 1 Octobre 1938, he obtained the same post at Goethe University. At the beginning of the Second World War he was an SS medical chief (from August 1939 to April 1941). During which time it took part in the Battle of France. He then became director of the new Institut d'anatomie de la Reichsuniversität Straßburg.

August Hirt was married and had a son and a daughter.

24.2 World War 2

Working with the Ahnenerbe division, Wolfram Sievers, Bruno Beger and Hirt together collected human corpses[1][2] from among the Dachau inmates in order to create an anatomical specimen collection specifically of Jews. In 1943, Hirt had 79 Jewish men, 30 Jewish women, 2 Poles, and 4 "Asians" selected among the inmates at Auschwitz. These people were sent to Natzweiler-Struthof on July 30, 1943. Here they were gassed, by Josef Kramer, on August 17 and August 19, 1943. Their bodies were returned to Hirt at the anatomical laboratory of the Reich University in Strasbourg for preparation as an anthropological display, where they were re-discovered after the liberation.

Hirt committed suicide before he could be tried for war crimes. Some of his records prepared for the trial are in possession of the US National Archives, including "Photocopies of certificates of proof of ancestry, in connection with research on prisoners in the Konzentrationslager Natzweiler, ...Feb. 9-Nov. 3, 1942. Partial copies of slips for the admittance of prisoners into the Konzentrationslager Natzweiler, medical examinations on prisoners, and a death certificate, Dec. 9, 1942-Aug. 9, 1944. Feb. 9, 1942-Aug. 9, 1944".[3]

24.2.1 The Jewish skeleton collection

The Ahnenerbe under the Third Reich was a society that organised "medical experiments" on prisoners, including a number of Jews at the Natzwiller-Struthof concentrations camp in Alsace, which August Hirt officiated. He also performed experiments on cadavers and collected human skulls.

Hirt wanted to create a collection of skulls for the Institute of Anatomy (of which he was the director since 1941) with skulls of "Judeo-Bolcheviks", as part of his research on race. According to him, the Jewish race was on the point of extinction and he wished to gather a collection of them while there was still time. Hirt sent his project to Heinrich Himmler. Hirt wrote of this project: "There are important collections of skulls of nearly all the races and peoples. Except for the Jews, of which science has so few skulls, so it is not possible to draw any meaningful inferences. The war in the East gives us the opportunity to fill the gap. We have the opportunity to acquire a tangible scientific document by procuring the skulls of Jewish-Bolsheviks who embody the disgusting but characteristic subhuman."

As part of its racial studies, Professor Hirt conceived the project of a collection of Jewish skeletons and so presented his research plan to Himmler. He approved the project so that Hirt could begin his "medical experiments." It is at this stage that men and women were selected in August 1943 at the Auschwitz camp by his assistant, the anthropologist Bruno Beger SS, before being sent to the Natzweiler-Struthof concentration camp in Alsace. Divided into four groups, they were

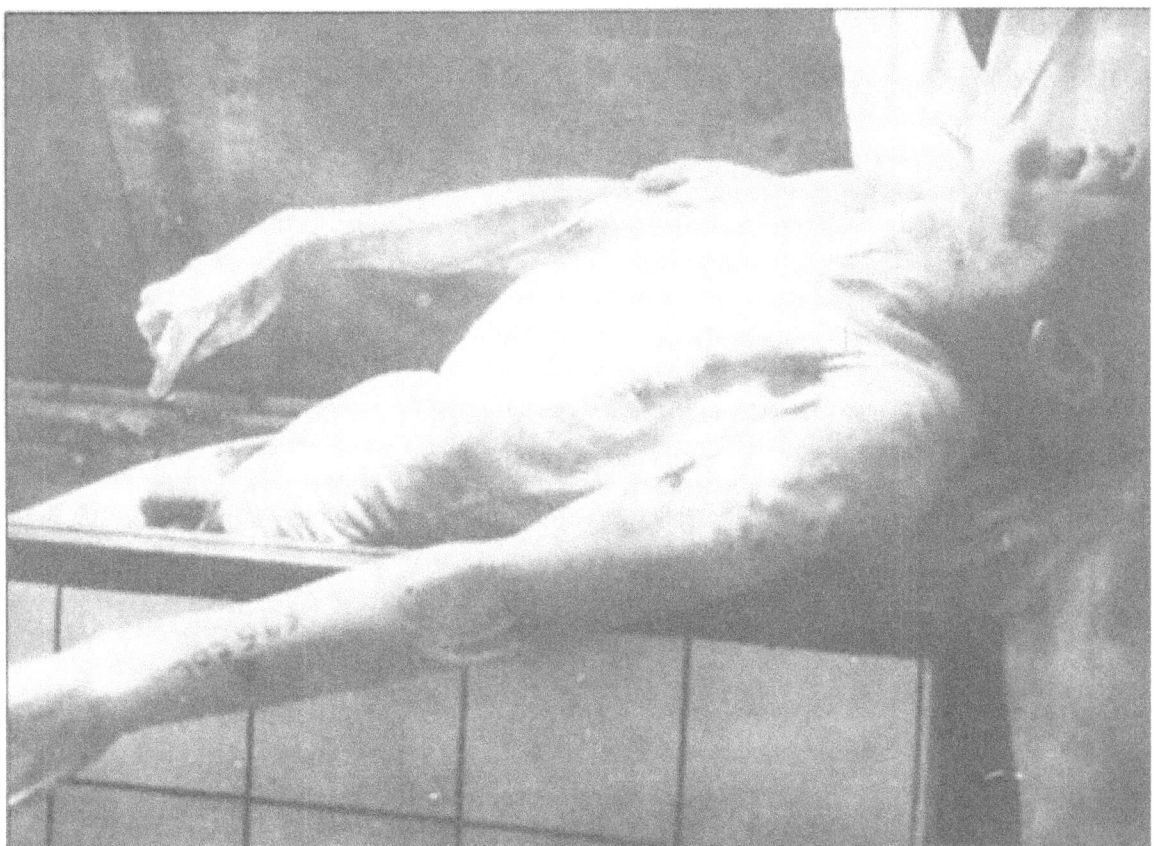

The cadaver of Menachem Taffel (b. July 21, 1900, Sedriczow, Russian Empire) a Berlin dairy merchant murdered 17 or 19 August, 1943 in the gas chamber at Natzweiler-Struthof

successively gassed a few days later and their bodies put at his disposal.

In September 1944, the rapid approach of the Allies led to the project being abandoned and Himmler ordered the destruction of all traces of this compromising collection. It failed. The remains of eighty-six bodies were later found and buried 23 October 1945 in the municipal cemetery of Strasbourg-Robertsau before being transferred in 1951 in the Jewish cemetery of Strasbourg-Cronenbourg.

August Hirt fled Strasbourg in September 1944, hiding in Tübingen in southern Germany. He committed suicide June 2, 1945 at Schönenbach, the Black Forest.

24.3   Posthumous

In the book, *Die Namen der Nummern* (2004, ISBN 978-3455094640.*The Names of the Numbers*), Hans-Joachim Lang describes this mass murder. He also recounts in detail the story of how he was able to determine the identities of 86 victims, 60 years after they were murdered. In 2015, a researcher, Raphael Toledano, identified tissue samples of victims in test tubes and a jar in the Strasbourg Medical Institute's closed collection. This followed his discovery of a 1952 letter from the then-director of the Institute, Camille Simonin, about the experiments directed by Hirt. The Strasbourg mayor's office said it hoped to return the remains to Strasbourg's Jewish community for eventual burial in the city.[4]

24.4   See also

- Block 10

- Anton Dilger

- Eduard Pernkopf

- Hermann Stieve

- Jewish skeleton collection

24.5   References

[1] http://holocaust-history.org/hirt/

[2] http://www.natzweiler-struthof.org/PhotographsofNatzweilerStruthof.htm

[3] http://www.archives.gov/research/captured-german-records/microfilm/t1021.pdf

[4] "Remains of victims of Nazi experiments found in France". *NZ Herald* (Paris). Associated Press. July 21, 2015. Retrieved July 21, 2015.

24.6   Further reading

- Courand, Raymond (2005). *Un camp de la mort en France: Struthof Natzweiler* (in French). Strasbourg: Ed. Hirlé. ISBN 2-914729-27-8.

- Lang, Hans-Joachim (2004). *Die Namen der Nummern; Wie Es Gelang, Die 86 Opfer eines NS-Verbrechens zu identifizieren* (in German). Hoffmann und Campe. ISBN 3-455-09464-3.

- Pressac, Jean-Claude (1985). *The Struthof album : study of the gassing at Natzweiler-Struthof of 86 Jews whose bodies were to constitute a collection of skeletons.* Serge Klarsfeld.

24.7   Documentary film

- Emmanuel Heyd, Raphael Toledano (2014). *The names of the 86 (Le nom des 86)* (in French, English, and German). France: Dora Films, 2014.

24.8   External links

- Auschwitz-Birkenau State Museum

- Die Namen der Nummern

- Holocaust History.org

Chapter 25

Waldemar Hoven

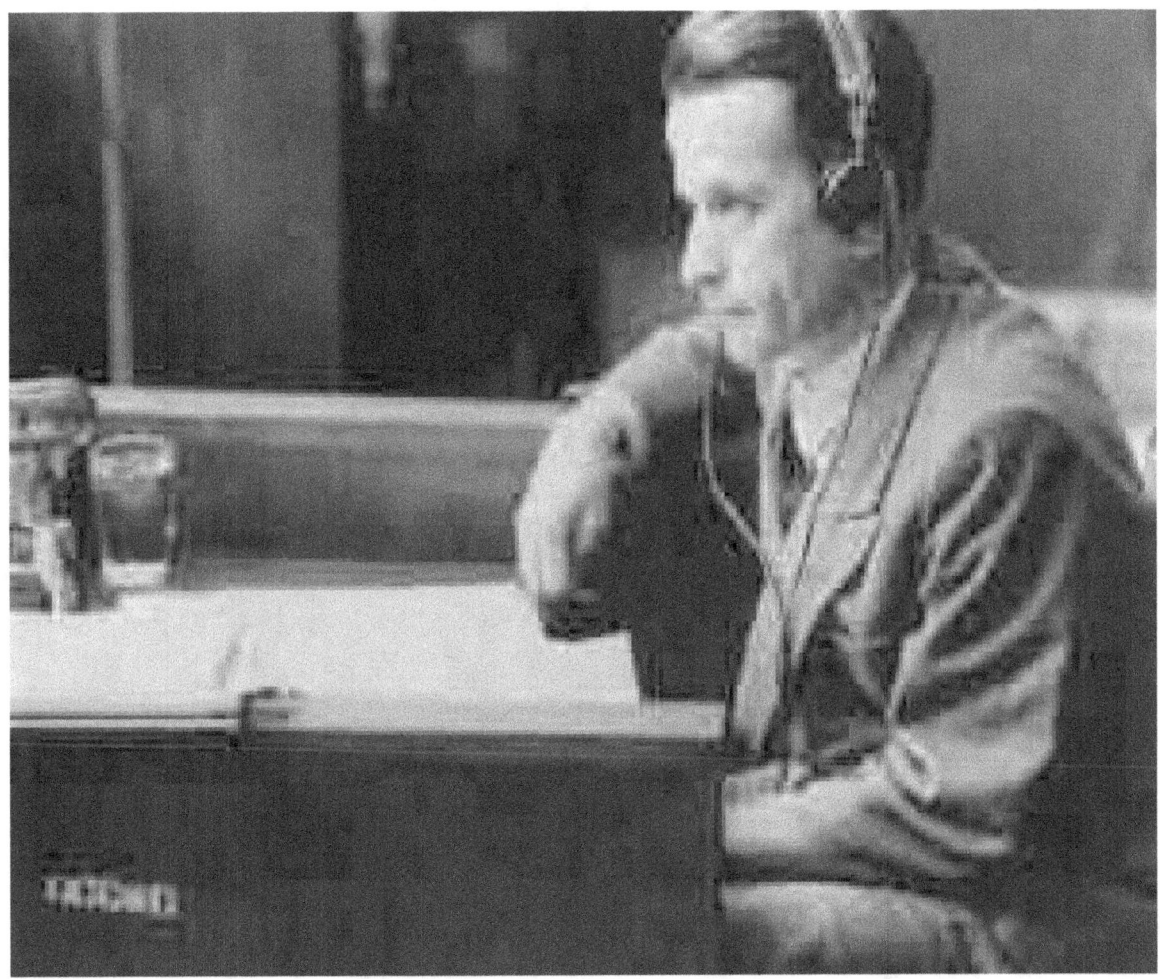

Hoven testifying during the trial

Waldemar Hoven (February 10, 1903 – June 2, 1948) was a Nazi and a physician at Buchenwald concentration camp.[1]

Hoven was born in Freiburg, Germany. Between the years 1919 and 1933, he visited Denmark, Sweden, the United States, and France, returning in 1933 to Freiburg, where he completed his high school studies. He then attended the Universities of Freiburg and Munich. In 1934, he joined the SS. In 1939, he concluded his medical studies and became

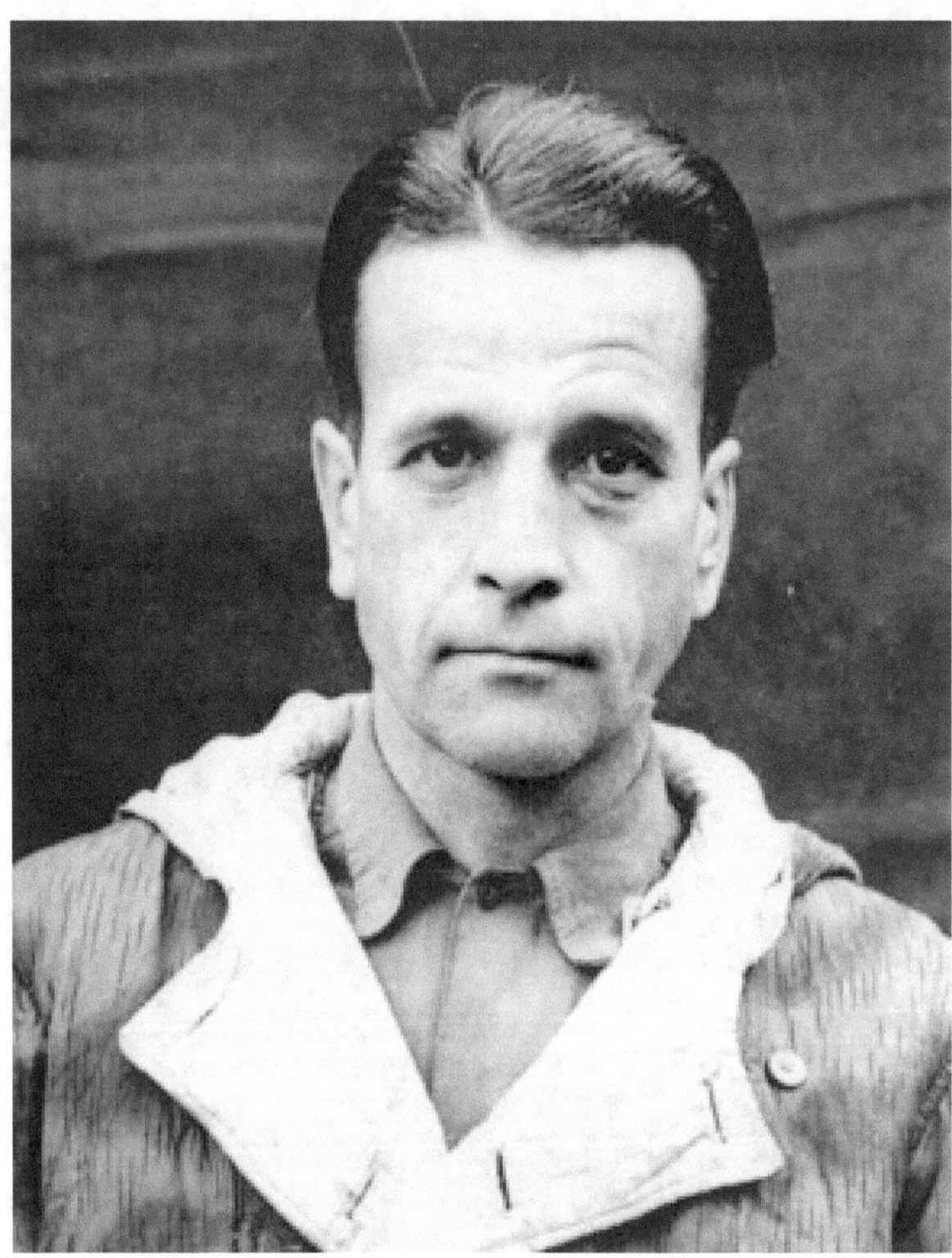

Hoven

a physician for the SS. Hoven rose to the rank of Hauptsturmführer (Captain) in the Waffen SS.[2]

Hoven was involved in the administration of medical experiments regarding typhus and the tolerance of serum containing phenol, and which led to the deaths of many inmates. He was also involved in Nazi euthanasia programs, during which people with disabilities were killed, along with Jewish people who were considered unfit for work.

He was arrested by the Nazis in 1943, accused of giving a lethal injection of phenol to an SS officer who was a potential witness in an investigation against Ilse Koch, with whom Hoven was rumoured to be having an affair. He was convicted and sentenced to death, although he was released in March 1945 due to the Nazi shortage of doctors.

25.1   Trial

Hoven was arrested at the end of World War II by the Allies and put on trial as a defendant at the Doctors' Trial (a part of the larger Nuremberg Trials). He was found guilty of war crimes, crimes against humanity and membership in a criminal organization. He was sentenced to death and hanged on June 2, 1948, at Landsberg prison in Bavaria.

25.2   References

[1] Klee, Ernst (2007). *Das Personenlexikon zum Dritten Reich* (in German) (2 ed.). Frankfurt am Main: Fischer Taschenbuch. p. 272. ISBN 978-3-596-16048-8.

[2] Affidavit of Walemar Hoven

- at nuremberg.law.Harvard.eduClosing brief for the United States of America against Waldemar Hoven

Chapter 26

Jewish skeleton collection

The **Jewish skeleton collection** was an attempt by the Nazis to create an anthropological display to showcase the alleged racial inferiority of the "Jewish race" and to emphasize the Jews' status as *Untermenschen* ("sub-humans"), in contrast to the German race which the Nazis considered to be Aryan *Übermenschen*. The collection was to be housed at the Anatomy Institute at the Reich University of Strasbourg in the annexed region of Alsace, where the initial preparation of the corpses was performed.

The collection was sanctioned by Reichsführer of the SS Heinrich Himmler, and under the direction of August Hirt with Rudolf Brandt and Wolfram Sievers, general manager of the Ahnenerbe, being responsible for procuring and preparing the corpses.

26.1   Selection

Originally the "specimens" to be used in the collection were to be Jewish commisars in the Red Army captured on the Eastern front by the Wehrmacht. The individuals ultimately chosen for the collection were obtained from among a pool of 115 Jewish inmates at Auschwitz concentration camp in Occupied Poland. They were chosen for their perceived stereotypical racial characteristics. The initial selections and preparations were carried out by SS-Hauptsturmführer Dr. Bruno Beger and Dr. Hans Fleischhacker, who arrived in Auschwitz in the first half of 1943 and finished the preliminary work by June 15, 1943.

Due to a typhus epidemic at Auschwitz, the candidates chosen for the skeleton collection were quarantined in order to prevent them from becoming ill and ruining their value as anatomical specimens. An excerpt from a letter written by Sievers in June 1943 reports on the preparation and the typhus epidemic: "Altogether 115 persons were worked on, 79 were Jews, 30 were Jewesses, 2 were Poles, and 4 were Asiatics. At the present time these prisoners are segregated by sex and are under quarantine in the two hospital buildings of Auschwitz."

In February 1942, Sievers submitted to Himmler, through Rudolf Brandt, a report from which the following is an extract read at the Nuremberg Doctors Trial by General Telford Taylor, Chief Counsel for the prosecution at Nuremberg: "We have a nearly complete collection of skulls of all races and peoples at our disposal. Only very few specimens of skulls of the Jewish race, however, are available with the result that it is impossible to arrive at precise conclusions from examining them. The war in the East now presents us with the opportunity to overcome this deficiency. By procuring the skulls of the Jewish-Bolshevik Commissars, who represent the prototype of the repulsive, but characteristic subhuman, we have the chance now to obtain a palpable, scientific document.

"The best, practical method for obtaining and collecting this skull material could be handled by directing the Wehrmacht to turn over alive all captured Jewish-Bolshevik Commissars to the Field Police. They in turn are to be given special directives to inform a certain office at regular intervals of the number and place of detention of these captured Jews and to give them special close attention and care until a special delegate arrives. This special delegate, who will be in charge of securing the 'material' has the job of taking a series of previously established photographs, anthropological measurements, and in addition has to determine, as far as possible, the background, date of birth, and other personal data of the prisoner.

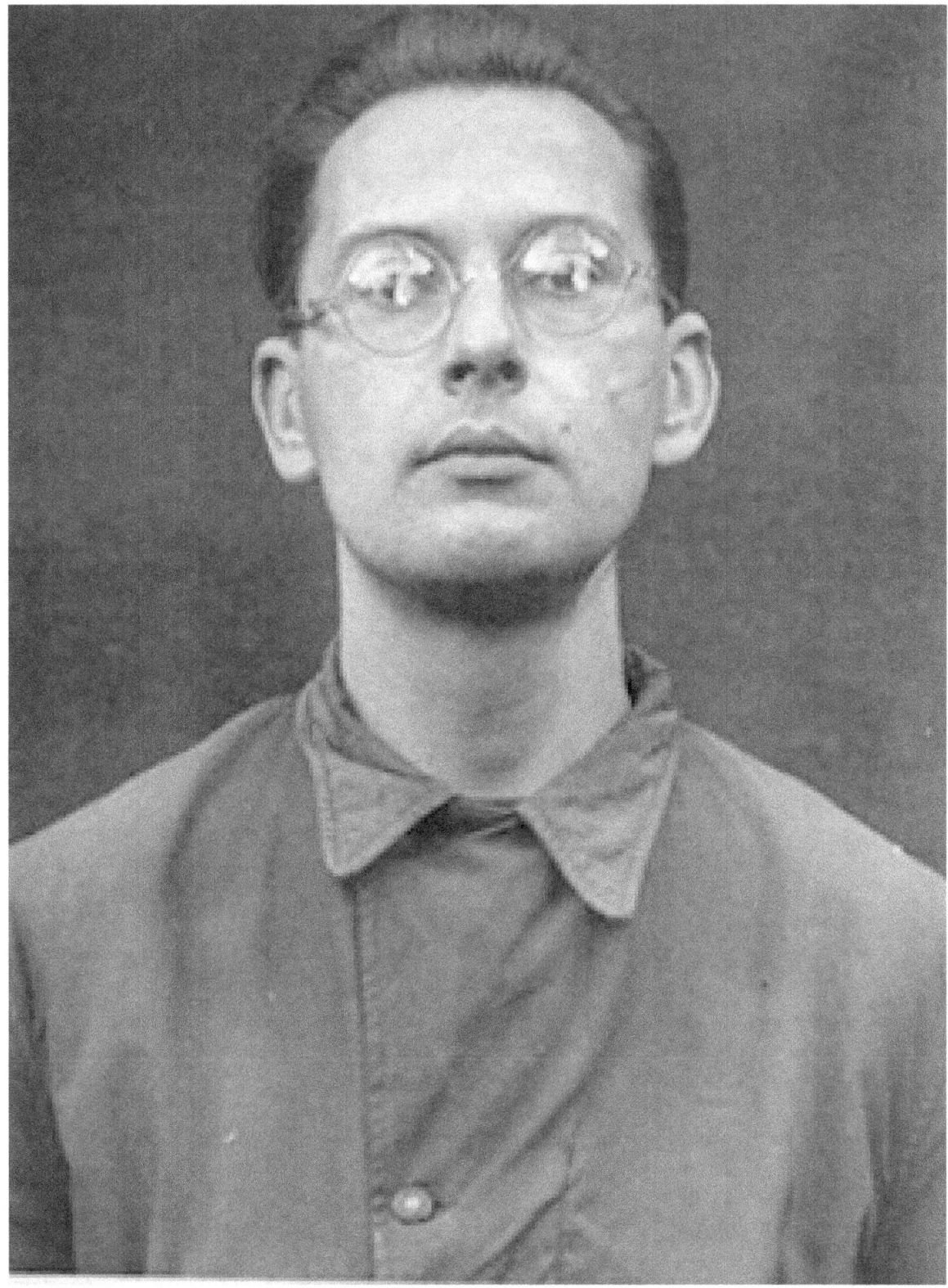

Mug shot of Rudolf Brandt, c. 1946

Following the subsequently induced death of the Jew, whose head should not be damaged, the delegate will separate

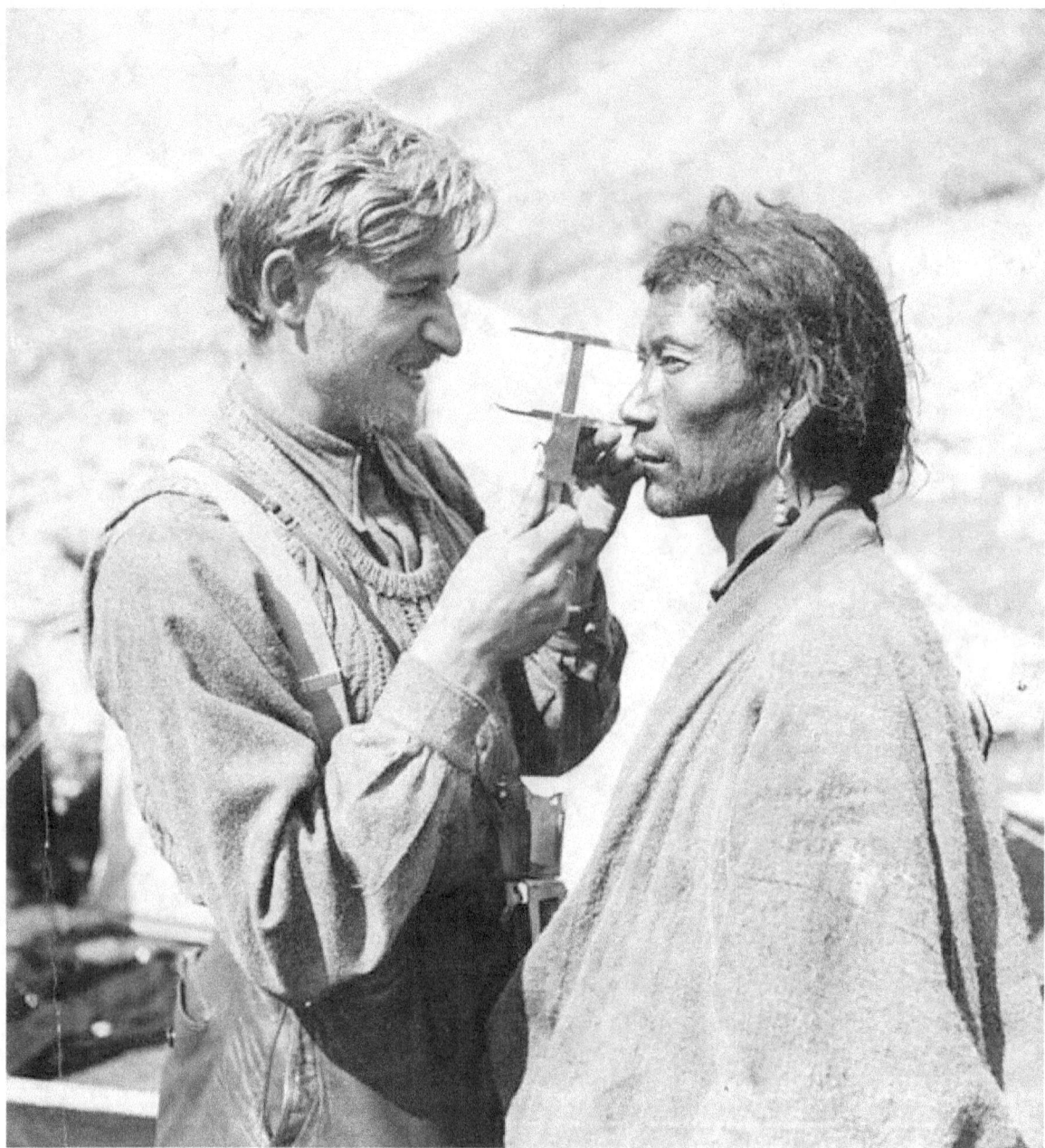

Beger conducting anthropometric studies in Sikkim, India.

the head from the body and will forward it to its proper point of destination in a hermetically sealed tin can especially produced for this purpose and filled with a conserving fluid.

"Having arrived at the laboratory, the comparison tests and anatomical research on the skull, as well as determination of the race membership of pathological features of the skull form, the form and size of the brain, etc., can proceed. The basis of these studies will be the photos, measurements, and other data supplied on the head, and finally the tests of the skull itself."

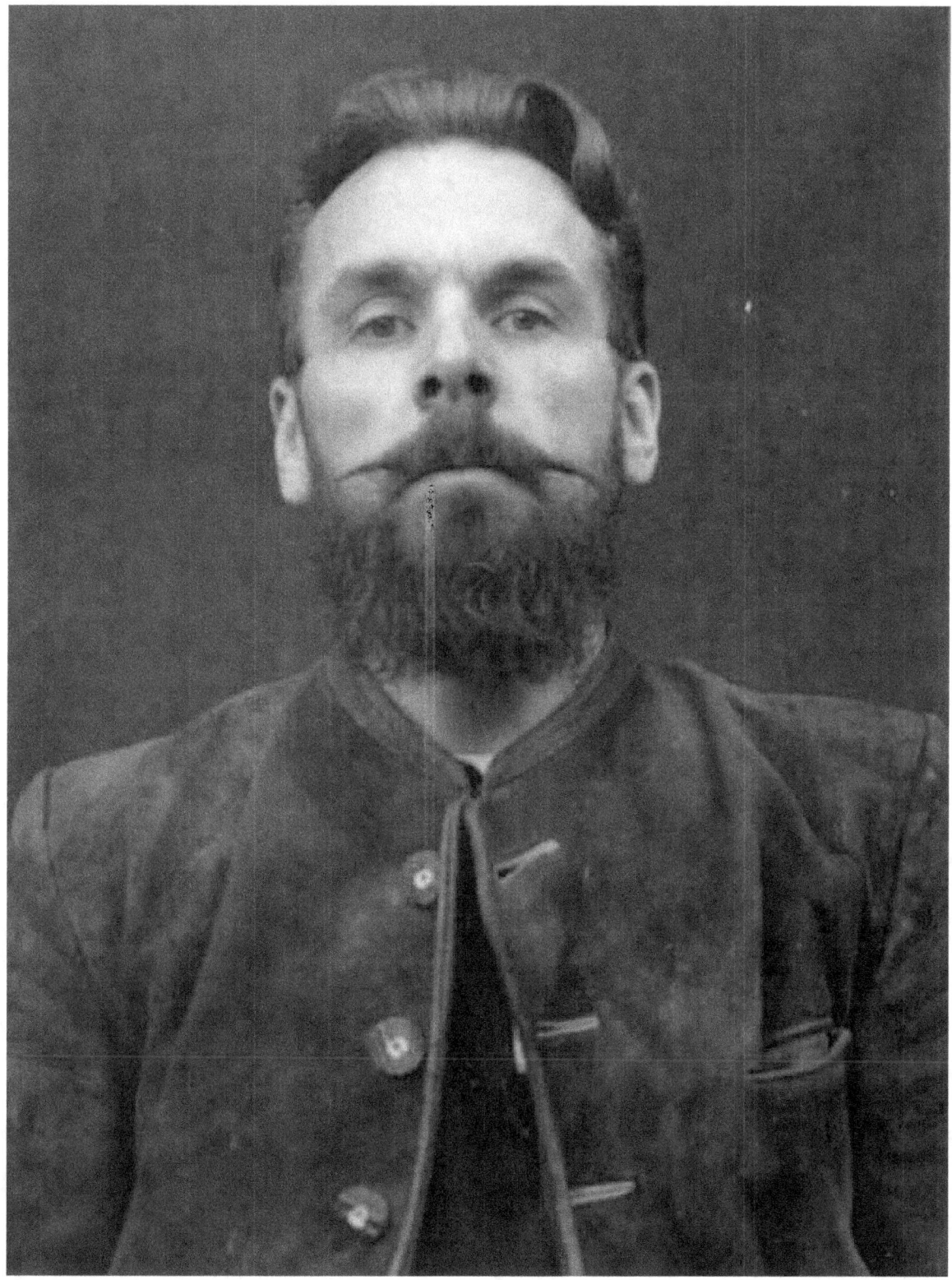

Wolfram Sievers

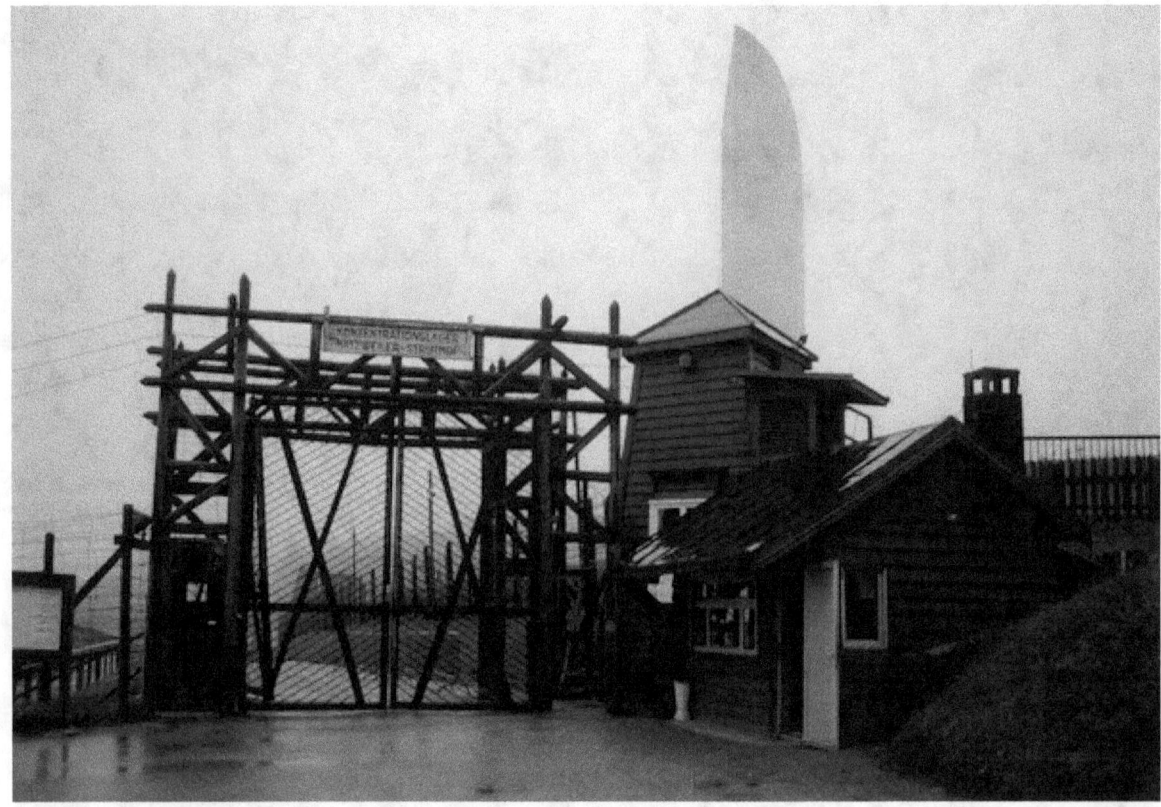

*Natzweiler-Struthof concentration camp entrance
(behind, the Monument to the Departed)*

26.2 Preparation

Ultimately 87 of the inmates were shipped to Natzweiler-Struthof, 46 of these individuals were originally from Thessaloniki, Greece. The deaths of 86 of these inmates were, in the words of Hirt, "induced" in an improvised gassing facility at Natzweiler-Struthof and their corpses, 57 men and 29 women, were sent to Strasbourg. One male victim was shot as he fought to keep from being gassed. Josef Kramer, acting commandant of Natzweiler-Struthof (who would become the commandant at Auschwitz and the last commandant of Bergen Belsen) personally carried out the gassing of 80 of these 86 victims.

The first part of the process for this "collection" was to make anatomical casts of the bodies prior to reducing them to skeletons. In 1944, with the approach of the allies, there was concern over the possibility that the corpses, which had still not been defleshed, could be discovered. In September 1944 Sievers telegrammed Brandt: "The collection can be defleshed and rendered unrecognizable. This, however, would mean that the whole work had been done for nothing-at least in part-and that this singular collection would be lost to science, since it would be impossible to make plaster casts afterwards."

26.3 Aftermath

Brandt and Sievers were indicted, tried and convicted in the Doctors' Trial in Nuremberg and both were hanged in Landsberg Prison on June 2, 1948. Hirt committed suicide in Schönenbach, Austria, on June 2, 1945 with a gunshot to the head. Josef Kramer was convicted of war crimes and hanged in Hamelin prison by noted British executioner Albert Pierrepoint on December 13, 1945. In 1974 Bruno Beger was convicted by a West German court as an accessory to 86 murders for his role in procuring the victims of the Jewish skeleton collection. He was sentenced to three years impris-

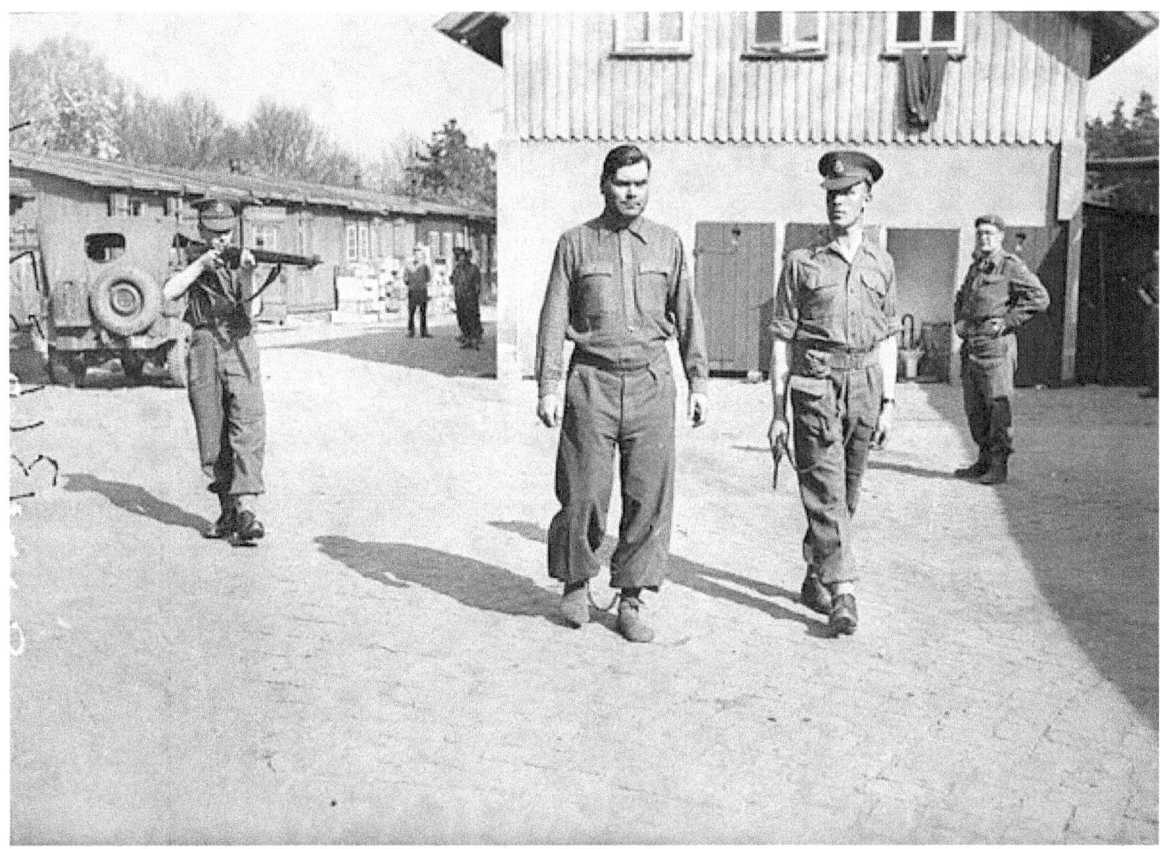

Josef Kramer, photographed in leg irons at Belsen concentration camp before being removed to the POW cage at Celle, 17 April 1945.

onment, the minimum sentence, but did not serve any time in prison. According to his family, Beger died in Königstein im Taunus on October 12, 2009.[1][2][3][4]

For many years only a single victim, Menachem Taffel (prisoner no. 107969), a Polish born Jew who had been living in Berlin, was positively identified through the efforts of Serge and Beate Klarsfeld. In 2003 Dr. Hans-Joachim Lang, a German professor at the University of Tübingen succeeded in identifying all the victims, by comparing a list of inmate numbers of the 86 corpses at Strasbourg, surreptitiously recorded by Hirt's French assistant Henri Henrypierre, with a list of numbers of inmates vaccinated at Auschwitz. The names and biographical information of the victims were published in the book *Die Namen der Nummern* (The Names of the Numbers).[5] In 1951 the remains of the 86 victims were reinterred in one location in the Cronenbourg-Strasbourg Jewish Cemetery. On December 11, 2005, memorial stones engraved with the names of the 86 victims were placed at the cemetery. One is at the site of the mass grave, the other along the wall of the cemetery. Another plaque honoring the victims was placed outside the Anatomy Institute at Strasbourg's University Hospital.

26.4   See also

- Ahnenerbe

- Bullenhuser Damm

- Kaiser Wilhelm Institute of Anthropology, Human Heredity, and Eugenics

- Nazi human experimentation

- Research Materials: Max Planck Society Archive

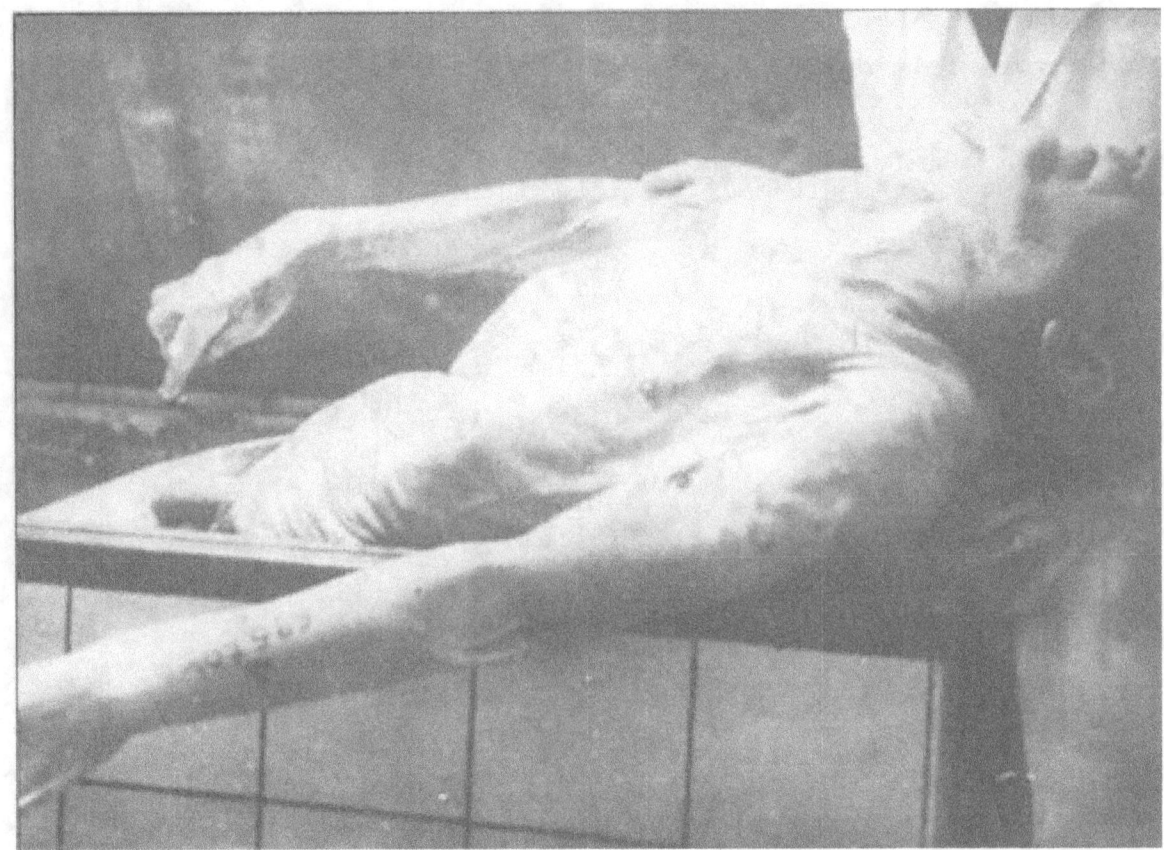

The cadaver of Berlin dairy merchant Menachem Taffel. Deported to Auschwitz in March 1943 along with his wife and child who were gassed upon arrival. He was chosen to be an anatomical specimen, shipped to Natzweiler-Struthof and executed in the gas chamber in August 1943

26.5 References

[1] "NS-Verbrechen - Die Spur der Skelette - SPIEGEL ONLINE". Einestages.spiegel.de. Retrieved 2012-10-09.

[2] "Bruno Beger". Die-namen-der-nummern.de.

[3] Doctors from Hell: the Horrific Account of Nazi Experiments on Humans. By Vivien Spitz Publisher: Sentient Publications (May 25, 2005) ISBN 1-59181-032-9 ISBN 978-1-59181-032-2 Pages 232-234

[4] Substantive and Procedural Aspects of International Criminal Law : The Experience of International and National Courts: Materials by Gabrielle Kirk McDonald Publisher: Springer; 1 edition (March 1, 2000) ISBN 90-411-1134-4 ISBN 9789041111340

[5] Die Namen der Nummern (Gebundene Ausgabe) von Hans-Joachim Lang (Autor) Publisher: Hoffmann + Campe Vlg GmbH (August 31, 2004) ISBN 3-455-09464-3 ISBN 978-3-455-09464-0

26.6 External links

- List and biographies of all 86 victims of the jewish skeleton collection in German - also in English, French, Dutch, Greek

- Jewish Skeleton Collection, Harvard Law School - Nuremberg Trials Project

- Names and information on the 46 Greek-Jewish victims from Theassaloniki, Greece

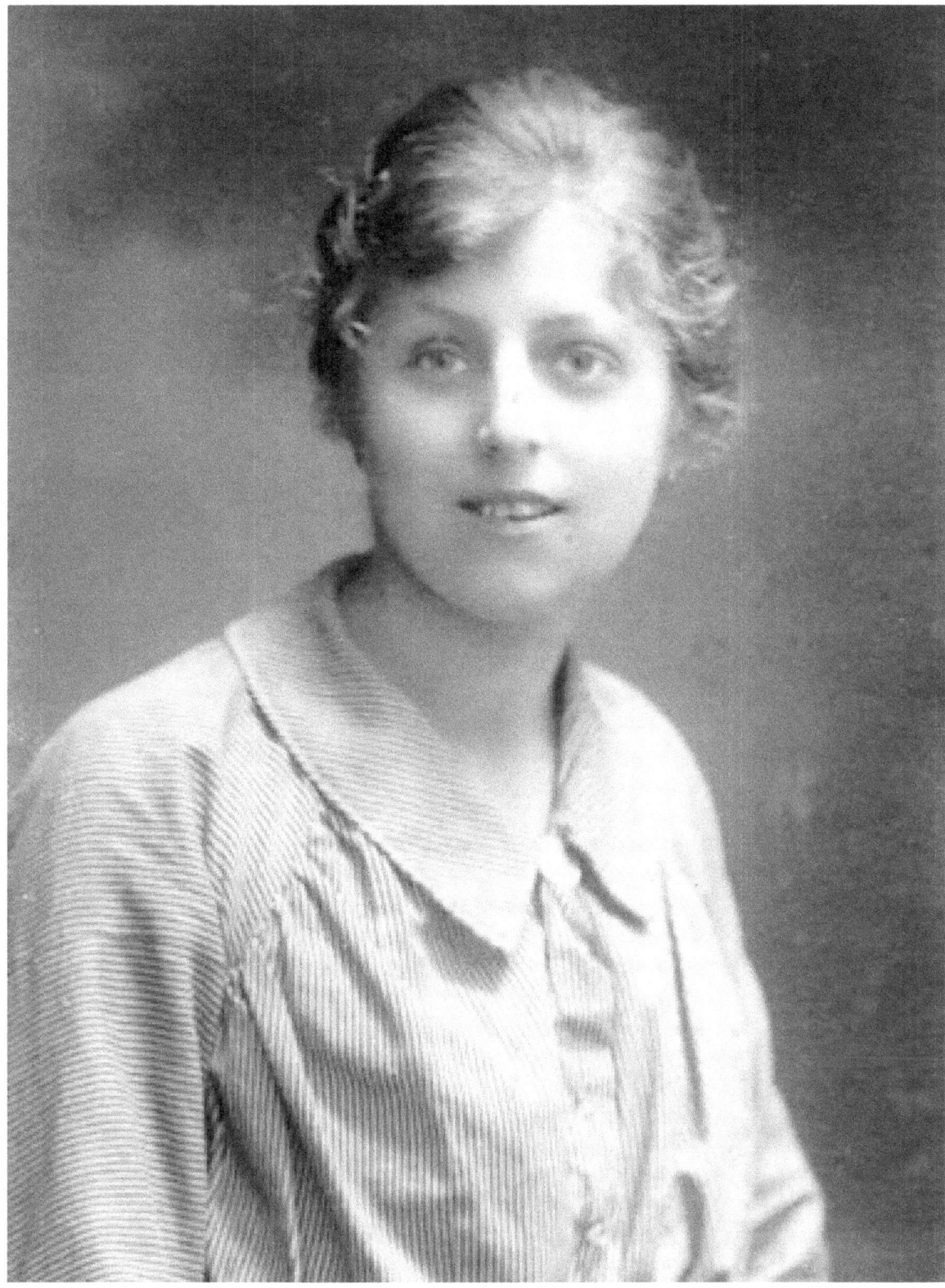

Victim Elisabeth Klein (b. 1901 Vienna, Austria), executed at the Natzweiler-Struthof concentration camp.

- the Struthof album - study of the gassing at Natzweiler-Struthof of 86 jews whose bodies were to constitute a collection of skeletons

- The Struthof-Natzweiler camp by Miloslav Bilik at The Holocaust History Project

- "The names of the 86" ("Le nom des 86"), documentary film directed by Emmanuel Heyd and Raphael Toledano (Dora films, 2014, Fr) - in French, English and German

Chapter 27

Emil Kaschub

Emil Kaschub was a German doctor who conducted experiments on Nazi concentration camp prisoners. On the instructions of the Wehrmacht, healthy prisoners were subjected to applications and injections of toxic substances. The subsequent wounds, often festering and blistered, were documented for "scientific" enlightenment.[1]

27.1 References

[1] *Auschwitz, A History in Photographs*; ed. Teresa Swiebocka; Auschwitz-Birkenau State Museum, 1990.

Chapter 28

Josef Klehr

Josef Klehr (October 17, 1904, Langenau, Upper Silesia – August 23, 1988, Leiferde) was an SS-*Oberscharführer*, supervisor in several Nazi concentration camps and head of the SS disinfection commando at Auschwitz concentration camp.

28.1   Life

Klehr was born as the son of a teacher. After attending the Volksschule in Wohlau until 1918 he got an apprenticeship with a cabinet maker, passing the exam in 1921 that allowed him to do it by trade.[1][2] As of 1934 he worked as a night porter in a community home, then subsequently as a nurse in a sanatorium.[1] From 1938 he was assistant sergeant at Wohlau prison.[3]

Klehr was a member of the Nazi Party and Allgemeine SS as of 1932. He participated in military exercises with the Wehrmacht and received training to become a medic. Shortly before the beginning of the war he was drafted into the Waffen-SS.[2] In August 1939 he was transferred to Buchenwald concentration camp as a guard, then to Dachau concentration camp as a medical orderly a year later.[3] In January, 1941 he was promoted to SS-Unterscharführer and transferred to Auschwitz, working as a medical orderly in the prisoners' infirmary.[2]

Klehr was renowned for killing by phenol injections into the heart, something he essentially took over as of some time in 1942.[4] He devised ways to optimise the speed of the killing process, such as experimenting with the positioning of prisoners before their injection.[4] Klehr occasionally conducted selections himself, and when he was informed that the camp doctor was unavailable, stated immediately, "Today I am the camp doctor."[4] Due to various descriptions of him standing against a background of corpses "wearing either a white coat or "a pink-rubber apron and rubber gloves" and "holding a 20-cc hypodermic with a long needle" in his hands, Klehr has been described as the "ultimate caricature of the omnipotent Auschwitz doctor."[4]

In 1943 Klehr became head of the disinfection squad (*Desinfektionskommando*).[2] As a handler of Zyklon B his tasks included not only delousing living quarters and clothes, but direct involvement in the mass gassing of prisoners.[2] Klehr was also one of those responsible for inserting the gas.[5] He was present during selections where those incapable of working were sent to the gas chambers, and drew up a schedule as to who under him was to insert the Zyklon B.[6]

On April 20, 1943 Klehr was awarded the War Merit Cross second class with swords. He was transferred to the Gleiwitz subcamp in 1944 where he was head of the prisoners' hospital and was medically responsible for Glewitz camps I to IV.

28.2   After the war

Upon the evacuation of Auschwitz Klehr guarded prisoners being transported to Gross-Rosen concentration camp, after which he was taken under command by an SS combat unit.[2] In the beginning of May 1945 he was taken prisoner in

Austria by Americans and was held until 1948.[2] He returned to his family in Braunschweig and resumed work as a cabinet maker. In April 1960 the Frankfurt prosecutor's office issued an arrest warrant which was executed in September after Klehr's whereabouts was determined.[2] On August 19, 1965 the court convicted him of murder in at least 475 cases, assistance in the joint murder of at least 2730 cases, and sentenced him to life imprisonment with an additional 15 years.[3] The witness Glowacki testified in court that Klehr killed the women who survived the massacre after the alleged uprising at the Budy female subcamp by phenol injection.[7][8]

While in prison, Klehr was interviewed by journalist and film-maker Ebbo Demant. When Demant brings up Holocaust denial, Klehr says:

On January 25, 1988, Klehr's sentence was suspended due to unfitness for custody (*Vollzugsuntauglichkeit*), and on June 10 he was ordered to serve the remainder on probation.[1] After seven months of freedom,[2] Klehr died at the age of 83.

28.3   Literature

- Demant, Ebbo (Hg.): *Auschwitz — "Direkt von der Rampe weg..." Kaduk, Erber, Klehr: Drei Täter geben zu Protokoll*: Hamburg: Rowohlt, 1979 ISBN 3-499-14438-7

- Ernst Klee: *Das Personenlexikon zum Dritten Reich: Wer war was vor und nach 1945.* Fischer-Taschenbuch-Verlag, Frankfurt am Main 2005. ISBN 3-596-16048-0

- Hermann Langbein: *Menschen in Auschwitz.* Frankfurt am Main, Berlin Wien, Ullstein-Verlag, 1980, ISBN 3-548-33014-2.

- Auschwitz-Birkenau State Museum: *Auschwitz in den Augen der SS.* Oswiecim 1998, ISBN 83-85047-35-2.

28.4   References

[1] "Josef Klehr" (in German). Retrieved 2008-11-29.

[2] "Josef Klehr Kurzportrait" (in German). Retrieved 2008-011-29. Check date values in: |access-date= (help)

[3] "Josef Klehr" (in German). Der Spiegel. January 29, 1979. Retrieved 2008-11-29.

[4] Lifton, Dr. Robert Jay. *The Nazi Doctors: Medical Killing and the Psychology of Genocide.* p. 265.

[5] "Karl Lill" (in German). Retrieved 2008-11-29.

[6] Naumann, Bernd. *Auschwitz* (NY:1966). pp 76-77.

[7] Kulka, Erich (1966). *Soudcové, žalobci, obhájci* (in Czech). Prague: Svoboda. p. 62.

[8] "The Budy Massacre - A grim anniversary". Auschwitz-Birkenau. Memorial and museum. 10 October 2007. Retrieved 9 December 2008.

[9] Demant, p. 114, cited in Jan van Pelt, Robert: *The case for Auschwitz.* Indiana University Press, 2002, p. 290-291.

Chapter 29

Hans Wilhelm König

Hans Wilhelm König (born 13 May 1912 in Stuttgart — date of death unknown) was an SS doctor assigned to the Auschwitz concentration camp during World War II. König was a medical service officer who often observed the experiments of Josef Mengele, reporting to various medical firms and authorities in Nazi Germany.

König joined the *Allgemeine-SS* in the mid to late 1930s, converting over to the *Waffen-SS* once World War II began. There are no records of König ever having served in combat, and the first significant mention of him in Nazi records occurred in September 1944 when he was assigned to Auschwitz.[1]

Initially, König worked at the main camp hospital at Auschwitz I. Here, he was known for experimenting with electroshock therapy on male camp inmates. He soon received an internal camp transfer, and was next assigned to the Birkenau camp where he became a medical liaison to Josef Mengele .

In her post-war memoirs, Eva Mozes Kor gives specific mention of König, specifying that he was often with Mengele during the latter's experimentation on twins.[2]

29.1   References

[1] Wagner, Bernd C., *IG Auschwitz. Zwangsarbeit und Vernichtung von Häftlingen des Lagers Monowitz 1941–1945* (Munich: Saur, 2000), p. 176

[2] "Surviving the Angel of Death", Eva Mozes Kor & Lisa Rojany Buccieri, Tanglewood Publishing (2009)

Chapter 30

Eduard Krebsbach

Eduard Krebsbach (8 August 1894 – 28 May 1947) was a former German physician and SS doctor in the Nazi concentration camp in Mauthausen from July 1941 to August 1943. He was executed for crimes against humanity committed at the Mauthausen camp.

30.1   Concentration camp career

In the autumn of 1941, Krebsbach became Standortarzt (garrison doctor) of Mauthausen concentration camp, tasked with supervising medical care and all medical personnel of the camp. He was responsible for initiating mass killing by lethal injection to the heart on handicapped and sick prisoners. Under his supervision approximately 900 Russian, Polish and Czech prisoners were murdered by lethal injections of gasoline. Because of this inmates nicknamed him 'Dr Spritzbach' (Dr Injection). Krebsbach was also responsible for the construction of a gas chamber in the basement of the hospital in the Mauthausen camp.

Krebsbach often inspected the prisoners and conducted selections for execution. A former inmate recalled Krebsbach's actions during such an inspection: "As the senior SS doctor in the camp, Dr Krebsbach sometimes came to block 5 and had the still surviving Jews paraded before him. He then asked if any of them were doctors. If there were, he would say: 'You Jewish pig, you're just an abortionist.' The next day they were done away with by the kapos. If a Jewish inmate was lying on the floor with a broken limb - a not uncommon occurrence at work - he was usually thrown over a wall by a kapo. If Dr Krebsbach were passing, he would say ironically: 'Yes, this broken foot is a hopeless case.'"

Josef Herzler, former Mauthausen inmate (AMM V/3/22).

Dr. Krebsbach was transferred to the Kaiserwald concentration camp in Latvia during the autumn of 1943, as it is believed he shot Josef Breitenfellner in his home. Breitenfellner was a German soldier from Langenstein on vacation when he and his friends awoke Krebsbach from his sleep on 22 May 1943.[1] Here he conducted selections and identified inmates to be gassed until the camps liquidation in August 1944.

Following the camp's closure, Krebsbach resumed a career as "Epidemic Inspector for Latvia, Estonia and Lithuania". Soon after he transferred to the regular army as a senior staff doctor, serving until late 1944. However this was short lived and at the end of 1944 he left the army and worked once again as a company doctor in a spinning mill in Kassel.

30.2   Dachau War Crime Trial

Following the end of World War II he was arrested and given the death penalty during the Dachau trials conducted by the US military on 13 May 1946 and was executed by hanging on 28 May 1947 at Landsberg Prison in Landsberg am Lech.

The following is from the court record of the Dachau trials (quoted in Hans Maršálek, "Die Geschichte des Konzentrationslagers Mauthausen", p. 174):

"Krebsbach: When I started work I was ordered by the head of Office III D to kill or have killed all those who were unable to work, and the incurably sick.

Prosecutor: And how did you carry out this order?

Krebsbach: Incurably sick inmates who were absolutely incapable of work were generally gassed. Some were also killed by gasonlie injection.

Prosecutor: To your knowledge, how many persons were killed in this way in your presence?

Krebsbach: (no answer)

Prosecutor: You were ordered to kill those unfit to live?

Krebsbach: Yes. I was ordered to have persons killed if I was of the opinion that they were a burden on the state.

Prosecutor: Did it never occur to you that these were human beings, people who had the misfortune to be inmates or who had been neglected?

Krebsbach: No. People are like animals. Animals that are born deformed or incapable of living are put down at birth. This should be done for humanitarian reasons with people as well. This would prevent a lot of misery and unhappiness.

Prosecutor: That is your opinion. The world does not agree with you. Did it never occur to you that killing a human being is a terrible crime?

Krebsbach: No. Every state is entitled to protect itself against asocial persons including those unfit to live.

Prosecutor: In other words, it never occurred to you that what you were doing was a crime?

Krebsbach: No. I carried out my work to the best of my knowledge and belief because I had to."

30.3 Literature

- Ernst Klee: *Auschwitz, die NS-Medizin und ihre Opfer*. 3. Auflage. S. Fischer Verlag, Frankfurt am Main, 1997, ISBN 3-596-14906-1.

- Ernst Klee: *Das Personenlexikon zum Dritten Reich: Wer war was vor und nach 1945*. Fischer-Taschenbuch-Verlag, Frankfurt am Main 2007, ISBN 978-3-596-16048-8.

- Hans Marsalek: *Geschichte des Konzentrationslagers Mauthausen*. Österreichische Lagergemeinschaft Mauthausen, Wien, 1980.

- Review and Recommendations of the Deputy Judge Advocate for War Crimes: United States of America vs. Hans Altfuldisch et al. - Case No. 000.50.5 Original document Mauthausen war crimes (pdf), 30. April 1947, in English.

- Florian Freund: Der Dachauer Mauthausenprozess, in: Dokumentationsarchiv des österreichischen Widerstandes. Jahrbuch 2001, Wien 2001, S. 35–66

30.4 References

[1] "Dr. Eduard Krebsbach - www.nizkor.org". 1998-12-05. Retrieved 2009-01-30.

30.5 External links

-
- Eduard Krebsbach in the German National Library catalogue
- Mauthausen Memorial: SS-site physician Dr. Eduard Krebsbach

Chapter 31

Johann Kremer

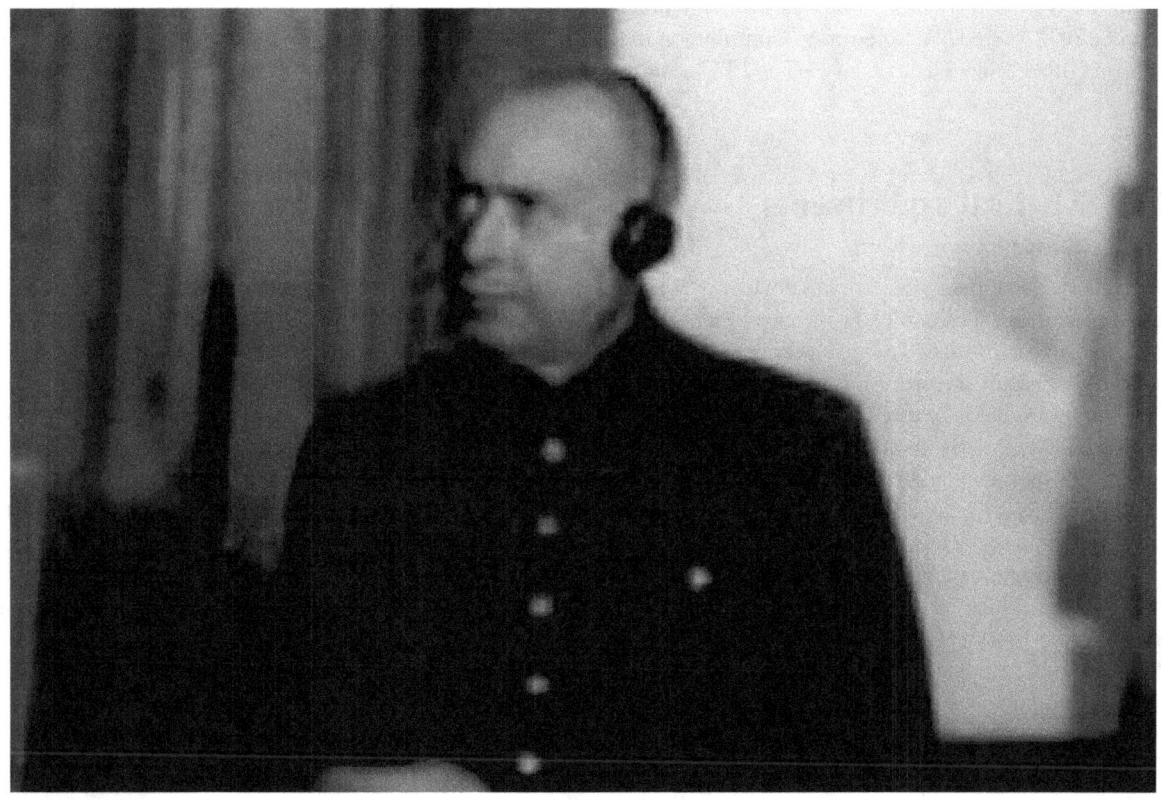

Kremer at the Auschwitz Trial in Kraków, 1947

Johann Paul Kremer (26 December 1883 – 8 January 1965) was a professor of anatomy and human genetics at Münster University who joined the Wehrmacht on May 20, 1941. He served in the SS in the Auschwitz concentration camp as a physician during World War II, from 30 August 1942 to 18 November 1942.

A member of the NSDAP, he was involved in Nazi human experimentation on the prisoners of Auschwitz-Birkenau. He was sentenced to death in the Auschwitz Trial, but this sentence was later commuted to one of life imprisonment. He was released in 1958.

Kremer received notoriety for his diary, which recounted mundane day to day activities interspersed with entries of his witnessing murder and depravity through gassings and *special actions*.

> September 5, 1942 : In the morning attended a special action from the women's concentration camp

(Muslims); the most dreadful of horrors. Obersturmführer Thilo (troop doctor) was right when he said to me that this is the anus mundi. In the evening towards 8:00 attended another special action from Holland [sic]. Because of the special rations they get a fifth of a liter of schnapps, 5 cigarettes, 100 g salami and bread, the men all clamor to take part in such actions. Today and tomorrow (Sunday) work.[1]

31.1 Life prior to Auschwitz

Kremer was born in Stellberg. He was a doctor of medicine as well as philosophy he also studied natural science and mathematics. He studied in Heidelberg, Strassburg as well as Berlin; he received his medical degree in 1919 and his philosophy degree in 1914. He was the "assistant surgeon at the surgical clinic of the University, Charité, the ward of internal diseases of the Municipal Hospital Berlin-Neukölln, the surgical clinic of the University of Cologne and prosector in the Institutes of Anatomy in Bonn and Münster. He became Dozent of anatomy in 1929 and was promoted there in 1936 to be professor in commission. At the same time he was commissioned to lecture on the science of human hereditariness."[2] He also did some writing, he mentions two articles that he wrote in the diary he kept, the first being "Inherited or Acquired? A Noteworthy Contribution to the Problem of Hereditariness of Traumatic Deformations" and the second titled "New Elements of Cell and Tissues Investigations".[2]

31.2 Medical experiments

The main priority of the SS doctors was not to provide basic medical services to prisoners, but rather to give the appearance of competent medical care. Mostly, they were busy with the camp exterminations, the selection of the newly arrived Jewish transports and the prisoners, as well as being present at the executions and gassings, conducting experiments and lastly, signing thousands of prisoners' death certificates with fabricated causes of death.[3] The experiments conducted by the SS Doctors were done for three main reasons: to improve the health of the soldiers, for post-war plans, and to support the bases of racial ideas. Some experiments were also done on the behalf of pharmaceutical companies and medical institutes, for their own interests and to benefit their personal careers.[3] Kremer was particularly interested in the effects starvation had on the body, especially on the liver, and seeing as Kremer was responsible for examining the prisoners that sought admission to the camp hospital, he was able to select the prisoners that he believed would make good test subjects. He often performed autopsies in order to extract samples from the liver, spleen and pancreas. On several occasions in his diary, he mentions the extraction of living-fresh material from various victims, such as on October 15, 1942, when he writes, "Living-fresh material of liver, spleen and pancreas taken from an abnormal individual."[2] Dr. Kremer mentions at least five more similar instances. Kremer states at his hearing on July 30, 1947 that "I observed the prisoners in this group [to be liquidated] carefully and whenever one of them particularly interested me because of his advanced stage of starvation, I ordered the medical orderly to reserve him and to inform me when this patient would be killed by injection."[1]

31.3 Special actions

All SS doctors were required to be present at what were called "special actions," which was when the mass gassings took place. The most common victims were children, the elderly, mothers with young children and any others considered unfit to work. During his trial, Kremer describes how a gassing was conducted and what his role as doctor was. The gassings were conducted in cabins located on the outskirts of the camp; the victims were transported by railway, and once "here people were first driven to barracks where the victims undressed and then went naked to the gas chambers. Very often no incidents occurred, as the SS men kept people quiet, maintaining that they were to bathe and be deloused. After driving all of them into the gas chamber the door was closed and an SS man in a gas mask threw the contents of a Cyclon tin through an opening in the side wall."[2] Kremer's role was to sit in a van along with a medical orderly ready to treat any officers that might succumb to the gas.

31.4   Executions and beatings

Throughout the doctor's diary there are multiple occasions where he mentions being in attendance at various executions and beatings. At least four instances can be found where he mentions executions either by gun, phenol injection or some other method not mentioned by him.[2] He mentions briefly no less than three instances where he oversaw the punishment of prisoners. The physicians were required to examine the victim before the punishment and to remain throughout. In general though, physicians never actually examined the victims and never objected to the punishments.[2]

31.5   Testimony and indictment

Johann Kremer was tried in the Auschwitz trials at the sitting of the Supreme Court National Tribune in Cracow throughout November and December 1947. Based on the contents of his diary and his own confessions, Kremer participated in fourteen gassings as well as multiple public executions and special actions, also known as gassings.[2] During his testimony, he describes the process by which he selected his victims, the process of gaining the necessary information required for his research, and he states that "after I had been given this information a medical orderly would come and kill the patient with an injection in the heart area. To my knowledge all these patients were killed with phenol injections. The patient died immediately after being given such an injection. I myself never administered fatal injections.".[1]

31.6   References

[1] Klee, Ernst, W. Dressen, V. Riess, eds. "The Good Old Days": The Holocaust as Seen by its Perpetrators and Bystanders. New York: The Free Press, 1991.

[2] Bezwińska, Jadwiga and Czech, Danuta. *KL Auschwitz seen by the SS*. New York: Howard Fertig Inc., 1984.

[3] Strzelecka, Irena. "Medicine in Auschwitz: Selection, executions, and experiments" Państwowe Muzeum Auschwitz-Birkenau w Oświęcimiu. Accessed November 14, 2012. www.en.auschwitz.org

Chapter 32

Elisabeth Marschall

Elisabeth Marschall (27 May 1886 – 3 May 1947) was the Head Nurse (*Oberschwester*) at the Ravensbrück concentration camp. Her duties included selecting prisoners for execution, overseeing medical experiments, and selecting which prisoners would be shipped to Auschwitz. At the Hamburg Ravensbrück Trials, she was found guilty and sentenced to death.

On 3 May 1947 she was hanged by British executioner Albert Pierrepoint on the gallows in Hameln prison. Aged 60, she was the oldest female Nazi to be executed.

32.1   References

- Patricia O'Brien D'Antonio, Barbra Mann Wall (2002). *Nursing History Review*. Springer Publishing Company. ISBN 0-8261-1478-4.

Chapter 33

Josef Mengele

"Mengele" redirects here. For other uses, see Mengele (disambiguation).

Josef Mengele (German: [ˈjoːzɛf ˈmɛŋələ]; 16 March 1911 – 7 February 1979) was a German *Schutzstaffel* (SS) officer and physician in Auschwitz concentration camp during World War II. Mengele was a notorious member of the team of doctors responsible for the selection of victims to be killed in the gas chambers and for performing deadly human experiments on prisoners. Arrivals deemed able to work were admitted into the camp, and those deemed unfit for labor were immediately killed in the gas chambers. Mengele left Auschwitz on 17 January 1945, shortly before the arrival of the liberating Red Army troops. After the war, he fled to South America, where he evaded capture for the rest of his life.

Mengele received doctorates in anthropology and medicine from Munich University and began a career as a researcher. He joined the Nazi Party in 1937 and the SS in 1938. Initially assigned as a battalion medical officer at the start of World War II, he transferred to the concentration camp service in early 1943 and was assigned to Auschwitz. There he saw the opportunity to conduct genetic research on human subjects. His subsequent experiments, focusing primarily on twins, had no regard for the health or safety of the victims.[2][3]

Assisted by a network of former SS members, Mengele sailed to Argentina in July 1949. He initially lived in and around Buenos Aires, then fled to Paraguay in 1959 and Brazil in 1960 while being sought by West Germany, Israel, and Nazi hunters such as Simon Wiesenthal so that he could be brought to trial. In spite of extradition requests by the West German government and clandestine operations by Mossad (the Israeli intelligence agency), Mengele eluded capture. He drowned while swimming off the Brazilian coast in 1979 and was buried under a false name. His remains were disinterred and positively identified by forensic examination in 1985.

33.1 Early life and education

Mengele was born the eldest of three children on 16 March 1911 to Karl and Walburga (Hupfauer) Mengele in Günzburg, Bavaria, Germany.[4] His younger brothers were Karl Jr and Alois. Mengele's father was founder of the Karl Mengele & Sons company, producers of farm machinery.[5] Mengele did well in school and developed an interest in music, art, and skiing.[6] He completed high school in April 1930 and went on to study medicine at Goethe University Frankfurt and philosophy at the University of Munich.[7] Munich was the headquarters of the Nazi Party.[8] In 1931 Mengele joined the *Stahlhelm, Bund der Frontsoldaten*, a paramilitary organisation that was in 1934 absorbed into the Nazi *Sturmabteilung* (Storm Detachment; SA).[9][7]

In 1935, Mengele earned a PhD in anthropology from the University of Munich.[7] In January 1937, at the Institute for Hereditary Biology and Racial Hygiene in Frankfurt, he became the assistant to Dr. Otmar Freiherr von Verschuer, a scientist conducting genetics research, with a particular interest in twins.[7] As an assistant to von Verschuer, Mengele focused on the genetic factors resulting in a cleft lip and palate or cleft chin.[10] His thesis on the subject earned him a *cum laude* doctorate in medicine in 1938.[11] Both of his degrees were later rescinded by the issuing universities.[12] In a letter of recommendation, von Verschuer praised Mengele's reliability and his ability to verbally present complex material in a clear manner.[13] The American author Robert Jay Lifton notes that Mengele's published works did not deviate much from the scientific mainstream of the time, and would probably have been viewed as valid scientific efforts even outside the borders of Nazi Germany.[13]

On 28 July 1939, Mengele married Irene Schönbein, whom he had met while working as a medical resident in Leipzig.[14] Their only son, Rolf, was born in 1944.[15]

33.2   Military service

The ideology of Nazism brought together elements of antisemitism, racial hygiene, and eugenics, and combined them with pan-Germanism and territorial expansionism with the goal of obtaining more *Lebensraum* (living space) for the Germanic people.[16] Nazi Germany attempted to obtain this new territory by attacking Poland and the Soviet Union, intending to deport or kill the Jews and Slavs living there, who were viewed as being inferior to the Aryan master race.[17]

Mengele joined the Nazi Party in 1937 and the *Schutzstaffel* (SS; protection squadron) in 1938. He received basic training in 1938 with the *Gebirgsjäger* (mountain infantry) and was called up for service in the Wehrmacht (German armed forces) in June 1940, some months after the outbreak of World War II. He soon volunteered for medical service in the *Waffen-SS*, the combat arm of the SS, where he served with the rank of SS-*Untersturmführer* (second lieutenant) in a medical reserve battalion until November 1940. He was next assigned to the *SS-Rasse- und Siedlungshauptamt* (SS Race and Resettlement Main Office) in Posen, evaluating candidates for Germanisation.[18][19]

In June 1941, Mengele was posted to Ukraine, where he was awarded the Iron Cross Second Class. In January 1942 he joined the 5th SS Panzer Division Wiking as a battalion medical officer. He rescued two German soldiers from a burning tank and was awarded the Iron Cross First Class, as well as the Wound Badge in Black and the Medal for the Care of the German People. He was seriously wounded in action near Rostov-on-Don in mid-1942 and was declared unfit for further active service. After recovery, he was transferred to the Race and Resettlement Office in Berlin. He also resumed his association with von Verschuer, who was at the Kaiser Wilhelm Institute for Anthropology, Human Genetics and Eugenics. Mengele was promoted to the rank of SS-*Hauptsturmführer* (captain) in April 1943.[20][21][22]

33.3   Auschwitz

In early 1943, encouraged by von Verschuer, Mengele applied for transfer to the concentration camp service, where he foresaw the opportunity to undertake genetic research on human subjects.[20][23] His application was accepted, and he was posted to Auschwitz concentration camp. He was appointed by SS-*Standortarzt* Eduard Wirths, chief medical officer at Auschwitz, to the position of chief physician of the *Zigeunerfamilienlager* (Romani family camp), located in the sub-camp at Birkenau.[20][23]

By late 1941 Hitler decided that the Jews of Europe were to be exterminated, so Birkenau, originally intended to house slave laborers, was re-purposed as a combination labor camp / extermination camp.[24][25] Prisoners were transported there by rail from all over German-occupied Europe, arriving in daily convoys.[26] By July 1942, the SS were conducting "selections". Incoming Jews were segregated; those deemed able to work were admitted into the camp, and those deemed unfit for labor were immediately killed in the gas chambers.[27] The group selected to die, about three-quarters of the total,[lower-alpha 1] included almost all children, women with small children, pregnant women, all the elderly, and all those who appeared on brief and superficial inspection by an SS doctor not to be completely fit.[29][30] Mengele, a member of the team of doctors assigned to do selections, undertook this work even when he was not assigned to do so in the hope of finding subjects for his experiments.[31] He was particularly interested in locating sets of twins.[32] In contrast to most of the doctors, who viewed undertaking selections as one of their most stressful and horrible duties, Mengele undertook the task with a flamboyant air, often smiling or whistling a tune.[33][34]

Mengele and other SS doctors did not treat inmates, but supervised the activities of inmate doctors forced to work in the camp medical service.[34] Mengele made weekly visits to the hospital barracks and sent to the gas chambers any prisoners who had not recovered after two weeks in bed.[35] He was also a member of the team of doctors responsible for supervising the administration of Zyklon B, the cyanide-based pesticide that was used to kill people in the gas chambers at Birkenau. He served in this capacity at the gas chambers located in crematoria IV and V.[36]

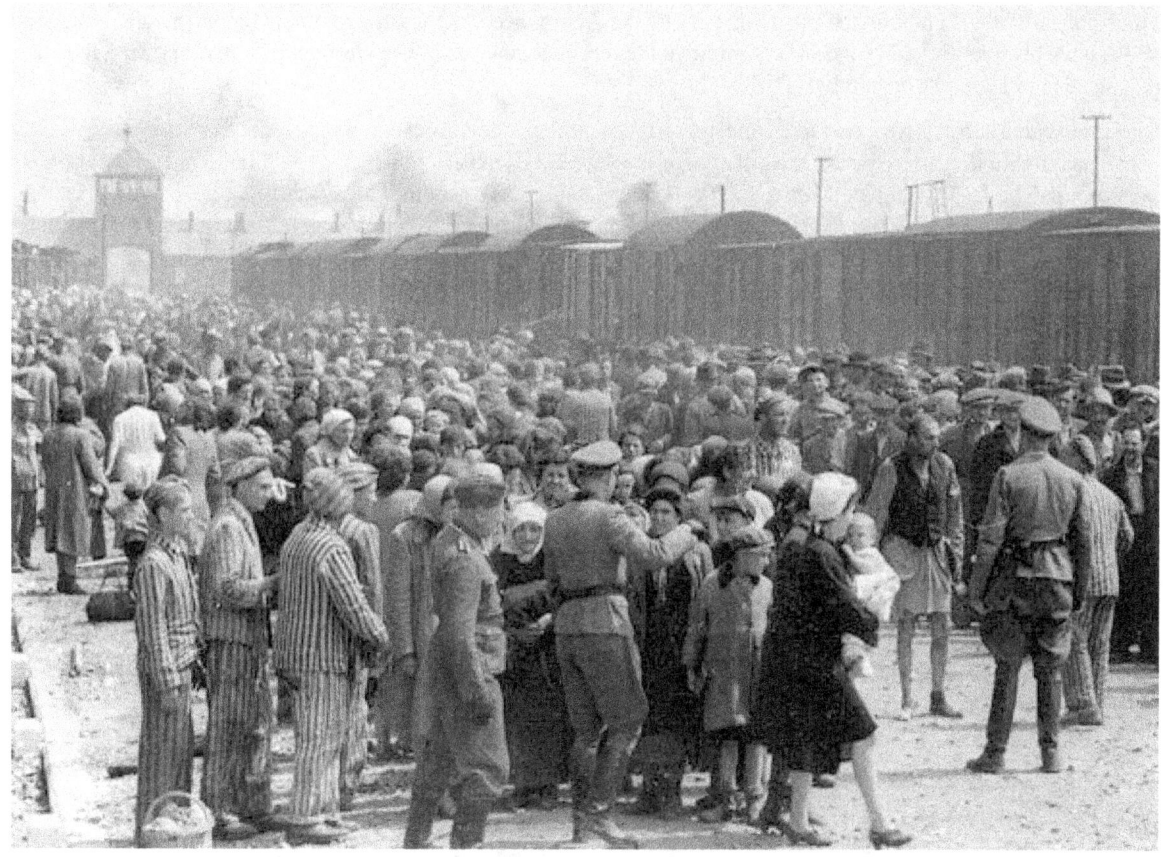

"Selection" of Hungarian Jews on the ramp at Auschwitz-II (Birkenau), May/June 1944

When an outbreak of noma (a gangrenous bacterial disease of the mouth and face) broke out in the Romani camp in 1943, Mengele initiated a study to determine the cause of the disease and develop a treatment. He enlisted the aid of prisoner Dr. Berthold Epstein, a Jewish pediatrician and professor at Prague University. Mengele isolated the patients in a separate barrack and had several afflicted children killed so that their preserved heads and organs could be sent to the SS Medical Academy in Graz and other facilities for study. The research was still ongoing when the Romani camp was liquidated and its remaining occupants killed in 1944.[2]

In response to a typhus epidemic in the women's camp, Mengele cleared one block of 600 Jewish women and sent them to the gas chamber. The building was then cleaned and disinfected, and the occupants of a neighboring block were bathed, de-loused, and given new clothing before being moved into the clean block. The process was repeated until all the barracks were disinfected. Similar disinfections were used for later epidemics of scarlet fever and other diseases, but with all the sick prisoners being sent to the gas chambers. For his efforts, Mengele was awarded the War Merit Cross (Second Class with Swords) and was promoted in 1944 to First Physician of the Birkenau subcamp.[37]

33.3.1 Human experimentation

Mengele used Auschwitz as an opportunity to continue his anthropological studies and research on heredity, using inmates for human experimentation.[2] The experiments had no regard for the health or safety of the victims.[2][3] He was particularly interested in identical twins, people with heterochromia iridum (eyes of two different colours), dwarfs, and people with physical abnormalities.[2] A grant was provided by the *Deutsche Forschungsgemeinschaft*, applied for by von Verschuer, who received regular reports and shipments of specimens from Mengele. The grant was used to build a pathology laboratory attached to Crematorium II at Auschwitz II-Birkenau.[38] Dr. Miklós Nyiszli, a Hungarian Jewish pathologist who arrived in Auschwitz on 29 May 1944, performed dissections and prepared specimens for shipment in this laboratory.[39] Mengele's twin research was in part intended to prove the supremacy of heredity over environment and thus bolster the Nazi premise of the superiority of the Aryan race.[40] Nyiszli and others report that the twins studies may also have been motivated by a desire to improve the reproduction rate of the German race by improving the chances of racially desirable people having twins.[41]

Mengele's research subjects were better fed and housed than other prisoners and temporarily safe from the gas chambers.[42] He established a kindergarten for children that were the subjects of experiments, along with all Romani children under the age of six. The facility provided better food and living conditions than other areas of the camp, and even included a playground.[43] When visiting his child subjects, he introduced himself as "Uncle Mengele" and offered them sweets.[44] But he was also personally responsible for the deaths of an unknown number of victims that he killed via lethal injection, shootings, beatings, and through selections and deadly experiments.[45] Lifton describes Mengele as sadistic, lacking empathy, and extremely antisemitic, believing the Jews should be eliminated entirely as an inferior and dangerous race.[46] Mengele's son Rolf said his father later showed no remorse for his wartime activities.[47]

A former Auschwitz prisoner doctor said:

> He was capable of being so kind to the children, to have them become fond of him, to bring them sugar, to think of small details in their daily lives, and to do things we would genuinely admire ... And then, next to that, ... the crematoria smoke, and these children, tomorrow or in a half-hour, he is going to send them there. Well, that is where the anomaly lay.[48]

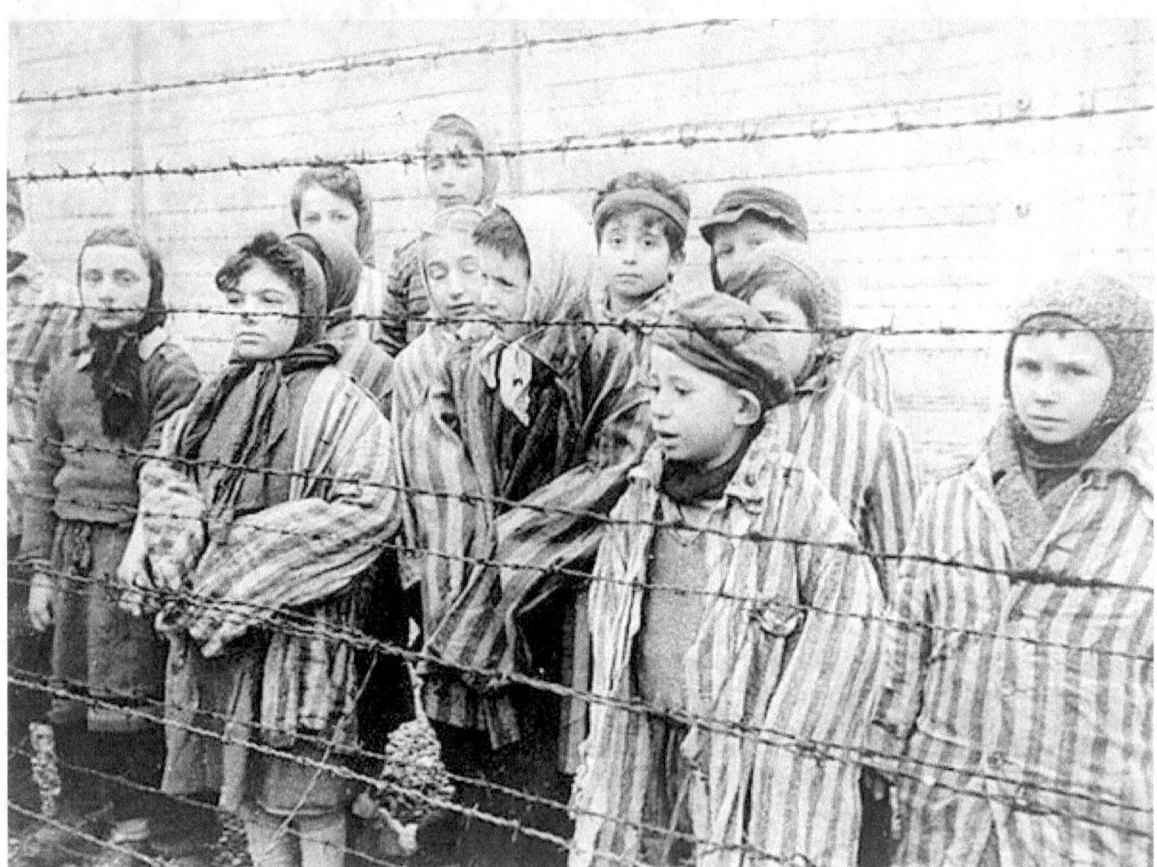

Jewish twins kept alive to be used in Mengele's medical experiments. These children were liberated from Auschwitz by the Red Army in January 1945.

Twins were subjected to weekly examinations and measurements of their physical attributes by Mengele or one of his assistants.[49] Experiments performed by Mengele on twins included unnecessary amputation of limbs, intentionally infecting one twin with typhus or other diseases, and transfusing the blood of one twin into the other. Many of the victims died while undergoing these procedures.[50] After an experiment was over, the twins were sometimes killed and their bodies dissected.[51] Nyiszli recalled one occasion where Mengele personally killed fourteen twins in one night via a chloroform injection to the heart.[34] If one twin died of disease, Mengele killed the other so that comparative post-mortem reports could be prepared.[52]

Mengele's experiments with eyes included attempts to change eye color by injecting chemicals into the eyes of living subjects and killing people with heterochromatic eyes so that the eyes could be removed and sent to Berlin for study.[53] His experiments on dwarfs and people with physical abnormalities included taking physical measurements, drawing blood, extracting healthy teeth, and treatment with unnecessary drugs and X-rays.[3] Many of the victims were sent to the gas chambers after about two weeks, and their skeletons were sent to Berlin for further study.[54] Mengele sought out pregnant women, on whom he would perform experiments before sending them to the gas chambers.[55] Witness Vera Alexander described how he sewed two Romani twins together back to back in an attempt to create conjoined twins.[50] The children died of gangrene after several days of suffering.[56]

33.4   After Auschwitz

Along with several other Auschwitz doctors, Mengele transferred to Gross-Rosen concentration camp in Lower Silesia on 17 January 1945. He brought along two boxes of specimens and records of his experiments. Most of the camp medical records had already been destroyed by the SS.[57][58] The Red Army captured Auschwitz on 27 January.[59] Mengele fled Gross Rosen on 18 February, a week before the Soviets arrived, and traveled westward disguised as a Wehrmacht officer to Saaz (now Žatec). Here he temporarily entrusted his incriminating Auschwitz documents to a nurse with whom he had struck up a relationship.[57] He and his unit hurried west to avoid being captured by the Soviets and were taken prisoner of war by the Americans in June. Mengele was initially registered under his own name, but because of the disorganization of the Allies regarding the distribution of wanted lists and the fact that Mengele did not have the usual SS blood group tattoo, he was not identified as being on the major war criminal list.[60] He was released at the end of July and obtained false papers under the name "Fritz Ullman", documents he later altered to read "Fritz Hollmann".[61]

After several months on the run, including a trip to the Soviet-occupied area to recover his Auschwitz records, Mengele found work near Rosenheim as a farmhand.[62] Worried that his capture would mean a trial and death sentence, he fled Germany on 17 April 1949.[63][64] Assisted by a network of former SS members, Mengele traveled to Genoa, where he obtained a passport under the alias "Helmut Gregor" from the International Committee of the Red Cross. He sailed to Argentina in July.[65] His wife refused to accompany him, and they divorced in 1954.[66]

33.5   In South America

In Buenos Aires, Argentina, Mengele worked as a carpenter while residing in a boarding house in the suburb of Vicente Lopez.[67] After a few weeks he moved to the house of a Nazi sympathiser in the more affluent neighborhood of Florida, Buenos Aires. He next worked as a salesman for his family's farm equipment company, and beginning in 1951 he made frequent trips to Paraguay as sales representative for that region.[68] An apartment in the center of Buenos Aires became his residence in 1953, the same year he used family funds to buy a part interest in a carpentry concern. In 1954 he rented a house in the suburb of Olivos.[69] Files released by the Argentine government in 1992 indicate that Mengele may have practiced medicine without a license, including performing abortions, while living in Buenos Aires.[70]

After obtaining a copy of his birth certificate through the West German embassy in 1956, Mengele was issued an Argentine foreign residence permit under his real name. He used this document to obtain a West German passport, also under his real name, and embarked for a visit to Europe.[71][72] He met up in Switzerland for a ski holiday with his son Rolf (who was told Mengele was his "Uncle Fritz"[73]) and his widowed sister-in-law Martha, and spent a week in his home town of Günzburg.[74][75] Upon his return to Argentina in September, Mengele began living under his real name. Martha and her son Karl Heinz followed about a month later, and the three took up residence together. The couple married while on holiday in Uruguay in 1958 and bought a house in Buenos Aires.[71][76] Business interests now included part ownership of Fadro Farm, a pharmaceutical company.[74] Along with several other doctors, Mengele was questioned and released in 1958 under suspicion of practicing medicine without a license after a teenage girl died following an abortion. Worried that the publicity would lead to his Nazi background and wartime activities being discovered, he took an extended business trip to Paraguay and was granted citizenship under the name José Mengele in 1959.[77] He returned to Buenos Aires several

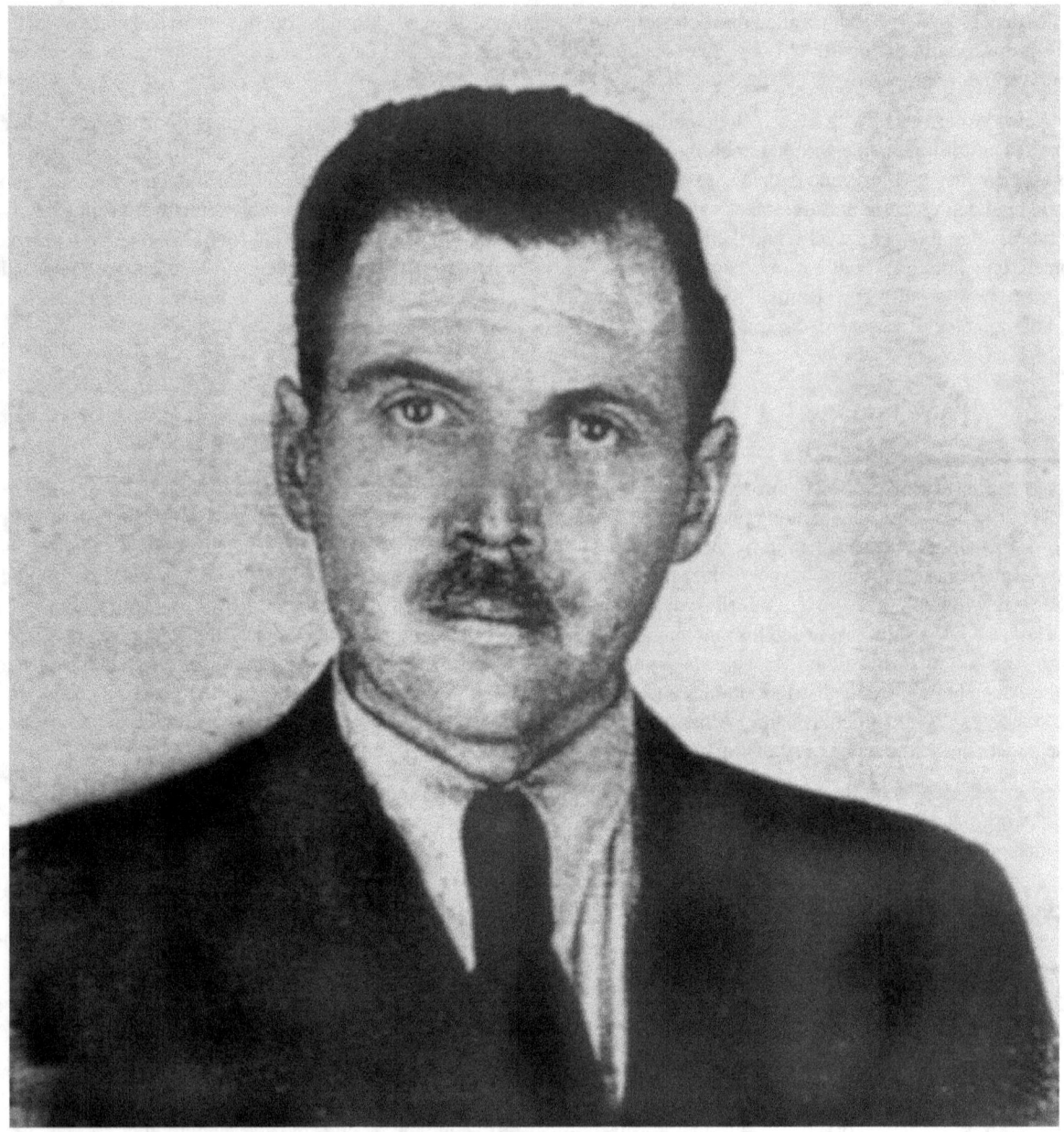

Photo from Mengele's Argentine identification document (1956)

times to wrap up his business affairs and visit his family. Martha and Karl Heinz lived in a boarding house in the city until December 1960, when they returned to Germany.[78]

Mengele's name was mentioned several times during the Nuremberg trials, but Allied forces were convinced that he was dead.[79] Irene and the family in Günzburg also said that he was dead.[80] Working in West Germany, Nazi hunters Simon Wiesenthal and Hermann Langbein collected information from witnesses as to Mengele's wartime activities. In a search of the public records, Langbein found Mengele's divorce papers listing an address in Buenos Aires. He and Wiesenthal pressured West German authorities into drawing up an arrest warrant on 5 June 1959, and starting extradition proceedings.[81][82] Initially Argentina turned down the request, because the fugitive was no longer living at the address given on the documents. By the time extradition was approved on 30 June 1960, Mengele had already fled to Paraguay, where he was living on a farm near the Argentine border.[83]

33.5.1   Efforts by the Mossad

In May 1960, Isser Harel, director of the Mossad (the Israeli intelligence agency), personally led the successful effort to capture Adolf Eichmann in Buenos Aires. He hoped to track down Mengele as well so he too could be brought to trial in Israel.[84] Under interrogation, Eichmann provided the address of a boarding house that had been used as a safe house for Nazi fugitives. Surveillance of the house did not reveal Mengele or any members of his family, and the neighborhood postman said that although Mengele had recently been receiving letters there under his real name, he had since relocated, leaving no forwarding address. Harel's inquiries at a machine shop where Mengele had been part owner did not turn up any leads either, so he had to give up.[85]

In spite of having provided Mengele with legal documents in his real name in 1956, thus enabling him to regularize his residency in Argentina, West Germany offered a reward for his capture. Ongoing newspaper coverage of his wartime activities (accompanied by photographs of the fugitive) led Mengele to relocate again in 1960. Former bomber pilot Hans-Ulrich Rudel put him in touch with the Nazi supporter Wolfgang Gerhard, who helped Mengele get across the border into Brazil.[78][86] He stayed with Gerhard on his farm near São Paulo until more permanent accommodations were found with Hungarian expatriates Geza and Gitta Stammer. Helped by an investment from Mengele, the couple bought a farm in Nova Europa, and Mengele was given the job of manager. In 1962 the three bought a coffee and cattle farm in Serra Negra, with Mengele owning a half interest.[87] Initially, Gerhard told the couple that Mengele's name was "Peter Hochbichler", but they discovered his true identity in 1963. Gerhard convinced them not to report Mengele's location to the authorities, saying they could themselves get in trouble for harboring the fugitive.[88] West Germany, tipped off to the possibility that Mengele had relocated there, widened its extradition request to include Brazil in February 1961.[89]

Meanwhile, Zvi Aharoni, one of the Mossad agents who had been involved in the Eichmann capture, was placed in charge of a team of agents tasked with locating Mengele and bringing him to trial in Israel. Inquiries in Paraguay gave no clues as to his whereabouts, and they were unable to intercept any correspondence between Mengele and his wife Martha, then living in Italy. Agents following Rudel's movements did not produce any leads.[90] Aharoni and his team followed Gerhard to a rural area near São Paulo, where they located a European man believed to be Mengele.[91] Aharoni reported his findings to Harel, but the logistics of staging a capture, budgetary constraints, and the need to focus on the nation's deteriorating relationship with Egypt led the Mossad chief to call a halt to the operation in 1962.[92]

33.5.2   Later life and death

Mengele and the Stammers bought a house on a farm in Caieiras in 1969, with Mengele as half owner.[93] When Wolfgang Gerhard returned to Germany in 1971 to seek medical treatment for his seriously ill wife and son, he gave his identity card to Mengele.[94] The Stammers had a falling out with Mengele in late 1974 and bought a house in São Paulo; Mengele was not invited.[lower-alpha 2] The Stammers bought a bungalow in Eldorado, São Paulo, which they rented out to Mengele.[97] Rolf, who had not seen his father since the ski holiday in 1956, visited him there in 1977 and found an unrepentant Nazi who claimed he had never personally harmed anyone and had only done his duty.[98]

Mengele's health had been steadily deteriorating since 1972, and he had a stroke in 1976.[99] He had high blood pressure and an ear infection that had an impact on his balance. While visiting his friends Wolfram and Liselotte Bossert in the coastal resort of Bertioga on 7 February 1979, he suffered another stroke while swimming and drowned.[100] Mengele was buried in Embu das Artes under the name "Wolfgang Gerhard", whose identification card he had been using since 1971.[101]

Other pseudonyms used by Mengele included Dr. Fausto Rindón and S. Josi Alvers Aspiazu.[102]

33.6   Exhumation

Meanwhile, Mengele sightings were reported all over the world. Wiesenthal claimed to have information that placed Mengele on the Greek island of Kythnos in 1960,[103] Cairo in 1961,[104] in Spain in 1971,[105] and in Paraguay in 1978, eighteen years after he had left.[106] He insisted as late as 1985—six years after Mengele's death—that he was still alive, in 1982 offering a reward of $100,000 for his capture.[107] Worldwide interest in the case was raised by a mock trial held in Jerusalem in February 1985 featuring the testimony of over a hundred victims of Mengele's experiments. Shortly afterwards, the governments of West Germany, Israel, and the United States launched a coordinated effort to determine Mengele's whereabouts. Rewards for his capture were offered by the Israeli and West German governments, *The Washington Times*, and the Simon Wiesenthal Center.[108]

On 31 May 1985, acting on a tip received by the West German prosecutor's office, police raided the house of Hans Sedlmeier, a lifelong friend of Mengele and sales manager of the family firm in Günzburg.[109] They found a coded address book and copies of letters to and from Mengele. Among the papers was a letter from Bossert notifying Sedlmeier of Mengele's death.[110] German authorities notified the police in São Paulo, who contacted the Bosserts. Under interrogation, they revealed the location of the grave.[111] The remains were exhumed on 6 June 1985, and extensive forensic examination confirmed with a high degree of probability that the body was Mengele's.[112] Rolf Mengele issued a statement on 10 June admitting the body was his father's. He said the news of his father's death had been kept quiet to protect the people who had sheltered his father for so many years.[113] In 1992, DNA testing verified Mengele's identity.[114] The family refused to have the remains repatriated to Germany, and they remain stored at the São Paulo Institute for Forensic Medicine.[115]

33.7 Legacy

Mengele's life was the inspiration for a novel and movie titled *The Boys from Brazil* (1978), where a fictional Mengele (portrayed by Gregory Peck[116]) produces clones of Hitler in a clinic in Brazil. [117] In 2007, the United States Holocaust Memorial Museum received as a donation the Höcker Album, an album of photographs of Auschwitz staff taken by Karl-Friedrich Höcker. Eight of the photographs include Mengele.[118]

In February 2010, a 180-page volume of Mengele's diary sold at auction for an undisclosed sum to the grandson of a Holocaust survivor. The unidentified previous owner, who acquired the journals in Brazil, was reported to be close to the Mengele family. A Holocaust survivors' organization described the sale as "a cynical act of exploitation aimed at profiting from the writings of one of the most heinous Nazi criminals."[119] Rabbi Marvin Hier of the Simon Wiesenthal Center was glad to see the diary fall into Jewish hands. "At a time when Ahmadinejad's Iran regularly denies the Holocaust and anti-Semitism and hatred of Jews is back in vogue, this acquisition is especially significant," he said.[120] In 2011, a further 31 volumes of Mengele's diaries were sold—again amidst protests—by the same auction house to an undisclosed collector of World War II memorabilia for $245,000.[121]

33.8 Summary of SS career

- SS number: 317,885

- Nazi Party number: 5,574,974

- Primary positions: *WVHA*, Medical Physician (Auschwitz Concentration Camp)

- *Waffen-SS* Service:

  - Medical Staff Officer, *Waffen-SS* Medical Inspectorate (1940)

  - Medical Officer, Pioneer Battalion No. 5, 5th SS Panzer Division Wiking (1941–1943)

  - Medical Officer, Battalion "Ost", 3rd SS Division Totenkopf (1943)

Dates of rank

Awards

- Iron Cross (First and Second Class)

- War Merit Cross (Second Class with Swords)

- Eastern Front Medal

- Wound Badge (Black)

- Social Welfare Decoration

- German Sports Badge (Bronze)

- Honour Chevron for the Old Guard[lower-alpha 4]

33.9   Journal articles

- *Racial-Morphological Examinations of the Anterior Portion of the Lower Jaw in Four Racial Groups.* This dissertation, completed in 1935 and first published in 1937, earned him a PhD in anthropology from Munich University. In this work Mengele sought to demonstrate that there were structural differences in the lower jaws of individuals from different ethnic groups, and that racial distinctions could be made based on these differences.[7][123]

- *Genealogical Studies in the Cases of Cleft Lip-Jaw-Palate* (1938), his medical dissertation, earned him a doctorate in medicine from Frankfurt University. Studying the influence of genetics as a factor in the occurrence of this deformity, Mengele conducted research on families who exhibited these traits in multiple generations. The work also included notes on other abnormalities found in these family lines.[7][124]

- *Hereditary Transmission of Fistulae Auris.* This journal article, published in *Der Erbarzt* (The Genetic Physician), focuses on fistula auris (an abnormal fissure on the external ear) as a hereditary trait. Mengele noted that individuals who have this trait also tend to have a dimple on their chin.[13]

33.10   See also

- Nazi eugenics

- Shirō Ishii, director of Imperial Japan's Unit 731 facility in World War II, involved in illegal human experimentation

33.11   Notes

[1] Of the Hungarians who arrived in mid-1944, 85 percent were killed immediately.[28]

[2] Based on entries in Mengele's journals and interviews with his friends, historians such as Gerald Posner and Gerald Astor believe he had a sexual relationship with Gitta Stammer.[95][96]

[3] Mengele's enlisted service is mentioned on only a single document of his official SS file. His entry date into the SS is stated to have occurred in early 1938, and by the date of his commissioning in 1940, Mengele was serving as an SS-First Sergeant in the *Waffen-SS* Reserve.[122]

[4] Mengele's SS service record indicates this decoration, even though he was not a Nazi Party or SS member prior to 1933, which was a primary requirement for the Old Guard Chevron.[122]

33.12   References

[1] Levy 2006, p. 242.

[2] Kubica 1998, p. 320.

[3] Astor 1985, p. 102.

[4] Astor 1985, p. 12.

[5] Posner & Ware 1986, pp. 4–5.

[6] Posner & Ware 1986, pp. 6–7.

[7] Kubica 1998, p. 318.

[8] Kershaw 2008, p. 81.

[9] Posner & Ware 1986, pp. 8, 10.

[10] Weindling 2002, p. 53.

[11] Allison 2011, p. 52.

[12] Levy 2006, p. 234 (footnote).

[13] Lifton 1986, p. 340.

[14] Posner & Ware 1986, p. 11.

[15] Posner & Ware 1986, p. 54.

[16] Evans 2008, p. 7.

[17] Longerich 2010, p. 132.

[18] Posner & Ware 1986, p. 16.

[19] Kubica 1998, pp. 318–319.

[20] Kubica 1998, p. 319.

[21] Posner & Ware 1986, pp. 16–18.

[22] Astor 1985, p. 27.

[23] Allison 2011, p. 53.

[24] Steinbacher 2005, p. 94.

[25] Longerich 2010, pp. 282–283.

[26] Steinbacher 2005, pp. 104–105.

[27] Rees 2005, p. 100.

[28] Steinbacher 2005, p. 109.

[29] Levy 2006, pp. 235–237.

[30] Astor 1985, p. 80.

[31] Levy 2006, pp. 248–249.

[32] Posner & Ware 1986, p. 29.

[33] Posner & Ware 1986, p. 27.

[34] Lifton 1985.

[35] Astor 1985, p. 78.

[36] Piper 1998, pp. 170, 172.

[37] Kubica 1998, pp. 328–329.

[38] Posner & Ware 1986, p. 33.

[39] Posner & Ware 1986, pp. 33–34.

[40] Steinbacher 2005, p. 114.

[41] Lifton 1986, pp. 358–359.

[42] Nyiszli 2011, p. 57.

[43] Kubica 1998, pp. 320–321.

[44] Lagnado & Dekel 1991, p. 9.

[45] Lifton 1986, p. 341.

[46] Lifton 1986, pp. 376–377.

[47] Posner & Ware 1986, p. 48.

[48] Lifton 1985, p. 337.

[49] Lifton 1986, p. 350.

[50] Posner & Ware 1986, p. 37.

[51] Lifton 1986, p. 351.

[52] Lifton 1986, pp. 347, 353.

[53] Lifton 1986, p. 362.

[54] Lifton 1986, p. 360.

[55] Brozan 1982.

[56] Mozes-Kor 1992, p. 57.

[57] Levy 2006, p. 255.

[58] Posner & Ware 1986, p. 57.

[59] Steinbacher 2005, p. 128.

[60] Posner & Ware 1986, p. 63.

[61] Posner & Ware 1986, pp. 63, 68.

[62] Posner & Ware 1986, pp. 68, 88.

[63] Posner & Ware 1986, p. 87.

[64] Levy 2006, p. 263.

[65] Levy 2006, p. 264–265.

[66] Posner & Ware 1986, pp. 88,108.

[67] Posner & Ware 1986, p. 95.

[68] Posner & Ware 1986, pp. 104–105.

[69] Posner & Ware 1986, pp. 107–108.

[70] Nash 1992.

[71] Levy 2006, p. 267.

[72] Astor 1985, p. 166.

[73] Posner & Ware 1986, p. 2.

[74] Astor 1985, p. 167.

[75] Posner & Ware 1986, p. 111.

[76] Posner & Ware 1986, p. 112.

[77] Levy 2006, pp. 269–270.

[78] Levy 2006, p. 273.

[79] Posner & Ware 1986, pp. 76, 82.

[80] Levy 2006, p. 261.

[81] Levy 2006, p. 271.

[82] Posner & Ware 1986, p. 121.

[83] Levy 2006, pp. 269–270, 272.

[84] Posner & Ware 1986, p. 139.

[85] Posner & Ware 1986, pp. 142–143.

[86] Posner & Ware 1986, p. 162.

[87] Levy 2006, pp. 279–281.

[88] Levy 2006, pp. 280, 282.

[89] Posner & Ware 1986, p. 168.

[90] Posner & Ware 1986, pp. 166–167.

[91] Posner & Ware 1986, pp. 184–186.

[92] Posner & Ware 1986, pp. 184, 187–188.

[93] Posner & Ware 1986, p. 223.

[94] Levy 2006, p. 289.

[95] Posner & Ware 1986, pp. 178–179.

[96] Astor 1985, p. 224.

[97] Levy 2006, pp. 242–243.

[98] Posner & Ware 1986, pp. 2, 279.

[99] Levy 2006, pp. 289, 291.

[100] Levy 2006, pp. 294–295.

[101] Blumenthal 1985, p. 1.

[102] Zentner & Bedürftig 1991, p. 586.

[103] Segev 2010, p. 167.

[104] Walters 2009, p. 317.

[105] Walters 2009, p. 370.

[106] Levy 2006, p. 296.

[107] Levy 2006, pp. 297, 301.

[108] Posner & Ware 1986, pp. 306–308.

[109] Posner & Ware 1986, pp. 89, 313.

[110] Levy 2006, p. 302.

[111] Posner & Ware 1986, pp. 315, 317.

[112] Posner & Ware 1986, pp. 319–321.

[113] Posner & Ware 1986, p. 322.

[114] Saad 2005.

[115] Simons 1988.

[116] Turner 2003.

[117] Levy 2006, p. 287.

[118] USHMM website.

[119] Oster 2010.

[120] Hier 2010.

[121] Aderet 2011.

[122] SS service record, NARA.

[123] Lifton 1986, p. 339.

[124] Lifton 1986, pp. 339–340.

33.13 Sources

- Aderet, Ofer (22 July 2011). "Ultra-Orthodox man buys diaries of Nazi doctor Mengele for $245,000". *Haaretz*. Retrieved 2 February 2014.

- Allison, Kirk C. (2011). "Eugenics, race hygiene, and the Holocaust: Antecedents and consolidations". In Friedman, Jonathan C. *Routledge History of the Holocaust*. Milton Park; New York: Taylor & Francis. pp. 45–58. ISBN 978-0-415-77956-2.

- Astor, Gerald (1985). *Last Nazi: Life and Times of Dr Joseph Mengele*. New York: Donald I. Fine. ISBN 0-917657-46-2.

- Blumenthal, Ralph (22 July 1985). "Scientists Decide Brazil Skeleton Is Josef Mengele". *New York Times* (Arthur Ochs Sulzberger, Jr.). Retrieved 1 February 2014.

- Brozan, Nadine (15 November 1982). "Out of Death, a Zest for Life". *The New York Times*.

- Evans, Richard J. (2008). *The Third Reich at War*. New York: Penguin. ISBN 978-0-14-311671-4.

- Hier, Marvin (2010). "Wiesenthal Center Praises Acquisition of Mengele's Diary". Simpn Wiesenthal Center. Retrieved 2 February 2014.

- Kershaw, Ian (2008). *Hitler: A Biography*. New York: W. W. Norton & Company. ISBN 978-0-393-06757-6.

- Kubica, Helena (1998) [1994]. "The Crimes of Josef Mengele". In Gutman, Yisrael; Berenbaum, Michael. *Anatomy of the Auschwitz Death Camp*. Bloomington, Indiana: Indiana University Press. pp. 317–337. ISBN 978-0-253-20884-2.

- Lagnado, Lucette Matalon; Dekel, Sheila Cohn (1991). *Children of the Flames: Dr Josef Mengele and the Untold Story of the Twins of Auschwitz*. New York: William Morrow. ISBN 0-688-09695-6.

- Levy, Alan (2006) [1993]. *Nazi Hunter: The Wiesenthal File* (Revised 2002 ed.). London: Constable & Robinson. ISBN 978-1-84119-607-7.

- Lifton, Robert Jay (21 July 1985). "What Made This Man? Mengele". *The New York Times*. Retrieved 11 January 2014.

- Lifton, Robert Jay (1986). *The Nazi Doctors: Medical Killing and the Psychology of Genocide*. New York: Basic Books. ISBN 978-0-465-04905-9.

- Longerich, Peter (2010). *Holocaust: The Nazi Persecution and Murder of the Jews*. Oxford; New York: Oxford University Press. ISBN 978-0-19-280436-5.

- Mozes-Kor, Eva (1992). "Mengele Twins and Human Experimentation: A Personal Account". In Annas, George J.; Grodin, Michael A. *The Nazi Doctors and the Nuremberg Code: Human Rights in Human Experimentation*. New York: Oxford University Press. pp. 53–59. ISBN 978-0-19-510106-5.

- Nash, Nathaniel C. (11 February 1992). "Mengele an Abortionist, Argentine Files Suggest". *The New York Times*. Retrieved 31 August 2014.

- Nyiszli, Miklós (2011) [1960]. *Auschwitz: A Doctor's Eyewitness Account*. New York: Arcade Publishing. ISBN 978-1-61145-011-8.

- Oster, Marcy (3 February 2010). "Survivor's grandson buys Mengele diary". Jewish Telegraphic Agency. Retrieved 2 February 2014.

- Piper, Franciszek (1998) [1994]. "Gas Chambers and Crematoria". In Gutman, Yisrael; Berenbaum, Michael. *Anatomy of the Auschwitz Death Camp*. Bloomington, Indiana: Indiana University Press. pp. 157–182. ISBN 978-0-253-20884-2.

- Posner, Gerald L.; Ware, John (1986). *Mengele: The Complete Story*. New York: McGraw-Hill. ISBN 0-07-050598-5.

- Rees, Laurence (2005). *Auschwitz: A New History*. New York: Public Affairs. ISBN 1-58648-303-X.

- Saad, Rana (1 April 2005). "Discovery, development, and current applications of DNA identity testing". *Baylor University Medical Center Proceedings* **18** (2): 130–133. PMC 1200713. PMID 16200161.

- Segev, Tom (2010). *Simon Wiesenthal: The Life and Legends*. New York: Doubleday. ISBN 978-0-385-51946-5.

- Simons, Marlise (17 March 1988). "Remains of Mengele Rest Uneasily in Brazil". *The New York Times*. Retrieved 2 February 2014.

- "SS service record of Josef Mengele". College Park, Maryland: National Archives and Records Administration.

- Steinbacher, Sybille (2005) [2004]. *Auschwitz: A History*. Munich: Verlag C. H. Beck. ISBN 0-06-082581-2.

- "The Album". United States Holocaust Memorial Museum. 2007. Retrieved 2 February 2014.

- Turner, Adrian (14 June 2003). "Gregory Peck: Elder statesman of the screen who stood for nobility, honour and decency". *The Independent*. Retrieved 1 September 2015.

- Walters, Guy (2009). *Hunting Evil: The Nazi War Criminals Who Escaped and the Quest to Bring Them to Justice*. New York: Broadway Books. ISBN 978-0-7679-2873-1.

- Weindling, Paul (2002). "The Ethical Legacy of Nazi Medical War Crimes: Origins, Human Experiments, and International Justice". In Burley, Justine; Harris, John. *A Companion to Genethics*. Blackwell Companions to Philosophy. Malden, MA; Oxford: Blackwell. pp. 53–69. doi:10.1002/9780470756423.ch5. ISBN 0-631-20698-1.

- Zentner, Christian; Bedürftig, Friedemann (1991). *The Encyclopedia of the Third Reich*. New York: Macmillan. ISBN 0-02-897502-2.

33.14   Further reading

- Harel, Isser (1975). *The House on Garibaldi Street: the First Full Account of the Capture of Adolf Eichmann.* New York: Viking Press. ISBN 0-670-38028-8.

- Levin, Ira (1991). *The Boys from Brazil.* London: Bantam. ISBN 0-553-29004-5.

- Lieberman, Herbert A. (1978). *The Climate of Hell.* New York: Simon and Schuster. ISBN 0-671-82236-5.

33.15   External links

- Breitman, Richard (April 2001). "Historical Analysis of 20 Name Files from CIA Records". US National Archives.

- Office of Special Investigations, Criminal Division (October 1992). "In the Matter of Josef Mengele: A Report to the Attorney General of the United States" (PDF). United States Department of Justice.

- Papanayotou, Vivi (18 September 2005). "Skeletons in the Closet of German Science". Deutsche Welle.

- Posner, Gerald; Ware, John (18 May 1986). "How Nazi war criminal Josef Mengele cheated justice for 34 years". *Chicago Tribune Magazine.*

Chapter 34

Joachim Mrugowsky

Joachim Mrugowsky (15 August 1905 in Rathenow, Brandenburg – 2 June 1948, Landsberg Prison, Landsberg am Lech) was a German hygienist. He was Associate Professor, Medical Doctorate, Chief of Hygiene Institute of the Waffen-SS, Senior Hygienist at the Reich, SS-Physician, SS and Waffen-SS Colonel, and defendant in the Doctors' Trial.

34.1 Early life and education

Mrugowsky's father was a general practitioner, who was killed at the beginning of World War I. In 1925, Mrugowsky began his studies of natural sciences and medicine in Halle. He completed the studies in 1930-1931 with a medical doctorate and a doctorate of natural sciences. 1930-1931 he was the *Hochschulgruppenführer* (University group leader) of the National Socialist German Students' League branch at the University of Halle. After a two-year internship, he became an assistant at the Hygiene Institute of the University of Halle.

Mrugowsky was made an associate professor in the area of hygiene at the University of Berlin, September 1944.

34.2 Career in the Third Reich

Since 1930, Mrugowsky had been involved in the Nazi ideology, first being the group leader of a local National Socialist German Students' Association then the NSDAP party member (No. 210,049). In 1931, he joined the SS, where he achieved the rank of *Oberführer* in both the General SS and the Waffen SS.

Mrugowsky coordinated human experimentation at the Sachsenhausen concentration camp near Berlin. This included testing of biological warfare agents, including poisoned bullets.

In 1940, as the troop physician of an SS "Das Reich" Division hospital company, Mrugowsky participated in the conquest of Western Europe.

34.3 Trial and execution

He was implicated in all medical experiments, with the exception of the aviation ones, which were conducted on concentration camp prisoners. Mrugowsky was condemned to death in August 1947, and executed on June 2, 1948.

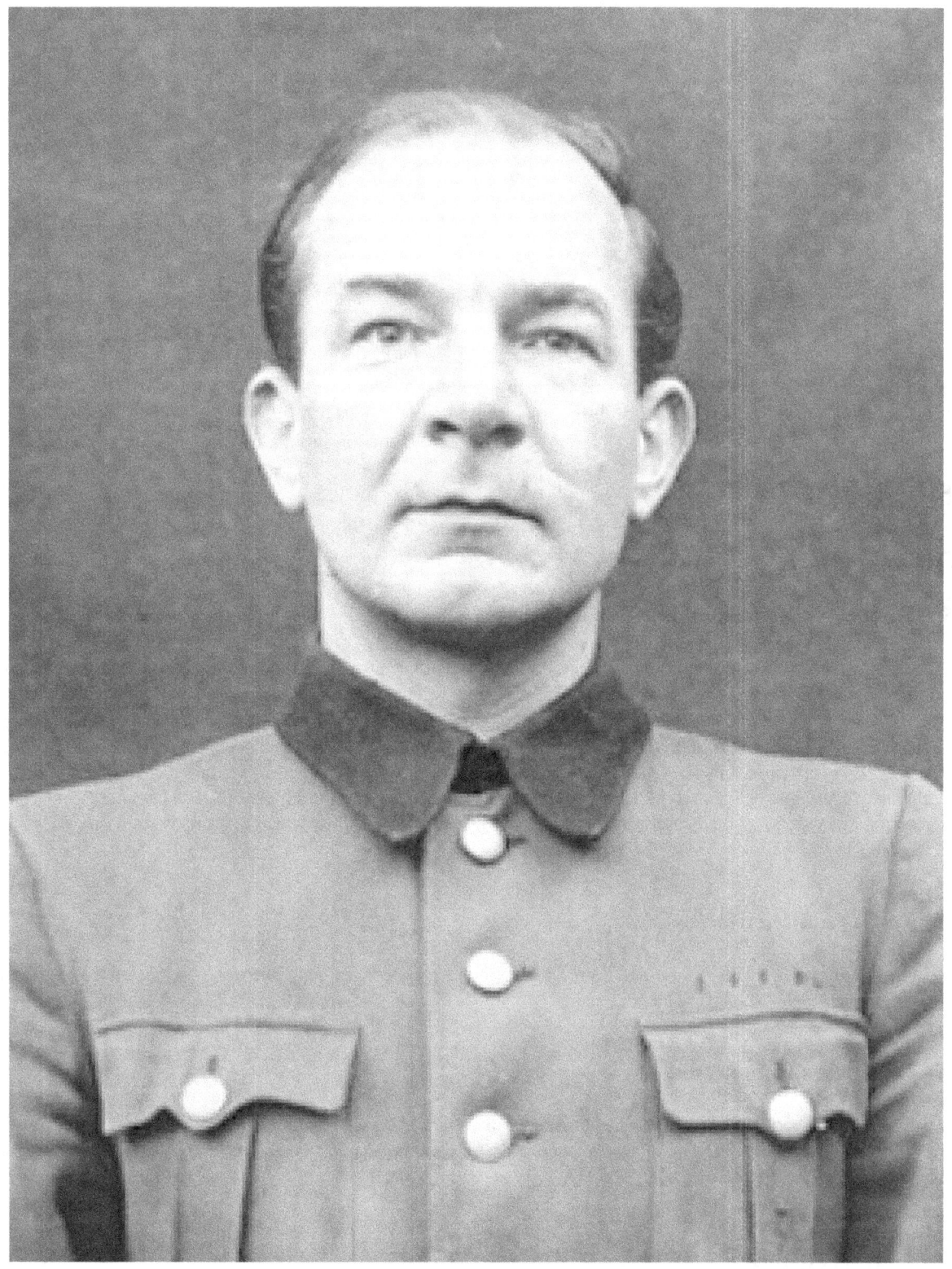

Joachim Mrugowsky as a defendant in the Doctors' Trial.

Chapter 35

Herta Oberheuser

Herta Oberheuser (15 May 1911 in Cologne, German Empire – 24 January 1978 in Linz am Rhein, West Germany) was a Nazi physician at the Auschwitz and Ravensbrück concentration camps from 1940 until 1943.

35.1 Biography

35.1.1 Youth and education

35.1.2 Medical experiments

Oberheuser worked at concentration camps under the supervision of Dr. Karl Gebhardt, participating in gruesome medical experiments (sulfanilamide as well as bone, muscle, and nerve regeneration and bone transplantation) conducted on 86 women, 74 of whom were Polish political prisoners in the camp. She killed healthy children with oil and evipan injections, then removed their limbs and vital organs. The time from the injection to death was between three and five minutes, with the person being fully conscious until the last moment. She performed some of the most gruesome and painful medical experiments, focusing on deliberately inflicting wounds on the subjects. In order to simulate the combat wounds of German soldiers fighting in the war, Oberheuser rubbed foreign objects, such as wood, rusty nails, slivers of glass, dirt, or sawdust into the cuts.

35.1.3 Nuremberg trials

Herta Oberheuser was the only female defendant in the Nuremberg Medical Trial, where she was sentenced to 20 years in jail. It was later reduced to 10 years in prison.

35.1.4 Release from prison

She was released in April 1952 for good behavior and became a family doctor in Stocksee, Germany. She lost her position in 1956, after a Ravensbrück survivor recognized her, and her license to practice medicine was revoked in 1958. She died in January 1978 at the age of 66.

35.2 External links

- Herta Oberheuser

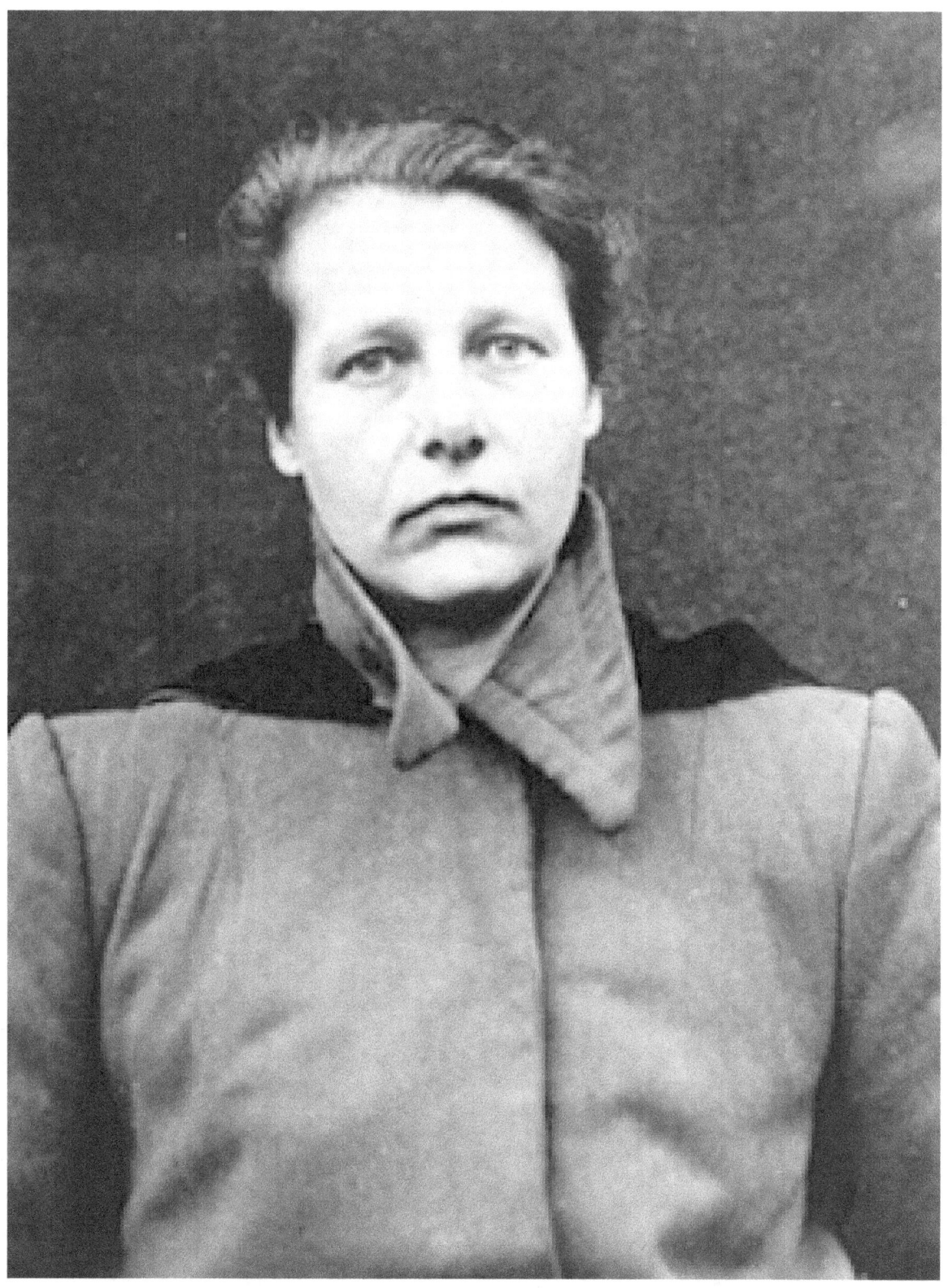

Oberheuser in 1946 or '47.

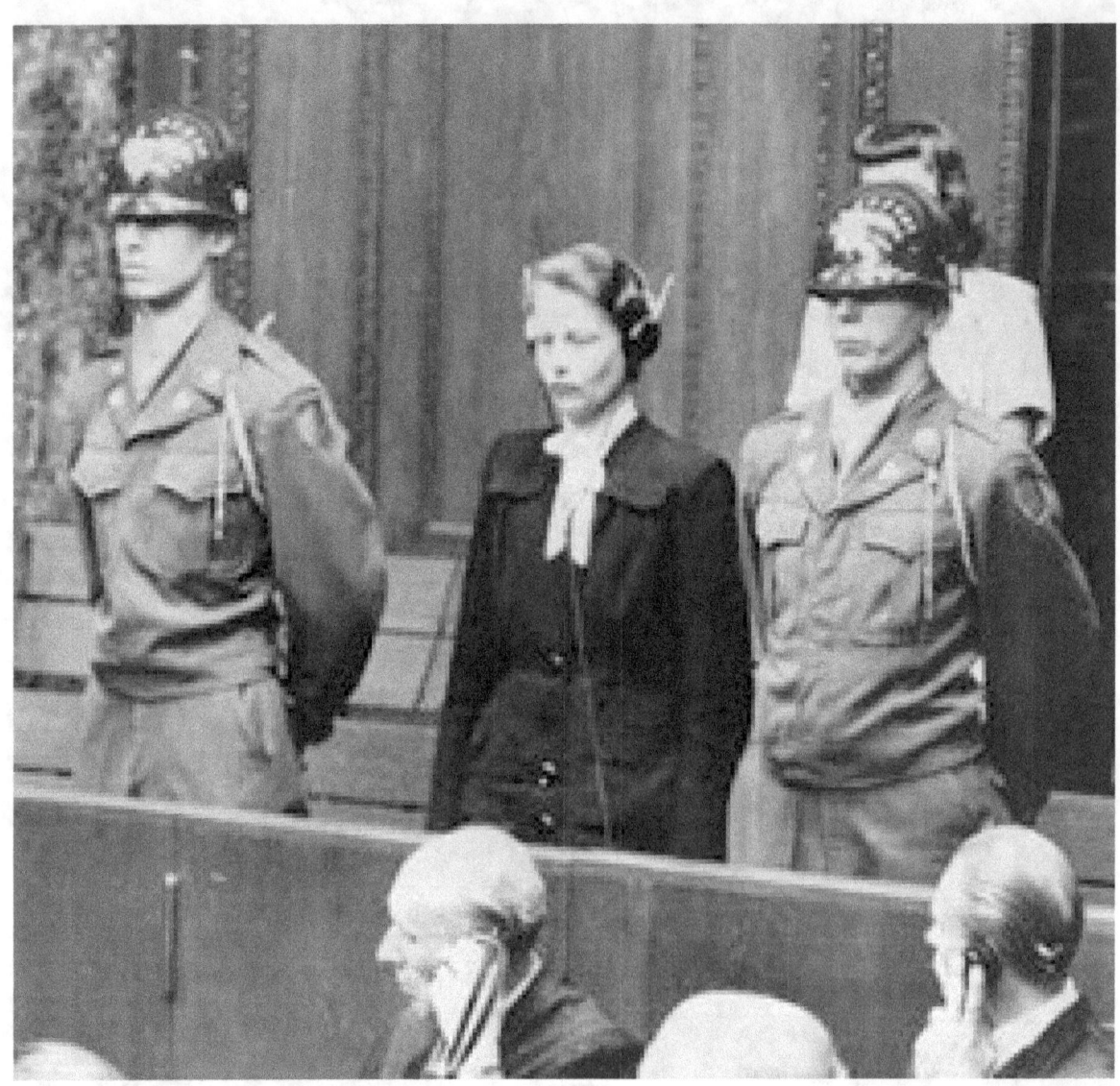

Oberheuser is sentenced to 20 years' imprisonment at the Doctors' Trial.

Chapter 36

Kurt Plötner

Kurt Friedrich Plötner (19 October 1905 – 26 February 1984) was a Nazi Party member and doctor who conducted human experimentation on Jews and Soviet prisoners of war in German concentration camps. American intelligence recruited him to work for the United States in 1945. He returned to the medical field as a professor at the University of Freiburg in West Germany after working for the Americans and living under an alias.

36.1 Biography

Kurt Friedrich Plötner was born in Hermsdorf on October 19, 1905. A devoted Nazi as well as a Leipzig lecturer and researcher, he joined the SS as a physician in the 1930s, reaching the SS rank of Sturmbannführer.

Plötner participated in a series of research tasks involving human experimentation at the Dachau concentration camp during the Second World War II. These included participation in the malaria experiments of Claus Schilling, in which prisoners were injected with drugs at lethal doses. In 1944, he was given Dachau physician Sigmund Rascher's role as head of the "Department R" of the Ahnenerbe project for carrying out experimental work on living subjects.[1] Plötner also administered the hallucinogen mescaline to Jews and Russian prisoners, watching them display schizophrenic behavior, as part of the Nazi search for a truth serum that could be employed as an aid in interrogations.[2]

Plötner's work in the concentration camps came to the attention of Boris Pash, an American intelligence officer who would go on to work in the CIA at the time of Operation BLUEBIRD in the late 1940s, and the United States Navy's intelligence officers recruited him in 1945, permitting him to continue his interrogation research.[3][4] Plötner proceeded to live under the name of "Schmitt" in Schleswig-Holstein into the early 1950s.[5]

Despite Plötner's actual residence in this western German zone, when the French government sought to have Plötner prosecuted in 1946 and appealed to the United States for assistance, the Americans replied that he could not be located, and was probably being shielded by the Soviet Union. He subsequently was able to quietly resume his real identity in 1952, at which time he was hired by the University of Freiburg in West Germany.[6] He became an associate professor in 1954.[5]

Plötner died on February 26, 1984.

36.2 See also

- Nazi human experimentation

- Operation Paperclip

36.3 References

[1] Kater, Michael H. *Das 'Ahnenerbe' der SS 1935- 1945: Ein Beitrag zur Kulturpolitik des dritten Reiches*, Studien zur Zeitgeschichte Volume 6. Munich: Oldenbourg Wissenschaftsverlag, 2006. ISBN 3-486-57950-9, ISBN 978-3-486-57950-5. P. 467. (German)

[2] Cockburn, Alexander & Jeffrey St. Clair. *Whiteout: The CIA, Drugs, and the Press.* London: Verso, 1998. ISBN 1-85984-139-2, ISBN 978-1-85984-139-6. P. 51.

[3] Blackman, Shane J. *Chilling Out: The Cultural Politics of Substance Consumption, Youth and Drug Policy.* Maidenhead, Berkshire: Open University Press, 2004. ISBN 0-335-20072-9, ISBN 978-0-335-20072-6. P. 33.

[4] Cockburn, Alexander. "The Wide World of Torture". *The Nation.* 8 November 2001. Retrieved 11 November 2009.

[5] Schmid, Hans. "Psychopathen, Psychiater und Psychonauten". *Telepolis.* 8 August 2009. Retrieved 11 November 2009. (German)

[6] Klee, Ernst. "Silke Seemann: Die politischen Säuberungen des Lehrkörpers der Freiburger Universität nach dem Ende des Zweiten Weltkrieges (1945–1957)". *Deutsches Ärzteblatt.* 27 June 2003. Retrieved 11 November 2009. (German)

Chapter 37

Helmut Poppendick

Helmut Poppendick (January 6, 1902[1]-January 11, 1994) was a German doctor who served in the SS during World War II. He was an internist and worked in the Medical Doctorate, as Chief of the Personal Staff of the *Reich* Physician SS and Police. After the war he was a defendant in the Doctors' Trial.

He studied medicine from 1919-1926 in Göttingen, Munich, and Berlin. Poppendick received his medical license on 1 February 1928. Then, he worked for four years as a clinical assistant at the First Medical Clinic of Charité in Berlin. From June 1933-October 1934, he was the assistant medical director at Virchow Hospital in Berlin.

In 1935, he completed training as an expert for "race hygiene" at the Kaiser Wilhelm Institute for Anthropology, Human Genetics and Eugenics. After this, he became the adjutant of the ministerial director Arthur Gütt at the *Reich* Ministry of the Interior. He was also the chief of staff at the SS Office for Population Politics and Genetic Health Care, which in 1937 became the SS Main Race and Settlement Office. Poppendick was departmental head and staff leader of the Genealogical Office.

At the beginning of World War II, he was drafted as an adjutant to a medical department of the army and took part in the attack on Belgium, France and the Netherlands. In November 1941, Poppendick was accepted into the *Waffen-SS*. In 1943, Ernst-Robert Grawitz of the *Reich* Physician SS appointed him to lead his personal staff. Poppendick joined the NSDAP in 1932 (party member No. 998607) and the SS (No. 36345). He reached the rank of *Oberführer* in the SS.

Poppendick was implicated in a series of medical experiments done on concentration camp prisoners, including the medical experiments done in Ravensbrück. At the American Military Tribunal No. I on August 20, 1947, he was acquitted from being criminally implicated in medical experiments, but was sentenced to 10 years imprisonment for membership in a criminal organization, the SS. He was released on January 31, 1951. Later on, Poppendick managed to get his medical services paid by insurance, in Oldenburg.

37.1 See also

- Doctor's Trial

- Ex-Nazis

- Nazi human experimentation

37.2 References

[1] *Nuremberg Trials Project: A Digital Document Collection*, "Helmut Poppendick Affidavit, 14 January 1947", Harvard Law School Library Item No. 849.

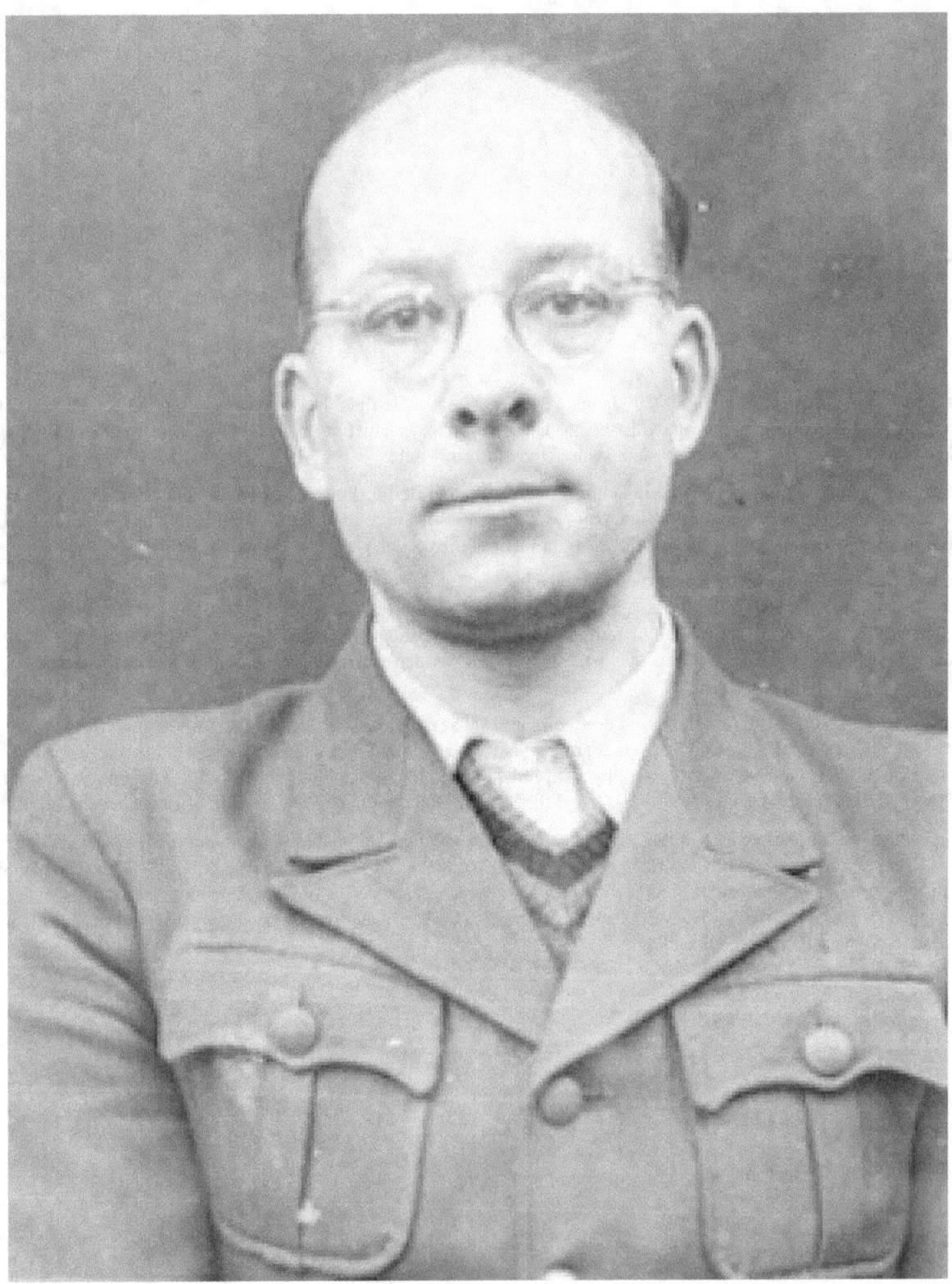

Helmut Poppendick.

Chapter 38

Sigmund Rascher

Sigmund Rascher (12 February 1909 – 26 April 1945) was a German SS doctor. His deadly experiments on humans, which were carried out in the Nazi concentration camp of Dachau, were judged inhumane and criminal during the Nuremberg Trials.[1]

38.1   Early life and career

Rascher was born the third child of Hanns-August Rascher (1880–1952), a physician, and completed his secondary education in Konstanz in 1930 or 1931 (this is uncertain, as he himself used both dates). His father was an avid follower of Rudolf Steiner, and Sigmund attended a Waldorf School which was based on Steiner's approach to education.[2] In 1933 he began studying medicine in Munich, where he also joined the NSDAP. The exact day of his joining is also uncertain, as there are two dates given: Rascher insisted that it was on March 1, whereas the documents show May 1. This is relevant in that the first date is before the Nazi victory in the election of 5th March 1933, where as the second date is after Hitler had consolidated power on 23rd March with his Enabling Act.[3]

After his *Praktikum* (internship), he worked with his now divorced father in Basel, Switzerland, and also continued his studies there, joining the Swiss Voluntary Work Forces. In 1934 he moved to Munich to finish his studies, and received his doctorate in 1936.

In May 1936 year Rascher joined the SA. In 1939 he transferred to the SS with the rank of SS-Mann (Private).

In Munich Rascher worked with Prof. Trumpp from 1936 to 1938 on cancer diagnostics, supported by a stipend, and until 1939 was an assistant physician at Munich's Schwabinger Krankenhaus hospital.[4]

38.2   Career with the SS

In 1939 Rascher denounced his father, joined the SS, and was conscripted into the Luftwaffe. A relationship and eventually marriage to former singer Karoline "Nini" Diehl gained him direct access to Reichsführer-SS Heinrich Himmler. Rascher's connection with Himmler gave him immense influence, even over his superiors.[5] Diehl may have been a former lover of Himmler; she frequently corresponded with him and interceded with him on her husband's behalf.[6]

A week after first meeting Himmler, Rascher presented a paper, "Report on the Development and Solution to Some of the Reichsfuehrer's Assigned Tasks During a Discussion Held on April 24, 1939".[5] Rascher became involved in testing a plant extract as a cancer treatment. Kurt Blome, deputy of the Reich Health Leader (Reichsgesundheitsführer) and Plenipotentiary for Cancer Research in the Reich Research Council, favoured testing the extract on rodents, but Rascher insisted on using human test subjects. Himmler took Rascher's side and a Human Cancer Testing Station was established at Dachau. Blome worked on the project.[5]

38.2.1 High altitude experiments

Rascher suggested in early 1941, while a captain in the Luftwaffe's Medical Service, that high-altitude/low-pressure experiments be carried out on human beings.[7] While taking a course in aviation medicine at Munich, he wrote Himmler a letter in which he said that his course included research into high-altitude flight and it was regretted that no tests with humans had been possible as such experiments were highly dangerous and nobody volunteered for them. Rascher asked Himmler to place human subjects at his disposal, stating quite frankly that the experiments might prove fatal, but that previous tests made with monkeys had been unsatisfactory. The letter was answered by Rudolf Brandt, Himmler's adjutant, who informed Rascher that prisoners would be made available.[8][9]

Rascher subsequently wrote back to Brandt, asking for permission to carry out his experiments at Dachau, and plans for the experiments were developed at a conference in early 1942 attended by Rascher and members of the Luftwaffe Medical Service. The experiments were carried out in the spring and summer of the same year, using a portable pressure chamber supplied by the Luftwaffe. The victims were locked in the chamber, the interior pressure of which was then lowered to a level corresponding to very high altitudes. The pressure could be very quickly altered, allowing Rascher to simulate the conditions which would be experienced by a pilot freefalling from altitude without oxygen. After viewing a report of one of the fatal experiments, Himmler remarked that if a subject should survive such treatment, he should be "pardoned" to life imprisonment. Rascher replied to Himmler that the victims had to date been merely Poles and Russians, and that he believed they should be given no amnesty of any sort.[8]

38.2.2 Freezing experiments

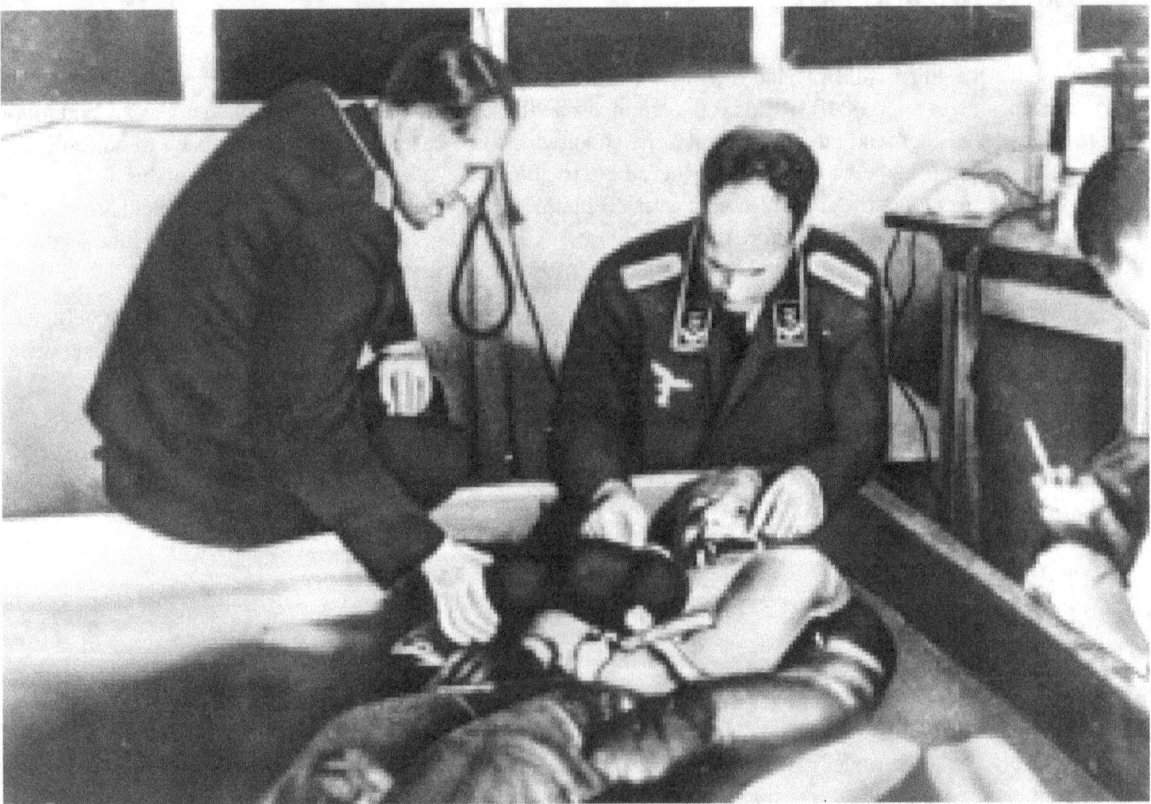

A cold water immersion experiment at Dachau concentration camp presided over by Professor Ernst Holzlöhner (left) and Dr. Sigmund Rascher (right). The subject is wearing an experimental Luftwaffe garment

Rascher also conducted so-called "freezing experiments" on behalf of the Luftwaffe, in which 300 test subjects were used against their will. These were also conducted at Dachau after the high-altitude experiments had concluded. The purpose was to determine the best way of warming German pilots who had been forced down in the North Sea and suffered

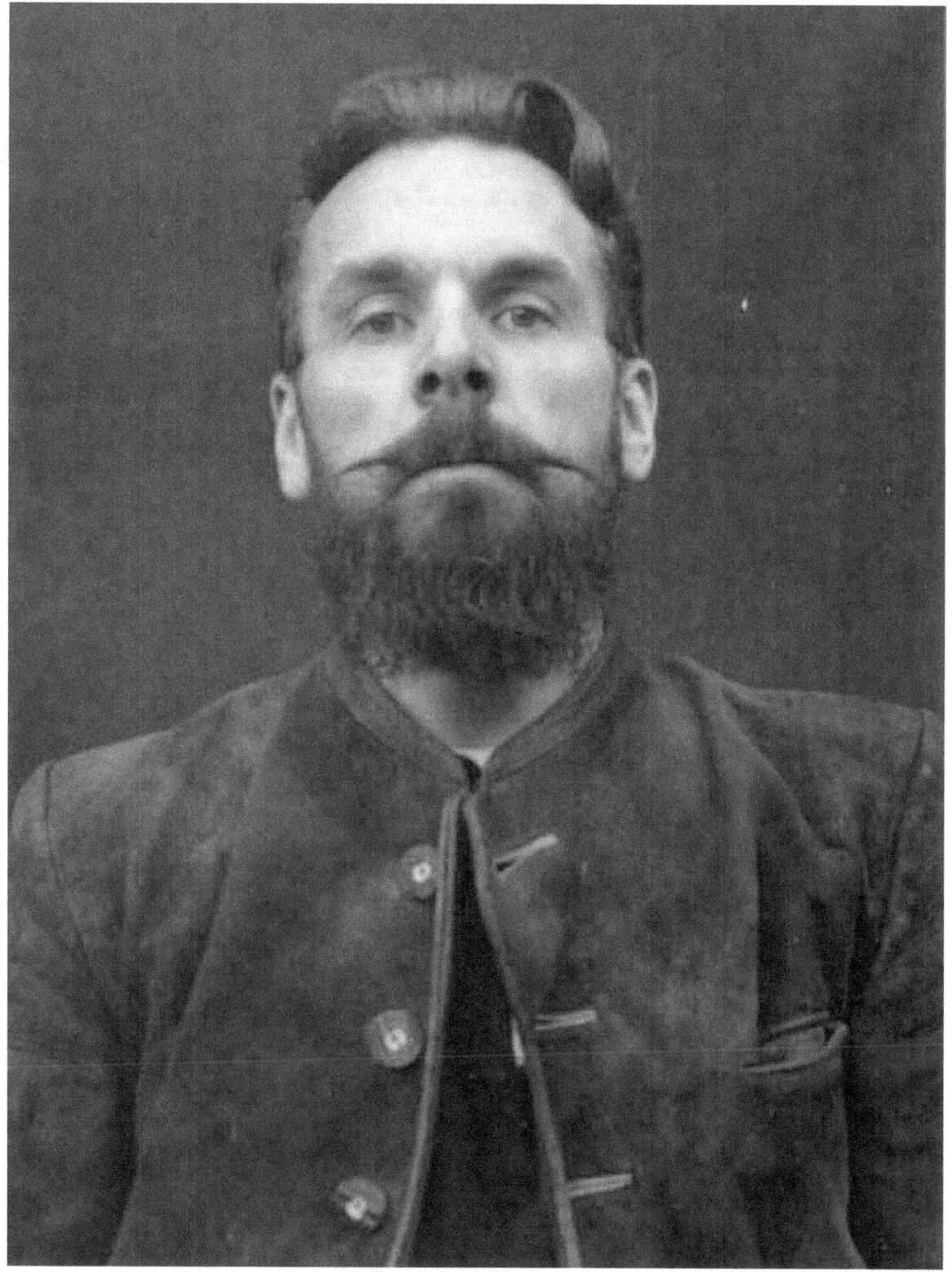

Mugshot of Wolfram Sievers, taken by American authorities after his arrest

hypothermia. Rascher's victims were forced to remain outdoors naked in freezing weather for up to 14 hours, or kept in a tank of icewater for 3 hours, their pulse and internal temperature measured through a series of electrodes. Warming of the victims was then attempted by different methods, most usually and successfully by immersion in hot water.

General Dr. Erich Hippke, chief of the Luftwaffe medical service, was the actual source of the idea for the so-called "freezing experiments" which were undertaken on behalf of the Luftwaffe and conducted at Dachau concentration camp by Sigmund Rascher.[10][11][12]

Himmler attended some of the experiments, and told Rascher he should go the North Sea and find out how the ordinary people there warmed victims of extreme cold. Himmler reportedly said he thought "that a fisherwoman could well take her half-frozen husband into her bed and revive him in that manner" and added that everyone believed "animal warmth" had a different effect than artificial warmth.[13] Four Romani women were sent from Ravensbrück concentration camp and warming was attempted by placing the hypothermic victim between two naked women.[14][15]

A medical conference was held in Nuremberg in October 1942, at which the results of the experiments were presented under the headings "Prevention and Treatment of Freezing", and "Warming Up After Freezing to the Danger Point".[16]

Rascher, who had by now been transferred to the Waffen-SS, was eager to obtain the academic credentials necessary for a high-level university position. A habilitation which was to be based on his research failed, however, at Munich, Marburg, and Frankfurt, due to the formal requirement that results be made available for public scrutiny.[17] US investigators later concluded that Rascher had been merely a convenient front for Luftwaffe chief surgeon Erich Hippke, who had been the true source of the ideas for Rascher's experiments.[6]

Similar experiments were conducted from July to September 1944, as the Ahnenerbe provided space and materials to doctors at Dachau to undertake "seawater experiments", chiefly through Wolfram Sievers. Sievers is known to have visited Dachau on 20 July 1944, to speak with Kurt Plötner and the non-Ahnenerbe Wilhelm Beiglboeck, who ultimately carried out the experiments.

While at Dachau, Rascher developed the standard cyanide capsules, which could be easily bitten through, either deliberately or accidentally.[18]

38.2.3 Blood coagulation experiments

Rascher experimented with the effects of *Polygal*, a substance made from beet and apple pectin, which aided blood clotting. He predicted that the preventive use of Polygal tablets would reduce bleeding from gunshot wounds sustained during combat or during surgery. Subjects were given a Polygal tablet, and shot through the neck or chest, or their limbs amputated without anaesthesia. Rascher published an article on his experience of using Polygal, without detailing the nature of the human trials and also set up a company to manufacture the substance, staffed by prisoners.[19]

38.3 Personal life and execution

In an attempt to please Himmler by demonstrating that population growth could be accelerated by extending the child-bearing age, Rascher publicized the fact that his wife had given birth to three children even after becoming 48 years of age, and Himmler used a photograph of Rascher's family as propaganda material. However, during her fourth "pregnancy", Mrs. Rascher was arrested for trying to kidnap a baby and an investigation revealed that her other three children had been either bought or kidnapped. Himmler felt betrayed by this conduct, and Rascher was arrested in April 1944. As well as complicity in the kidnappings of the three infants, Rascher was also accused of financial irregularities, the murder of his former lab assistant, and scientific fraud. Both Rascher and his wife were hastily condemned without trial to the concentration camps.[20] Rascher was imprisoned at Buchenwald following his arrest in 1944 until the camp's evacuation in April 1945. He and other prisoners were then taken to Dachau where Rascher was executed by firing squad on April 26, 1945; just three days before the camp was liberated by American troops.[21]

38.4 Literature

Hubert Rehm: The Fall of the House of Rascher. The bizarre life and death of the SS-doctor Sigmund Rascher.

38.5   Notes

[1] Heller, Kevin (2011). Oxford University Press, ed. *The Nuremberg Military Tribunals and the Origins of International Criminal Law*. ISBN 978-0199554317.

[2] Sardar, Ziauddin ,; Yassin-Kassab, Robin. *Love and Death*. Oxford: Oxford University Press.

[3] "Hitler Becomes Dictator". *The History Place*. The History Place. Retrieved 27 October 2015.

[4] Kater, Michael H. (2000). *Doctors under Hitler*. UNC Press. p. 125. ISBN 0-8078-4858-1.

[5] Michalczyk, John J. (1994). *Medicine, Ethics, and the Third Reich: Historical and Contemporary Issues*. Rowman & Littlefield. p. 95. ISBN 1-55612-752-9.

[6] Moreno, Jonathan D. (2001). *Undue Risk: Secret State Experiments on Humans*. Routledge. pp. 60–61. ISBN 0-415-92835-4.

[7] Moreno, Jonathan D. (2000). *Undue Risk: Secret State Experiments on Humans*. Routledge. pp. 7–17. ISBN 978-0415928359.

[8] Annas, George J.; Michael A. Grodin (1995). *The Nazi doctors and the Nuremberg Code: human rights in human experimentation*. Oxford University Press US. pp. 71–73. ISBN 0-19-510106-5.

[9] Pringle, Heather, *The Master Plan: Himmler's Scholars and the Holocaust*, Hyperion, 2006.

[10] Moreno, Jonathan D. (2000). *Undue Risk: Secret State Experiments on Humans*. Routledge. pp. 7–17. ISBN 978-0415928359.

[11] Heller, Kevin (2011). Oxford University Press, ed. *The Nuremberg Military Tribunals and the Origins of International Criminal Law*. ISBN 978-0199554317.

[12] *Hippkes letter to Wolff of 6 March 1943*. In Facsimile at *Nuremberg Trials Project*. (Nürnberger Document NO-262).

[13] Mackowski, Maura Phillips (2006). *Testing the Limits: Aviation Medicine and the Origins of Manned Space Flight*. Texas A&M University Press. p. 94. ISBN 1-58544-439-1.

[14] Annas, p. 74

[15] Letter from Rascher to Himmler, 17 Feb 1943 from *Trials of War Criminals before the Nurenberg Military Tribunals, Vol. 1, Case 1: The Medical Case (Washington, DC: US Government Printing Office, 1949-1950), pp. 249-251*.

[16] Annas, p. 76

[17] Kater, pp. 125-126

[18] ALEXANDER L. (July 1949). "Medical science under dictatorship". *N. Engl. J. Med.* **241** (2): 39–47. doi:10.1056/NEJM194907142410201. PMID 18153643.

[19] Michalczyk, p. 96

[20] Michalczyk, p. 97

[21] *Doctors From Hell: The Horrific Account of Nazi Experiments on Humans* by Vivien Spitz, p. 225

Chapter 39

Hans Conrad Julius Reiter

For the Knight's Cross recipient, see Hans Reiter.

Hans Conrad Julius Reiter (February 26, 1881 – November 25, 1969) was a German physician convicted of war crimes for his medical experiments at the concentration camp at Buchenwald. He wrote a book on "racial hygiene" called *Deutsches Gold, Gesundes Leben - Frohes Schaffen*.

Reiter was born in Reudnitz near Leipzig in the German Empire. He studied medicine at Leipzig and Breslau (now Wrocław) and received a doctorate from Tübingen on the subject of tuberculosis. After receiving his doctorate, he went on to study at the hygiene institute in Berlin, the Pasteur Institute in Paris and St. Mary's Hospital in London, where he worked with Sir Almroth Wright for two years. Reiter was also known for implementing strict anti-smoking laws in Nazi Germany.

39.1 First World War

During the First World War, Hans Reiter worked as a military physician on the Western Front and in the Balkans, where he served in the 1st Hungarian Army. It was here in 1916 that he reported a German Lieutenant with non-gonococcal urethritis, arthritis and uveitis. He was not the first person to describe this syndrome, which would later become known as Reiter's syndrome (later renamed to Reactive arthritis when his Nazi affiliation came to light). In the same year, and quite separately, the triad was reported by Feissinger & Leroy, and the triad was first reported by Sir Benjamin Collins Brodie (English surgeon 1783-1862). However, the combination of two of the elements (arthritis and urethritis) had been known from the 16th century. Reiter erroneously thought the triad to be due to a spirochaete related to but distinct from the causative agent of syphilis. This error probably was influenced by his discovery of the spirochaete cause of leptospirosis and a nonpathogenic strain of treponema related to *T. pallidum* (the cause of syphilis). This "Reiter strain" of treponema enabled drug companies to later develop the "Reiter Complement Fixation Test" for syphilis.

39.2 1918–1939

After the war ended, Reiter became chief of the hygiene department at Rostock. Hans Reiter was a political man, and an enthusiastic supporter of the Nazi regime. His career was further boosted when, in 1932, he signed an oath of allegiance to Adolf Hitler. In 1933 he was made department director of the Kaiser Wilhelm Institute of Experimental Therapy. In 1936, his meteoric rise continued when he was made director of the health department of Mecklenberg-Schwerin and received an honorary professorship in Berlin. With Johann Breger he wrote a book on racial hygiene—*Deutsches Gold, Gesundes Leben—Frohes Schaffen* ("German Gold, Healthy Life—Glad Work"). He was also a strong supporter of Hitler's anti-smoking campaign, medically progressive at the time. Reiter was a talented teacher who was popular with his students.

39.3 Second World War

As a member of the SS during the Second World War, Hans Reiter designed typhus inoculation experiments that killed more than 250 prisoners at concentration camps like Buchenwald. He was an enthusiastic supporter of and participant in enforced racial sterilisation and euthanasia. After the Nazis were defeated, he was arrested by the Red Army in Soviet Union-occupied Germany and tried at Nuremberg, where he was found guilty of his involvement in the deaths of hundreds of inmates at Buchenwald. He was interned at an American prisoner-of-war camp.

39.4 Later life

After his release, Reiter went back to work in the field of medicine and research in rheumatology. He died, aged 88, in 1969 at his country estate in Kassel-Wilhelmshöhe.[1]

39.5 Controversy

In 1977 a group of doctors began a campaign to replace the term "Reiter's Syndrome" with "reactive arthritis". In addition to Reiter's war crimes, they pointed out that he was not the first to describe the syndrome, nor were his conclusions correct regarding its pathogenesis. The campaign has gradually gained momentum, and the term "Reiter's syndrome" has become increasingly anachronistic.[2]

39.6 References

[1] Obituary *Arthritis and Rheumatism*, Vol.**13**, No.3 (May–June 1970). pp.296-297. Retrieved 2011-10-08.

[2] Panush, RS; Wallace, DJ; Dorff, RE; Engleman, EP (2007). "Retraction of the suggestion to use the term "Reiter's syndrome" sixty-five years later: the legacy of Reiter, a war criminal, should not be eponymic honor but rather condemnation". *Arthritis Rheum* **56** (2): 693–694. doi:10.1002/art.22374. PMID 17265506.

39.7 External links

- Biography and photograph

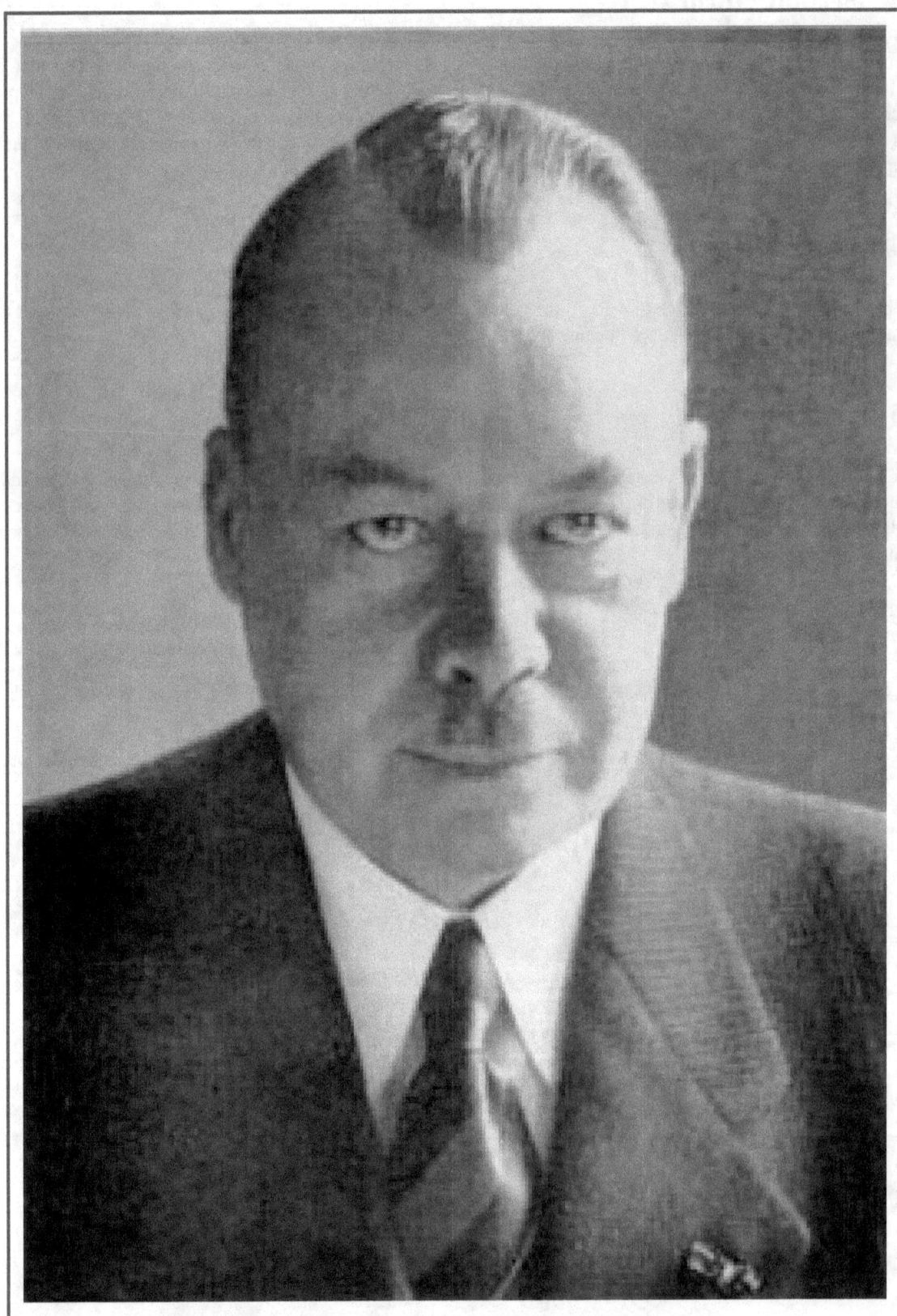

Hans Conrad Julius Reiter

Chapter 40

Gerhard Rose

Gerhard August Heinrich Rose (November 30, 1896 in Danzig – January 13, 1992 in Obernkirchen) was a German expert on tropical medicine who was tried for war crimes at the end of World War II.

Rose was born in Danzig (then part of Germany, now Gdańsk Poland). He studied at the University of Breslau and the University of Berlin. After completing his studies he worked at the Robert Koch Institute and Heidelberg University. He worked in China from 1929 to 1936.

In 1939, Rose became a member of the Luftwaffe medical corps, where he became a brigadier general. During the war, he carried out experiments on the prisoners in the Dachau concentration camp and Buchenwald, in which he investigated malaria and typhus. He also carried out tests of malaria drugs on mentally ill Russian prisoners of war in a psychiatric clinic in Thuringia.[1] He attempted to obtain a research position in the United States, but was arrested at war's end.

During the Doctors' Trial at Nuremberg, he was found guilty of war crimes and crimes against humanity. Sentenced to life imprisonment, he later had his sentence reduced to twenty years. He was released from Landsberg Prison in 1955.

40.1   See also

- Nazi human experimentation
- Doctors' Trial
- Ex-Nazis
- Kurt Blome
- Unit 731
- Yellow fever
- Erich Traub
- Claus Schilling

40.2   References

[1] http://www.ncbi.nlm.nih.gov/pubmed/11234332

- Hedy Epstein. "Gerhard Rose".
- "Gerhard Rose". *Nuremberg Trials Project.* Harvard Law School Library.

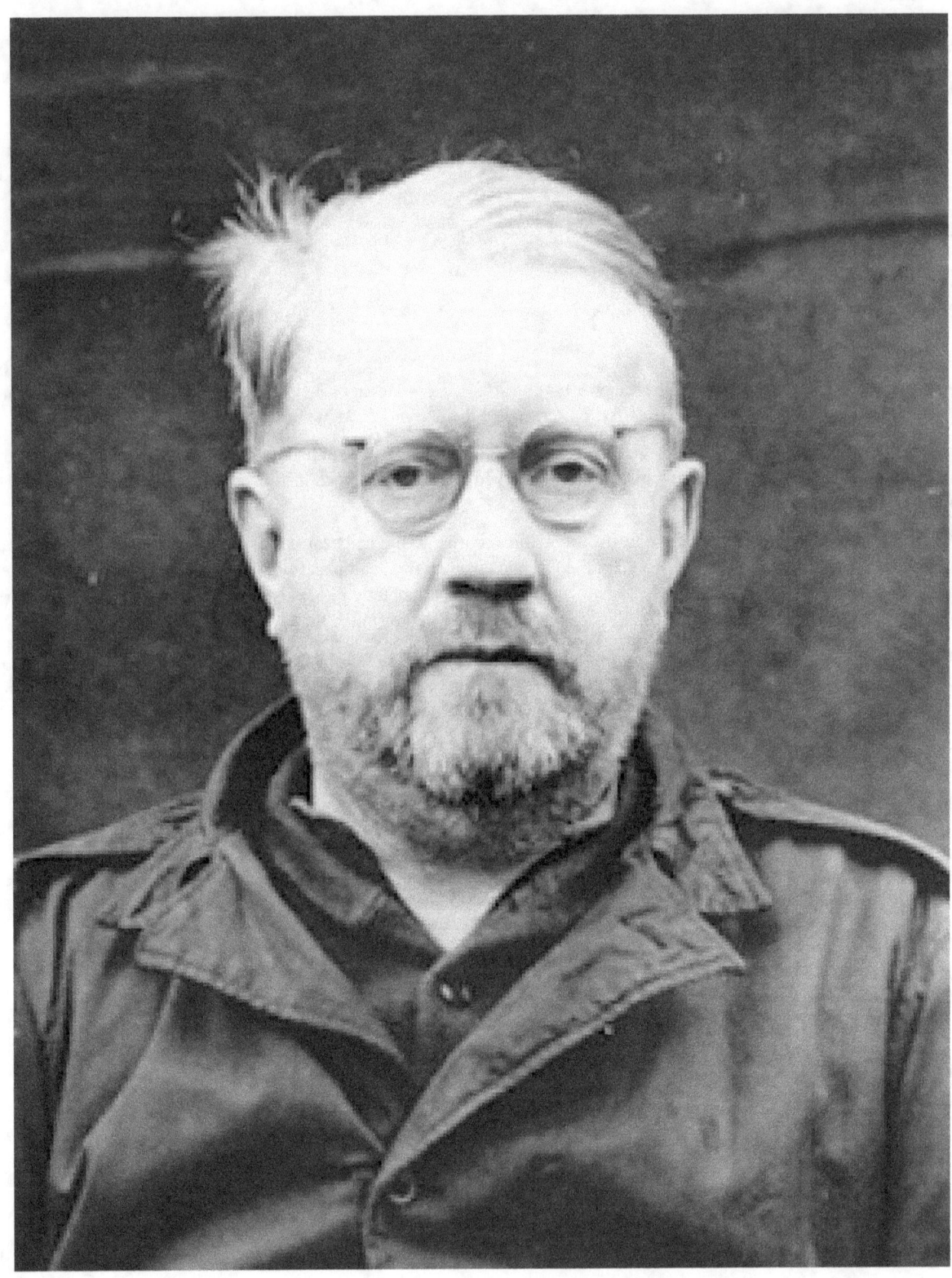

Gerhard Rose

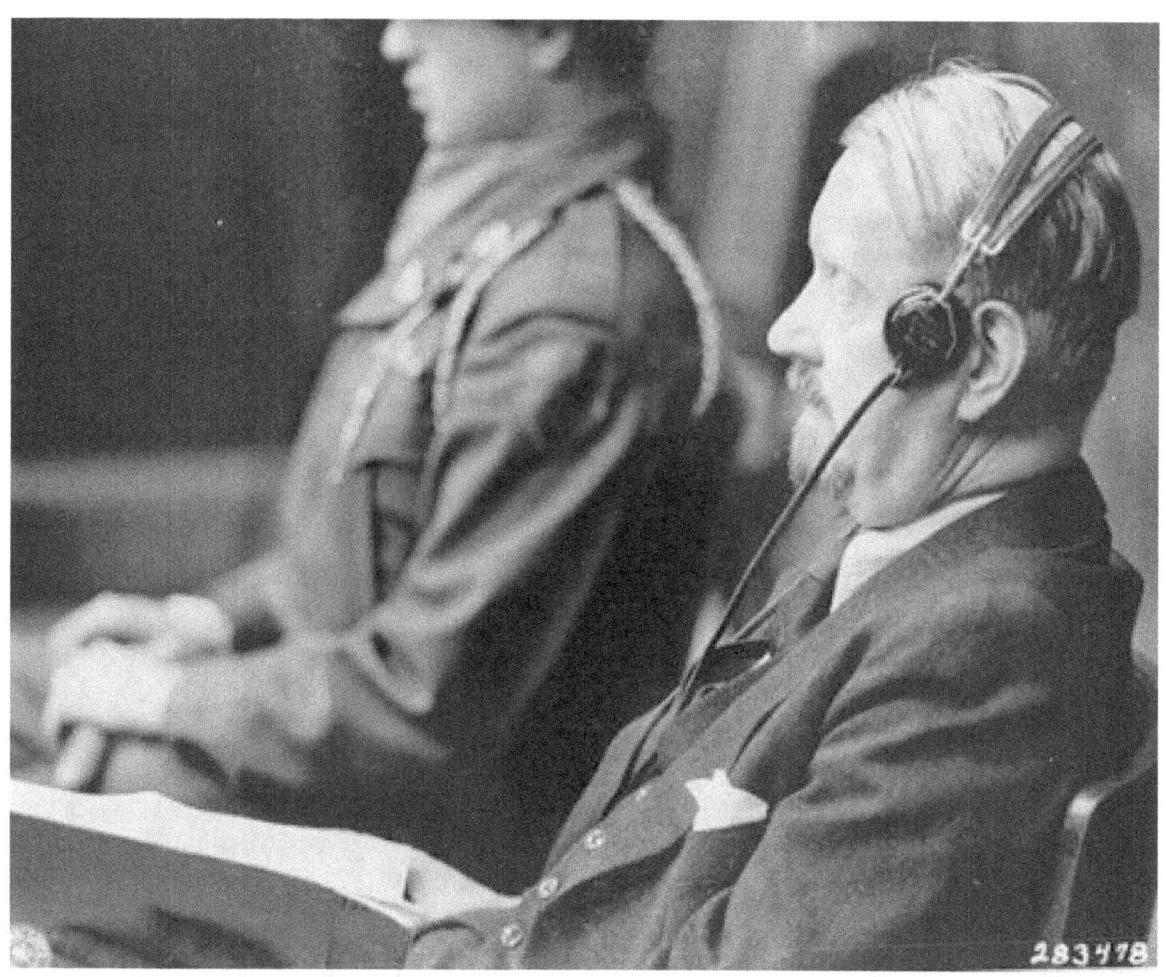

Gerhard Rose testifies in his own defense at the Doctors' Trial in Nuremberg in 1947

Chapter 41

Bernhard Rust

Bernhard Rust (30 September 1883 in Hanover – 8 May 1945) was Minister of Science, Education and National Culture (Reichserziehungsminister) in Nazi Germany.[1] A combination of school administrator and zealous Nazi, he issued decrees, often bizarre, at every level of the German educational system to immerse German youth in the National Socialist philosophy.

41.1   Early life

Rust was born in Hannover, and obtained a doctorate in German philology and philosophy. After passing the state teaching examination with the grade "*gut*" (i.e. *good*)[2] in 1908, he became a high school teacher at Hannover's Ratsgymnasium, then served in the army during World War I. He reached the rank of lieutenant and was awarded the Iron Cross for bravery.[3]

41.2   Political career

Rust joined the NSDAP in 1922, and eventually became the Gauleiter for the Gau of Süd-Hannover-Braunschweig. In 1930, he was elected to the Reichstag. When Hitler became Chancellor in 1933, Rust was appointed as the Prussian Minister for Cultural Affairs. On 1 June 1934, he was selected as Minister of Science, Education and National Culture (Reichsminister für Wissenschaft, Erziehung und Volksbildung), and set about to reshape the German educational system to conform to his ideals of National Socialism. Considered by many to be mentally unstable, Rust would spuriously create new regulations and then repeal them just as quickly. One noted example was in 1935, when he changed the traditional six-day school week to five days, with Saturday to be "Reich's Youth Day" when children in the Hitler Youth and the League of German Girls would be out of school for study and testing. He then ordered the creation of a "rolling week", with six days for study, followed by the "youth day" and a rest day, in 8-day periods. Thus, a rolling week starting on Monday would end with rest on the following Monday; the next rolling week would start on Tuesday and end 8 days later on the next Tuesday. When the 8-day week proved unworkable, Rust went back to the former system.[4]

It was Rust who, in 1933, issued a rule that students and teachers should greet each other with the Nazi salute "as a symbol of the new Germany". He added his opinion that it was "expected of every German" regardless of membership in the party.[5] Rust was instrumental in purging German universities of Jews and others regarded as enemies of the State, most notably at the University of Göttingen. Nazi Germany's future leaders received their instruction elsewhere, in an NPEA or "Napola" (NAtionalPOLitische erziehungsAnstalten), of which there were 30 in the nation, where they would receive training to become administrators of conquered provinces.[6]

He bluntly informed teachers that their aim was to educate ethnically aware Germans.[1] Rust also believed that non-Aryan science (such as Albert Einstein's "Jewish physics") was flawed, and had what he felt to be a rational explanation for this view. In an address to scientists, he said, "The problems of science do not present themselves in the same way to all men.

The Negro or the Jew will view the same world in a different light from the German investigator."[7] Erika Mann, the daughter of Thomas Mann, wrote an exposé of the Rust system in 1938 entitled *School for Barbarians*, followed in 1941 by Gregor Ziemer's *Education for Death*.

41.3 Death

Rust reportedly committed suicide on 8 May 1945 when Germany surrendered to Allied forces.

41.4 Spelling Reform

Rust prepared a reform of German orthography, and his fairly extensive version corresponded to the ideas of the spelling reformers of the 1970s (lower case common nouns, elimination of lengthening-symbols). This attempt met internal resistance of the Reich's ministry. The German orthography reform of 1944 also failed. Before these failures, the rules of the reform were printed in millions of copies intended for classroom use and published in numerous newspapers. The 1944 reform was postponed on the orders of Hitler because it was "not important for the war effort." Some of Rust's innovations had, however, found their way into the 1942 Duden, such as the spelling of the word *Kautsch* for *Couch*, which persisted into the 1980s. Many of the proposed changes were finally implemented with the German orthography reform of 1996.

41.5 References

[1] Claudia Koonz, *The Nazi Conscience*, p 134 ISBN 0-674-01172-4

[2] Hitlers Bildungsreformer: Das Reichsministerium für Wissenschaft, Erziehung und Volksbildung 1934-1945, by Anne C. Nagel, Fischer publishing house, 2012, ISBN 978-3596194254

[3] *Current Biography 1942*, pp725-27

[4] *Current Biography 1942*, pp725; "The Good Earth", *TIME* magazine, 30 September 1935

[5] "Sub-Dictator", *TIME* magazine, 21 August 1933

[6] "How Nazis are Trained", *TIME* magazine, 25 August 1941

[7] *Current Biography 1942*, p727

41.6 External links

- Short biography of Rust

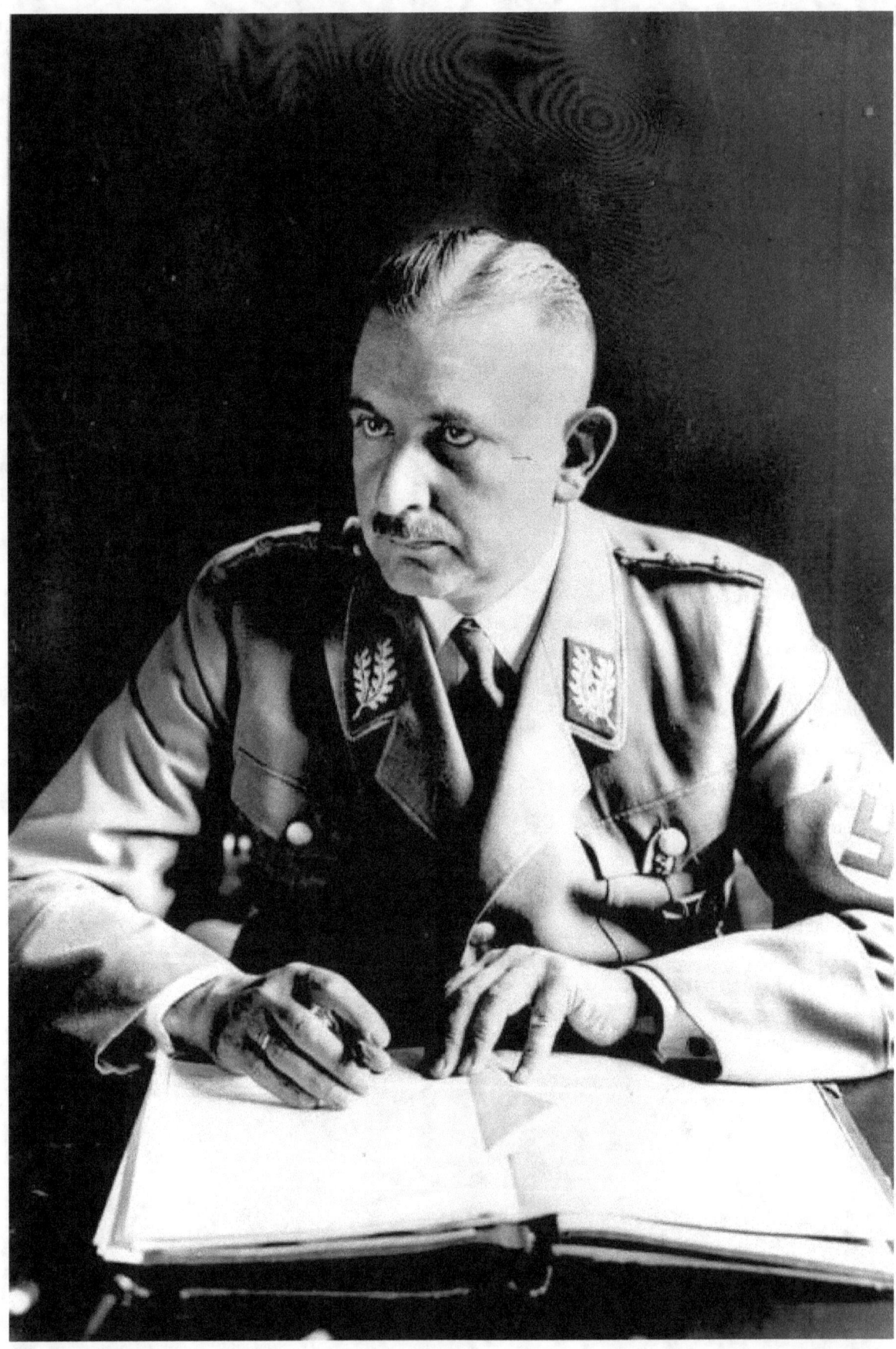

Bernhard Rust, 1934

Chapter 42

Claus Schilling

Claus Karl Schilling (born 5 July 1871 in Munich, Bavaria, Germany; died 28 May 1946 in Landsberg am Lech, Bavaria, West Germany), also recorded as **Klaus Schilling**, was a German tropical medicine specialist, particularly remembered for his infamous participation in the Nazi human experiments at the Dachau concentration camp during World War II.

Though never a member of the Nazi Party and a recognized researcher before the war, Schilling became notorious as a consequence of his enthusiastic participation in human research under both Fascist Italy and Nazi Germany. From 1942 to 1945, Schilling's research of malaria and attempts at fighting it using synthetic drugs resulted in over a thousand cases of human experimentation on camp prisoners.

Sentenced to death by hanging after the fall of Hitler's Germany, he was executed for his crimes against the Dachau prisoners in 1946.

42.1 Biography

Born in Munich on 5 July 1871, Schilling studied medicine in his native city, receiving a doctor's degree there in 1895. Within a few years, Schilling was practicing in the German colonial possessions in Africa. Recognized for his contributions in the field of tropical medicine, he was appointed the first-ever director of the tropical medicine division of the Robert Koch Institute in 1905, where he would remain for the subsequent three decades.

42.1.1 Italian research

Upon retirement from the Robert Koch Institute in 1936, Schilling moved to Benito Mussolini's Fascist Italy, where he was given the opportunity to conduct immunization experiments on inmates of the psychiatric asylums of Volterra and San Niccolò di Siena.[1] (The Italian authorities were concerned that troops faced malarial outbreaks in the course of the Italo-Ethiopian War.) As Schilling stressed the significance of the research for German interests, the Nazi government of Germany also supported him with a financial grant for his Italian experimentation.[1]

42.1.2 Dachau experiments

Schilling returned to Germany after a meeting with Leonardo Conti, the Nazis' Health Chief, in 1941, and by early 1942 he was provided with a special malaria research station at Dachau's concentration camp by Heinrich Himmler, the leader of the SS. Despite negative assessments from colleagues, Schilling would remain in charge of the malaria station for the duration of the war.[1]

Although in the 1930s Schilling had stressed the point that malaria research on human subjects could be performed in an entirely harmless fashion, the Dachau subjects included experimentees who were injected with synthetic drugs at doses ranging from high to lethal. Of the more than 1,000 prisoners used in the malaria experiments at Dachau during the war, between 300 and 400 died as a result; among survivors, a substantial number remained permanently damaged afterward.[1]

In the course of the Dachau Trials following the liberation of the camp at the close of the war, Schilling was tried by an American tribunal, with an October 1945 affidavit from Schilling being presented in the proceedings.[2]

The tribunal sentenced Schilling to death by hanging on 13 December 1945. His execution took place at Landsberg Prison in Landsberg am Lech on 28 May 1946. See Schilling execution

42.2 References

[1] Hulverscheidt, Marion. "German Malariology Experiments with Humans, Supported by the DFG Until 1945". *Man, Medicine, and the State: The Human Body as an Object of Government Sponsored Medical Research in the 20th Century*, Beiträge zur Geschichte der Deutschen Forschungsgemeinschaft Volume 2. Ed. Wolfgang Uwe Eckhart. Stuttgart: Franz Steiner Verlag, 2006. ISBN 3-515-08794-X, ISBN 978-3-515-08794-0, pp. 221–236.

[2] Spitz, Vivien. *Doctors from Hell: The Horrific Account of Nazi Experiments on Humans*. Boulder, Colorado: Sentient Publications, 2005. ISBN 1-59181-032-9, ISBN 978-1-59181-032-2, p. 105.

Chapter 43

Walter Schreiber

Dr. **Walter Paul Emil Schreiber** (21 March 1893 – 5 September 1970) was a German medical military officer in World War I, a brigadier-general (*Generalarzt*) of the Medical Service of the Wehrmacht and a key witness against Hermann Goering during the Nuremburg Trials.

43.1 Life

Walter Schreiber was born in Berlin to Paul Schreiber (a postal inspector) and his wife Gertrud Kettlitz. After completing gymnasium in Berlin, he studied medicine at the universities of Berlin, Tübingen, and Greifswald. In 1914, he enlisted voluntarily for military service and served with the 42nd Infantry Regiment in France. He was injured at the First Battle of the Marne. After his recovery, he continued with his studies and served as a provisional doctor on the Western Front until the end of the war in 1918, at which time he was decorated for valor and humanitarian service by three different countries, Finland, Switzerland and Germany. In 1920, he graduated Dr. med. from the University of Greifswald and began his field studies in epidemiology in Africa.

After WWI, the United States sought to assess the feasibility of using biological warfare agents in future military conflicts.[1] As a professor of Bacteriology and Hygiene at the University of Berlin and one of the foremost experts in epidemiology, Dr. Schreiber was invited to Walter Reed Army Medical Center, then known as Walter Reed General Hospital, in a scientific exchange between Germany and the United States. During this time, he learned of U.S. past and proposed plans for both defensive and offensive biological warfare research and the possibility of an official US biological warfare program. As a member of the medical branch of the Heer, and a representative of the Army Medical Inspectorate, he was charged with preventing the spread of infectious disease and developing vaccines, in particular to guard against potential biological warfare agents. In 1942 he wrote a memorandum expressing his objections to the Third Reich's own development of such weapons, stating during his witness testimony at the Nuremberg Trials, " I personally made a report to Generaloberstabsarzt Handloser... It was an extremely serious matter for us physicians, for if there really should be a plague epidemic it was clear that it would not stop at the fronts, but would come over to us too. We had to bear a very grave responsibility."[2][3] In October 1942, Schreiber attended the conference where the results of human experiments at Dachau were presented. In May 1943, he headed the third session of the advisory specialists of the Armed Forces. This led to a confrontation in which Dr. Schreiber spoke out against human experimentation in general, but especially with biological agents such as plague and typhus, testifying later that he "pointed out that bacteria were an unreliable and dangerous weapon" but that he was "confronted with a fait accompli", the decision had already been made, "the Fuhrer had given the Reichsmarschall (Hermann Goering) full powers, and so forth, for carrying out all the preparations."[2][4][5] In September 1943, Schreiber accepted the position of the commander of the Training Division C of the Military Medical Academy under which authority he denied permission for Kurt Blome, the head of the Posen research institute, to conduct his plague research in Sachsenburg. This was later overruled by Himmler.[2] In 1944, Dr Schreiber, who had grown increasingly aware of Hermann Goering's antagonism toward him, conferred with Dr. Karl Brandt, the attorney for health care, scientific advisory board.[4] In 1944, from May 16 to 18, Dr. Schreiber learned of research into gas gangrene experiments conducted by Dr. Karl Gebhardt at Hohenlychen Sanatorium. (Nuremberg document 619)[6]

On 30 April 1945, while caring for wounded in a makeshift hospital in Berlin, he was taken prisoner of war by the Red Army and transported to the Soviet Union.[2] On 26 August 1946, Schreiber appeared as a surprise witness at the Nuremberg Trials, giving evidence in support of the Soviet Chief Prosecutor, Roman Rudenko, against, Hermann Goering and Kurt Blome, who had been in charge of German offensive biological weapons development.[7][8] A recording of his testimony at the trial can be found at the online archive of the Imperial War Museum.[9] The transcript became part of the Nuremberg proceedings against German major war criminals.[4] Dr. Schreiber, whose long-standing record against the use of offensive biological warfare and human experimentation was well established, was himself never charged or considered for prosecution on war crimes charges.

In fall 1948, Dr. Schreiber reappeared in the West with his wife, his son and one of his adult daughters. In a press conference on 2 November, he explained that he had initially been held in Lubyanka Prison in the USSR where he became ill almost to death. Only when the captured former German ambassador to Russia, Norbert von Baumbach, became ill and refused care from anyone but Generalarzt, Dr. Schreiber, was the doctor's true identity discovered by Soviet authorities. Schreiber reported he was then given medical attention and moved to a series of safe houses in the Soviet Zone of Germany. There he remained to provide medical care to former Nazi generals. Still under Soviet custody, he was later given the rank of starshina, and was ultimately offered the position of Chief Medical Officer in the newly formed East German Police Force, the Volkspolizei. Rejecting this position, Schreiber reported that he was then offered a professorship at the University of Leipzig. However, in hopes of finding his family, requested the University of Berlin instead. In response, Soviet authorities reported they were holding Schreiber's family in the USSR, thereby convincing Dr. Schreiber to relocate and join other German scientists who had already been taken there (see Russian Alsos).[10] In the meantime, his daughter, who had presented herself to Allied military authorities in the American Occupation Zone, learned that the Soviets were transporting more German scientists to the Soviet Union, her father presumably among them. Boarding multiple trains, she walked the cars until she caught her father's attention. Seeing an opportunity, Dr. Schreiber evaded his handler and on 17 October took a train from Dresden to Berlin where he presented himself to the Allied Control Authority in West Berlin.[8][11] Dr. Schreiber was subsequently hired to work with the Counter Intelligence Corps and beginning in 1949 was employed as post physician at Camp King, a large clandestine POW interrogation center in Oberursel, Germany.[12]

43.1.1 Emigration

In 1951, Schreiber was taken to the United States as part of Operation Paperclip. He arrived in New York on September 17, 1951, on the USNS *General Maurice Rose* with his wife Olga Conrad Schreiber, his son Paul-Gerhard Schreiber, and his mother-in-law, Marie Schulz Conrad. The manifest of the ship does not list travel documents for them, but declares them to be "Paper Clips".[13]

On 7 October 1951 the *New York Times* reported that he was working at the Air Force School of Medicine at Randolph Air Force Base in Texas. A notice also appeared in a medical journal and was seen by Leopold Alexander, who had been an expert consultant at the Nuremberg Doctors' Trial. He contacted the *Boston Globe*, and the resulting publicity by Drew Pearson sensationalizing Schreiber's Nuremberg evidence and ties between him and the abusive experiments performed by Blome and others on concentration camp inmates, such as Janina Iwańska and the other "Ravensbrück rabbits", led to a public outcry.[8][14] Schreiber, consequently did not seek contract renewal. He left Texas for the Bay Area of California, where one of his daughters now lived. Thereafter the Joint Intelligence Objectives Agency arranged a visa for him through an Argentinian general and he was provided with moving funds for himself and his family. On 22 May 1952 they were flown on a military aircraft to New Orleans and from there to Buenos Aires where he joined another daughter.[15][16]

In Argentina, he worked as a physician and at an epidemiological research laboratory. He researched family history and compiled his journals. He died suddenly of a heart attack on 5 September 1970 in San Carlos de Bariloche, Río Negro, Argentina.[5][17]

43.2 Further reading

- McCoy, Alfred. "Science in Dachau's Shadow: Hebb, Beecher, and the Development of CIA Psychological Torture and Modern Medical Ethics". *Journal of the History of the Behavioral Sciences*, Volume 43 (4), 2007.

43.3   References

[1]

[2] http://avalon.law.yale.edu/imt/08-26-46.asp

[3] Annie Jacobsen, *Operation Paperclip: The Secret Intelligence Program that Brought Nazi Scientists to America*, New York: Little, Brown, 2014. ISBN 978-0-316-22105-4, pp. 7, 164–65.

[4] Transcripts, Trial of German Major War Criminals Nuremberg, Germany, August 26, 1946.

[5] Family tree, Ancestry.com.

[6] "Air Force Hires Nazi Doctor" The Free Lance Star. Feb 14, 1952

[7] Jacobsen, pp. 232–39.

[8] Linda Hunt, *Secret Agenda: The United States Government, Nazi Scientists, and Project Paperclip, 1945 to 1990*, New York: St. Martin's, 1991, ISBN 9780312055103, p. 89.

[9] International Military Tribunal, Nuremberg: Day 211 26/8/1946 Walter Schreiber questioned. Audio Recordings, Imperial War Museum, London.

[10] %20to%20USSR&f.

[11] Jacobsen, pp. 322–30.

[12] Jacobsen, pp. 331–33.

[13] Ancestry.com.

[14] Jacobsen, pp. 348–56.

[15] Jacobsen, pp. 361–63.

[16] Hunt, p. 90.

[17] Jacobsen, p. 363.

Chapter 44

Horst Schumann

Horst Schumann (1 May 1906 – 5 May 1983), *SS-Sturmbannführer* (major) and medical doctor, conducted sterilization and castration experiments at Auschwitz and was particularly interested in the mass sterilization of Jews by means of X-rays.

44.1   Early life

Schumann was born on 1 May 1906 in Halle an der Saale. His father, Paul Schumann, was also a doctor. Schumann entered the NSDAP in 1930 and joined the SA in 1932. In 1933, he received his medical degree after producing a thesis entitled "*Frage der Jodresorption und der therapeutischen Wirkung sog. Jodbäder*" ("The Question of Iodine Absorption and the Therapeutic Effects of so-called Iodine Baths"). He started his career as an assistant doctor in the Surgical Clinic of the clinic of Halle University.

44.2   Nazi doctor

From 1934, Schumann was employed in the Public Health Office in Halle. He was recruited to the air force as a physician in 1939. He joined the *Aktion* T4 Euthanasia program in early October 1939, after a meeting with Dr. Viktor Brack in Hitler's chancellery. In January 1940, Schumann became head of the Grafeneck euthanasia centre in Württemberg, where mentally ill people were gassed with carbon monoxide in the first gas chamber. In the early summer of 1940, he was ordered to the Sonnenstein Euthanasia Centre. Schumann also belonged to a commission of doctors called "Action 14f13", who transferred weak and sick prisoners from Auschwitz, Buchenwald, Dachau, Flossenbürg, Gross-Rosen, Mauthausen, Neuengamme and Niederhangen concentration camps to the euthanasia killing centers.

44.3   Auschwitz

On 28 July 1941, Schumann arrived in Auschwitz. He worked at Block 30 in the women's hospital, where he set up an x-ray station in 1942. Here men and women were forcibly sterilized by being positioned repeatedly for several minutes between two x-ray machines, the rays aiming at their sexual organs. Most subjects died after great suffering, or were gassed immediately because the radiation burns from which they suffered rendered them unfit for work. Men's testicles were removed and sent to Breslau for histopathological examination. Schumann "...chose his test persons himself. They were always young, healthy, good-looking Jewish men, women and girls who looked like old people afterwards. The parts of the body that were treated with the rays were burnt, suppurating. Often the intestines were also affected. Many died. Part of Schumann's control tests, to check whether the radiation had worked, was the so-called semen check: a stick covered with a rubber hose was inserted into the rectum of the victim and the glands stimulated until ejaculation occurred so that the ejaculate could be tested for sperm..." [1] Both kinds of samples were sent to the University of Breslau (today Wrocław) for examination.

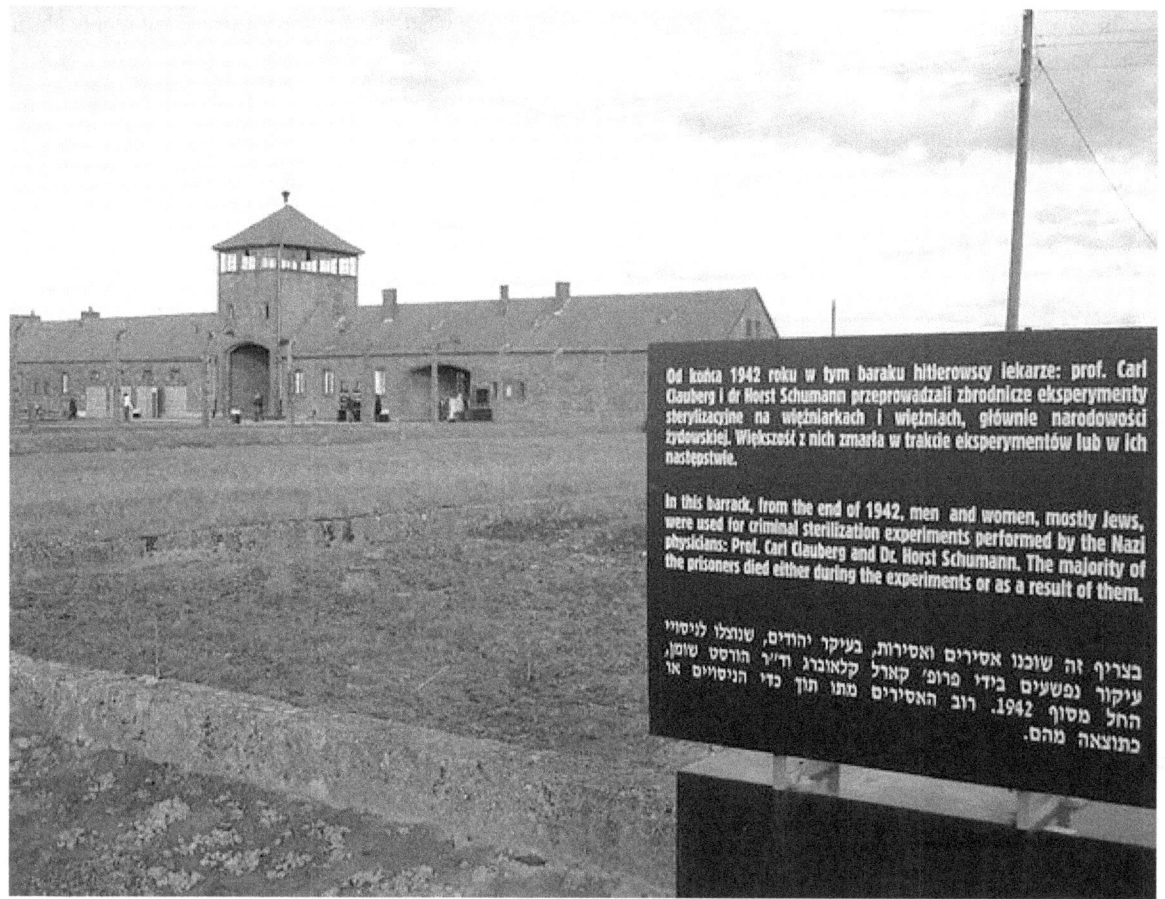

Remains of the building at Auschwitz II (Birkenau) where Schuman committed his medical atrocities.

Schumann selected some of the women in Block 10 in the main camp of Auschwitz. In this Block Jewish women had been imprisoned for human experiments. To control the radiation on women, prisoner doctors (Dr. Maximilian Samuel, Dr. Wladislaw Dering) had to remove an ovary.[2]

Schumann also performed typhus experiments by injecting people with blood from typhus patients and then attempting to cure the newly infected subjects. Schumann left Auschwitz in September 1944 and was appointed to the Sonnenstein Clinic in Saxony which had earlier been converted into a military hospital.

44.4   Medical career after the war

While serving as a military doctor on the Western Front, he was captured by the Americans in January 1945. He was released from captivity in October 1945. In April 1946, he began to work as a sports doctor for the city of Gladbeck. An application for a license for a hunting gun led to his being identified in 1951 so the GDR issued an arrest warrant. According to his own statement, Schumann served as a ship's doctor for three years and because he did not have a German passport, he applied for one in Japan in 1954 and received it under his own name. Schumann then fled, first to Egypt and eventually settled in Khartoum in the Sudan as head of a hospital. He was forced to flee from Sudan in 1962 after being recognized by an Auschwitz survivor. Then he went to Ghana, where he received the protection of the head of state, Kwame Nkrumah.

In 1966, he was extradited from Ghana to West Germany where the trial against him was opened in Frankfurt on 23

September 1970. However, Schumann was released from prison on 29 July 1972 due to his heart condition and generally deteriorating health. However, he did not die until 5 May 1983, 11 years after he had been released. As Robert Jay Lifton has observed "...Schumann has great importance for us because of what he did – intense involvement in both direct medical killing and unusually brutal Auschwitz experiments – and what he was – an ordinary, but highly Nazified man and doctor..." [3]

44.5 Footnotes

[1] Klee, 53

[2] Lang, 132-143

[3] Lipton, p. 284

44.6 See also

- The Holocaust

- Nazi human experimentation

- Josef Mengele

- Eduard Wirths

44.7 References

- Robert Jay Lifton, (1986) *The Nazi Doctors: Medical Killing and the Psychology of Genocide.* New York: Basic Books.

- Klee, Ernst. "Turning the tap on was no big deal", (1990) - The gassing doctors during the Nazi period and afterwards, Dachau Review 2, History of Nazi Concentration Camps, Studies, Reports, Documents, Volume 2. edited by Wolfgang Benz and Barbara Distel, published for the Comite International de Dachau, Brussels. Verlag Dachauer Hefte, Alte Roemerstrasse 75, 8060 Dachau.

- Klodzinski, Stanislaw: "Sterilisation und Kastration durch Röntgenstrahlen im Auschwitz-Lager. Verbrechen Horst Schumann" in Internationales Auschwitz-Komitee (Hrsg.) "Unmenschliche Medizin" Anthologie, Bd. 1, Teil 2, Warschau 1969.

- Mitscherlich, Alexander/Mielke, Fred: "Medizin ohne Menschlichkeit", Frankfurt a. M. 1978, [ISBN 3-596-22003-3]

- Lang, Hans-Joachim: *Die Frauen von Block 10. Medizinische Experimente in Auschwitz.* Hamburg 2011. ISBN 978-3-455-50222-0.

44.8 External links

- Biography of Dr. Horst Schumann

- "Medical Experiments at Auschwitz"

Chapter 45

Wolfram Sievers

Wolfram Sievers (Hildesheim, 10 July 1905 – Landsberg, 2 June 1948) was *Reichsgeschäftsführer*, or managing director, of the Ahnenerbe from 1935 to 1945.

45.1   Early life

Sievers was born in 1905 in Hildesheim in the Province of Hanover (now in Lower Saxony), the son of a Protestant church musician. It is reported that he was musically gifted, that he played the harpsichord, organ, and piano, and loved German baroque music. He was expelled from school for being active in the Deutschvölkischer Schutz und Trutzbund and went on to study history, philosophy, and religious studies at Stuttgart's Technical University while working as a salesman. A member of the Bündische Jugend, he became active in the *Artamanen-Gesellschaft* ("Artaman League"), a nationalist back-to-the-land movement.[1]

45.2   Ahnenerbe

Sievers joined the NSDAP in 1929. In 1933 he headed the *Externsteine-Stiftung* ("Externsteine Foundation"), which had been founded by Heinrich Himmler to study the Externsteine in the Teutoburger Wald. In 1935, having joined the SS that year, Sievers was appointed *Reichsgeschäftsführer*, or General Secretary, of the *Ahnenerbe*, by Himmler. He was the actual director of *Ahnenerbe* operations and was to rise to the rank of SS-Standartenführer by the end of the war.

In 1943 Sievers became director of the *Institut für Wehrwissenschaftliche Zweckforschung* (Institute for Military Scientific Research), which conducted extensive experiments using human subjects. He also assisted in assembling a collection of skulls and skeletons for August Hirt's study at the Reichsuniversität Straßburg as a part of which 112 Jewish prisoners were selected and killed, after being photographed and their anthropological measurements taken.[2]

45.3   Trial and execution

Sievers was tried during the Doctors' Trial at Nuremberg following the end of World War II, where he was dubbed "the Nazi Bluebeard" by journalist William L. Shirer because of his "thick, ink-black beard".[3] The Institute for Military Scientific Research had been set up as part of the Ahnenerbe, and the prosecution at Nuremberg laid the responsibility for the experiments on humans which had been conducted under its auspices on the Ahnenerbe. Sievers, as its highest administrative officer, was accused of actively aiding and promoting the criminal experiments.[4]

Sievers was charged with being a member of an organization declared criminal by the International Military Tribunal (the SS), and was implicated in the commission of war crimes and crimes against humanity. In his defense, he alleged that as early as 1933, he had been a member of an anti-Nazi resistance movement which planned to assassinate Hitler

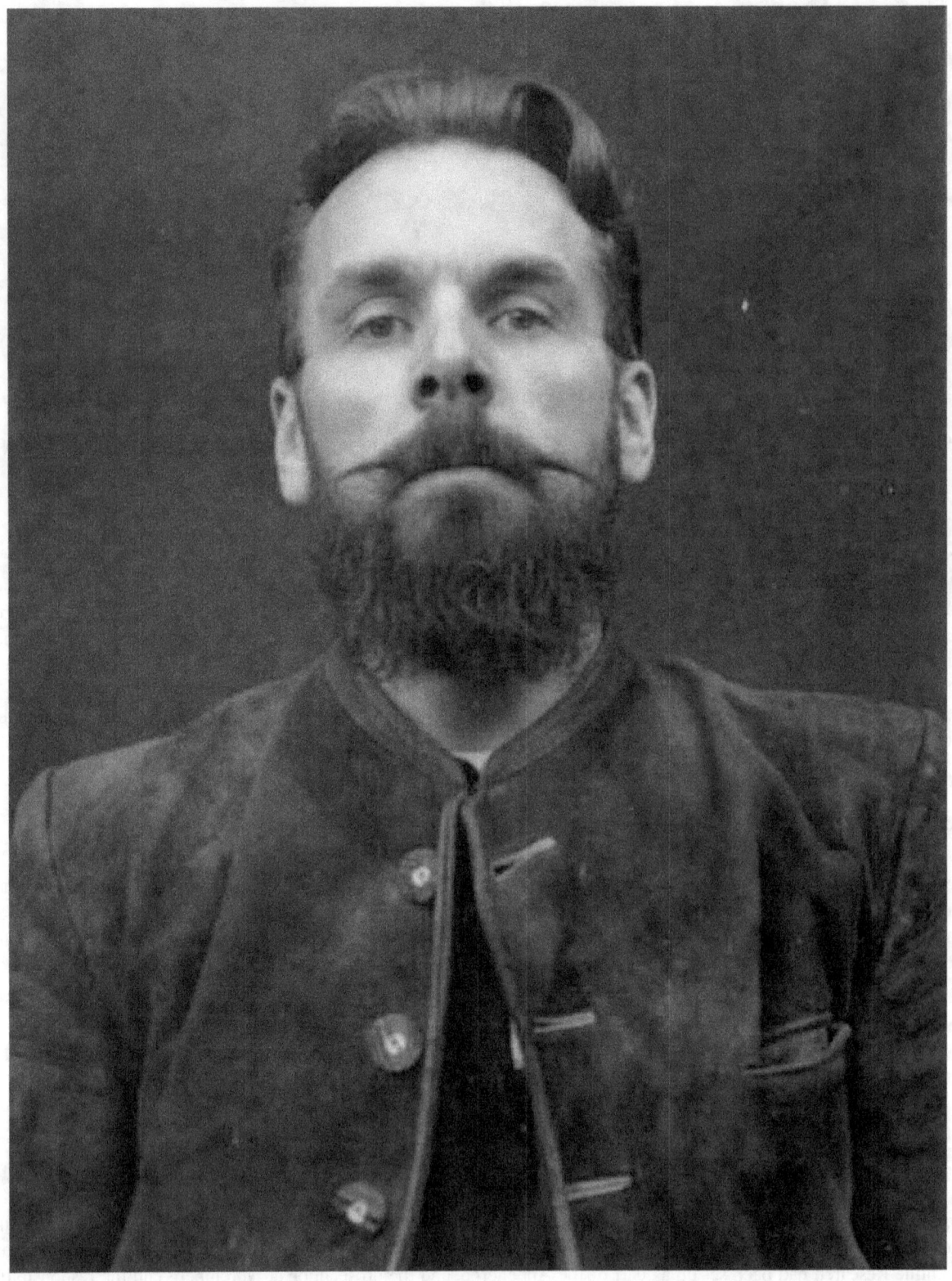

Mugshot of Wolfram Sievers, taken by American authorities after his arrest

and Himmler, and that he had obtained his appointment as Manager of the Ahnenerbe so as to get close to Himmler and observe his movements. He further claimed that he remained in the post on the advice of his resistance leader to gather vital information which would assist in the overthrow of the Nazi regime.[5]

Sievers was sentenced to death on 20 August 1947 for crimes against humanity, and hanged on 2 June 1948, at Landsberg prison in Bavaria.

45.4 References

[1] Lixfeld, Hannjost; James R. Dow (1994). *The Nazification of an Academic Discipline: Folklore in the Third Reich*. Indiana University Press. pp. 198–199. ISBN 0-253-31821-1.

[2] http://nuremberg.law.harvard.edu/

[3] Shirer, William L. (1960). *The Rise and Fall of the Third Reich*. Simon and Schuster. p. 981.

[4] Epstein, Fritz T., *War-Time Activities of the SS-Ahnenerbe* (in *On the Track of Tyranny: Essays Presented by the Wiener Library to Leonard G. Montefiore, on the Occasion of His Seventieth Birthday*. Ayer Publishing. 1971. pp. 79–81.)

[5] McDonald, Gabrielle Kirk; Olivia Swaak-Goldman (2000). *Substantive and Procedural Aspects of International Criminal Law: The Experience of International and National Courts*. BRILL. p. 1755. ISBN 90-411-1134-4.

45.5 External links

- Befragung beim Nürnberger Prozess (Englische Fassung)

- Kriegsverbrechergefängnis (WCP No 1) Landsberg

- Michael H. Kater: Das "Ahnenerbe" der SS 1935–1945. Oldenbourg Verlag, 2001, ISBN 3-486-56529-X

- Hans-Joachim Lang: Die Namen der Nummern. Hoffmann und Campe, 2004, ISBN 3-455-09464-3

- Emmanuel Heyd and Raphael Toledano, *The Names of the 86 ('Le Nom des 86" in french)* (in French, German, and English), dora films, 2014.

Chapter 46

Hugo Spatz

Hugo Spatz (2 September 1888 - 27 January 1969) was a German neuropathologist. In 1937, he was appointed director of the Kaiser Wilhelm Institute for Brain Research.[1] He was a member of the Nazi Party, and admitted to knowingly performing much of his controversial research on the brains of executed prisoners. Along with Julius Hallervorden, he is credited with the discovery of Hallervorden-Spatz syndrome (now, in light of revelations of his Nazi past, more commonly referred to as Pantothenate kinase-associated neurodegeneration).[2][3]

46.1   See also

- List of medical eponyms with Nazi associations

46.2   References

[1] "Hugo Spatz Papers 1940-1945". National Library of Medicine.

[2] Strous, Rael D.; Morris C. Edelman (March 2007). "Eponyms and the Nazi Era: Time to Remember and Time For Change" (PDF). *Israel Medical Association Journal* **9** (3): 207–214. Retrieved 2010-12-09.

[3] "Hugo Spatz". Who Named It?. Retrieved 2010-12-09.

Chapter 47

Ludwig Stumpfegger

SS-*Obersturmbannführer* (Lieutenant Colonel) **Ludwig Stumpfegger** (11 July 1910 – c. 2 May 1945) was a German SS doctor in World War II and Adolf Hitler's personal surgeon from 1944. Stumpfegger was present in the *Führerbunker* in Berlin in late April 1945.

47.1 Biography

Stumpfegger was born in Munich in Bavaria. He studied medicine from 1930 onwards. Stumpfegger joined the SS on 2 June 1933 and the Nazi Party on 1 May 1935. He initially worked as an assistant doctor under Professor Karl Gebhardt in the Sanatorium Hohenlychen, which specialised in sports accidents. As a result of this experience, he was part of the medical team, along with Gebhardt, at the 1936 Summer Olympics in Berlin and the Winter Olympics of the same year in Garmisch-Partenkirchen. In August 1937 Stumpfegger obtained his doctor's degree.[1]

After World War II began in Europe, the "Hohenlychen" was used by the SS as part of the war effort. Working under the supervision of Gebhardt, Dr. Fritz Fischer and Dr. Herta Oberheuser, he participated in medical experiments, the subjects of which were women from the concentration camp at Ravensbrück. On 1 November 1939, transferred to the surgical department of the SS hospital in Berlin. He was transferred back to the "Hohenlychen" as adjutant to Gebhardt in March 1940. On 20 April 1943, he was promoted to SS-*Obersturmbannführer*. Upon Himmler's recommendation, he was transferred to "Wolfsschanze" Führer headquarters as the resident doctor on 9 October 1944.[1]

47.1.1 Berlin 1945

In 1945, Stumpfegger started working directly for Hitler in the *Führerbunker* in Berlin under the direction of Dr. Theodor Morell. At Hitler's request, he provided a cyanide capsule for Blondi, the German Shepherd dog which was a past gift from Martin Bormann, to see how quickly and effectively it worked. As the Red Army advanced towards the bunker complex, some sources report that he helped Magda Goebbels kill her children as they slept in the *Vorbunker*, before she and her husband Joseph Goebbels committed suicide.[2]

On 30 April 1945, just before committing suicide, Hitler signed the order to allow a breakout. On 1 May, Stumpfegger left *Führerbunker* in a breakout group that included Martin Bormann, Werner Naumann and Hitler Youth leader Artur Axmann.[3] They were one of ten groups attempting to break out of the Soviet encirclement. At the Weidendammer Bridge, a Tiger tank spearheaded the first attempt by the Germans to storm across the bridge, but it was destroyed. Bormann and Stumpfegger were "knocked over" when the tank was hit.[3] On the third attempt, made around 01:00, Stumpfegger and his group from the Reich Chancellery crossed the Spree.[3] Leaving the rest of their group, Bormann, Stumpfegger, and Axmann walked along railroad tracks to Lehrter station, where Axmann decided to go alone in the opposite direction of his two companions.[4] When he encountered a Red Army patrol, Axmann doubled back. He saw two bodies, which he later identified as Bormann and Stumpfegger, on a bridge near the railway switching yard; the moonlight clearly illuminating their faces.[4][5] He did not have time to check the bodies, so he did not know what killed them.[6]

47.1.2 Discovery of remains

In 1963, a retired postal worker named Albert Krumnow told police that around 8 May 1945 the Soviets had ordered him and his colleagues to bury two bodies found near the railway bridge near Lehrter station. One was dressed in a *Wehrmacht* uniform and the other was clad only in his underwear.[7] Krumnow's colleague Wagenpfohl found an SS doctor's paybook on the second body identifying him as Dr. Ludwig Stumpfegger.[8] He gave the paybook to his boss, postal chief Berndt, who turned it over to the Soviets. They in turn destroyed it. He wrote to Stumpfegger's wife on 14 August 1945 and told her that her husband's body was "... interred with the bodies of several other dead soldiers in the grounds of the Alpendorf in Berlin NW 40, Invalidenstrasse 63."[9]

Excavations on 20–21 July 1965 at the site specified by Axmann and Krumnow failed to locate the bodies.[10] However, on 7 December 1972, construction workers uncovered human remains near Lehrter station in West Berlin just 12 m (39 ft) from the spot where Krumnow claimed he had buried them.[11] Upon autopsy, fragments of glass found in the jawbones of both skeletons led to the conclusion that they had committed suicide by biting cyanide capsules to avoid capture.[12][13] Dental records, reconstructed from memory in 1945 by Dr. Hugo Blaschke, along with forensic examiners determined that the size of the skeleton and shape of the skull were identical to Bormann's.[11][12] Likewise, the second skeleton was deemed to be Stumpfegger's, since it was of similar height to his last known proportions.[11] Composite photographs, where images of the skulls were overlaid on photographs of the two men's faces, were completely congruent.[12] Facial reconstruction was undertaken in early 1973 on both skulls to confirm the identities of the bodies of Stumpfegger and Bormann.[14] Any lingering doubt as to Bormann's identity was removed when confirmed by DNA testing in 1999.[15]

47.2 Portrayal in the media

Ludwig Stumpfegger has been portrayed by the following actors in film and television productions.

- Erwin Felgenhauer in the 1971 Eastern Bloc co-production *Liberation: The Final Assault*.

- John Barron in the 1973 British film *Hitler: The Last Ten Days*.[16]

- Peter Blythe in the 1973 British television production *The Death of Adolf Hitler*.[17]

- Thorsten Krohn in the 2004 German film *Downfall (Der Untergang)*.[18]

47.3 Notes

[1] Joachimsthaler 1999, p. 290.

[2] Beevor 2002, pp. 380-382.

[3] Beevor 2002, pp. 382–383.

[4] Le Tissier 2010, p. 188.

[5] Trevor-Roper 1992, p. 245.

[6] Beevor 2002, p. 383.

[7] Lang 1979, p. 417.

[8] Whiting 1996, p. 200.

[9] Whiting 1996, pp. 136–137.

[10] Lang 1979, pp. 421–422.

[11] Whiting 1996, pp. 217–218.

[12] Lang 1979, p. 432.

[13] Sweeting 2002.

[14] Lang 1979, p. 436.

[15] Miller 2006, p. 154.

[16] "Hitler: The Last Ten Days (1973)". IMDb.com. Retrieved May 8, 2008.

[17] "The Death of Adolf Hitler (1973) (TV)". IMDb.com. Retrieved May 8, 2008.

[18] "Untergang, Der (2004)". IMDb.com. Retrieved May 8, 2008.

47.4 References

- Beevor, Antony (2002). *Berlin: The Downfall 1945*. London: Viking-Penguin Books. ISBN 0-670-03041-4.

- Joachimsthaler, Anton (1999) [1995]. *The Last Days of Hitler: The Legends, the Evidence, the Truth.* Trans. Helmut Bögler. London: Brockhampton Press. ISBN 978-1-86019-902-8.

- Lang, Jochen von (1979). *The Secretary. Martin Bormann: The Man Who Manipulated Hitler.* New York: Random House. ISBN 978-0-394-50321-9.

- Le Tissier, Tony (2010) [1999]. *Race for the Reichstag: The 1945 Battle for Berlin.* Pen and Sword. ISBN 978-1-84884-230-4.

- Miller, Michael (2006). *Leaders of the SS and German Police, Vol. 1.* San Jose, CA: R. James Bender. ISBN 978-93-297-0037-2.

- Sweeting, C. G. *Hitler's Personal Pilot - The Life and Times of Hans Baur.* ISBN 1-57488-288-0.

- Trevor-Roper, Hugh (1992) [1947]. *The Last Days of Hitler.* University Of Chicago Press. ISBN 0-226-81224-3.

- Whiting, Charles (1996) [1973]. *The Hunt for Martin Bormann: The Truth.* London: Pen & Sword. ISBN 0-85052-527-6.

Chapter 48

Alfred Trzebinski

Alfred Trzebinski (29 August 1902 – 8 October 1946) was an SS-physician at the Auschwitz, Majdanek and Neuengamme concentration camps in Nazi Germany. He was sentenced to death and executed for his involvement in war crimes committed at the Neuengamme subcamps.

48.1   Life

Trzebinski was born in Jutroschin, Province of Posen (now Rawicz County). After his study and graduation he became a physician in Saxony. Trzebinski was a member of the Nazi Party and SS. Trzebinski was a *camp physician* (German: *Lagerarzt*) at Auschwitz concentration camp from July 1941 to October 1941, and from October 1941 to September 1943 at the Majdanek camp. He was then transferred to Neuengamme concentration camp. At Neuengamme he was the supervisor for SS physician Kurt Heissmeyer. Heißmeier had done medical experiments on adult concentration camp prisoners and children. Trzebinski was liable for the medical care of the inmates of the Neuengamme camp and all its subcamps. Of 100,000 inmates, at least 42,900 died between 1938 and 1945.[1]

48.2   Murder of children

Trzebinski was involved in the murder of 20 children at the subcamp *Bullenhuser Damm*, a former school partly destroyed during the bombing of Hamburg in World War II. Heißmeyer had ordered 20 Jewish children (10 boys and 10 girls) from Auschwitz to continue his experiments. His purpose had been to inject tuberculosis bacteria and to excise the axillary lymph nodes. On the night of 20 April 1945, Trzebinski injected morphine into the children (to sedate them) after which they were hanged in the basement of the *Bullenhuser Damm* school. That same night, 28 adults died as well, mostly Soviet prisoners.[2]

48.3   Trial and execution

Trzebinski was able to escape at the end of the Second World War. On February 1, 1946 he was arrested—after working for the British forces in the POW camp Neumünster—because of the persistency of Walter Freud, a grandchild of Sigmund Freud. Trzebinski was sentenced to death during the "Curiohaus processes" in Rotherbaum in March 1946, also for his complicity in the homicide of the children.[2] At his trial he confessed[3] freely and frankly, saying, "If I had acted as a hero the children might have died a little later, but their fate could no longer be averted" and admitted "you cannot execute children, you can only murder them" but they were "only" Jews.[4] Trzebinski was executed by hanging on 8 October 1946[2][5] by Albert Pierrepoint at Hamelin Prison.

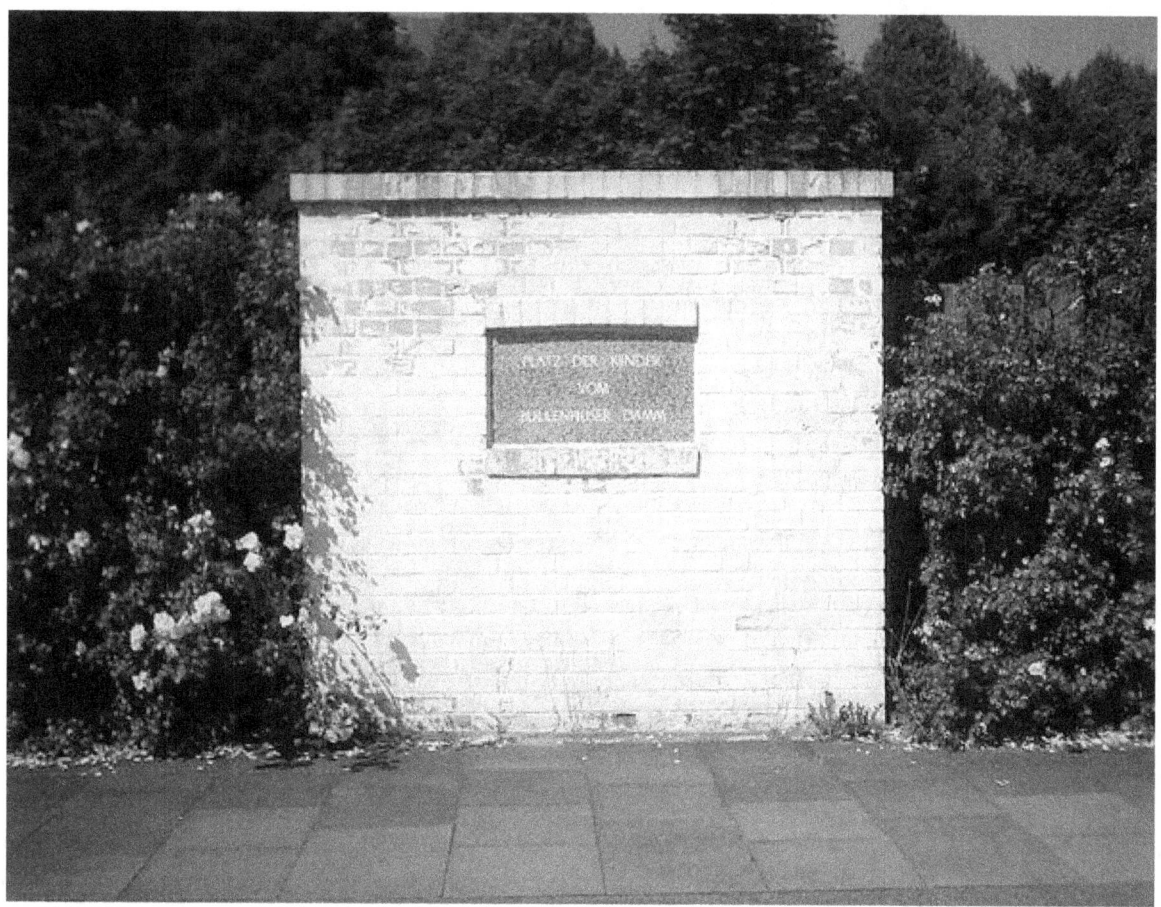

Place of children from Bullenhuser Damm *in Hamburg, Germany*

48.4   References

[1] "Geschichte" (in German). Memorial site Neuengamme. Archived from the original on 4 October 2008. Retrieved 2008-10-12.

[2] "Die Kinder vom Bullenhuser Damm" (in German). Hamburger Abendblatt. 2005-04-20. Archived from the original on 22 October 2008. Retrieved 2008-10-11.

[3] Neumann, Klaus (2000). *Shifting memories: the Nazi past in the new Germany. Social history, popular culture, and politics in Germany.* Ann Arbor: University of Michigan Press. ISBN 978-0-472-11147-3.

[4] Langer, Lawrence L (1996). *Admitting the Holocaust: collected essays.* New York: Oxford University Press. p. 67. ISBN 0-19-510648-2.

[5] "Axis History Factbook: Neuengamme Trial". Retrieved 2008-10-11.

Chapter 49

Carl Værnet

Carl Peter Værnet (April 28, 1893 – November 25, 1965) was a Danish physician, SS-Sturmbannfuhrer (major) and a medical research officer at the Buchenwald concentration camp. He experimented extensively with hormone therapy as a possible means of overriding homosexuality or bisexuality[3] in men. Værnet injected testosterone and other synthetic hormones into the testicles of live human test subjects.[4] His research was under the authority of Reichsführer-SS Heinrich Himmler. Following the war Værnet escaped prosecution for war crimes by fleeing to South America.[5]

49.1   Life

Værnet had trained as a physician at the University of Copenhagen and set up his first practice in the city. He took further courses in Germany, France, and the Netherlands, where he developed a special interest in hormone treatments. Although he had been a member of the Danish Nazi Party since the late 1930s, his private medical career only began to suffer after the German-occupation during World War II as he came to be considered a collaborator in his native country. In order to further his hormone research, he was introduced to SS-Obergruppenfuhrer Dr. Ernst-Robert Grawitz, chief physician of the SS and Police services, by the operatic tenor Helge Rosvaenge. He would later meet with the leader of the SS, Heinrich Himmler, and was given a prominent medical post with the SS in Prague in early 1944.

Between June and December 1944, Carl Værnet experimented on 17 male inmates at Buchenwald who were forced to undergo an operation with an artificial gland. Although none of the inmates died as a direct result of his research, at least two contracted infections which proved fatal. His research proved inconclusive and he quickly lost favour with his Nazi benefactors. After the war, he was arrested in Copenhagen and interrogated at Alsgades School. Although the Danish authorities wanted to press charges of his SS involvement, he feigned heart trouble and escaped. It appears he tried to sell the hormone research to DuPont in 1946. He later fled to Brazil and then to Buenos Aires, Argentina, where he died in 1965.

49.2   See also

- Ex-Nazis

- Homophobia

49.3   References

[1] Potthoff, Herbert. "Hans Davidsen-Nielsen / Niels Høiby / Niels-Birger Danielsen / Jakob Rubin: Carl Værnet. Der dänische SS-Arzt im KZ Buchenwald". Site FHG - Invertito. Retrieved 2015.

[2] Würdemann, Ulrich. "Vaernets Experimente in Buchenwald". Site OndaMaris. Retrieved 2015.

[3] http://pills52.com/2014/2578012/

[4] David A Hackett (1995). *The Buchenwald report.* ISBN 0-8133-1777-0.

[5] Louis-Georges Tin (2008). *Dictionary of Homophobia: A Global History of Gay and Lesbian Experience.* ISBN 1-55152-229-2.

Chapter 50

Werner Villinger

Werner Villinger (9 October 1887 in Besigheim – 8 August 1961 near Innsbruck) was a Nazi German psychiatrist, neurologist, eugenicist and the leading physician at the Bethel Institution ("Anstalt Bethel"). Villinger's specialities included juvenile delinquency, child guidance and group therapy. He was a Professor of Psychiatry at the Philipps University of Marburg and a leading member of the World Federation for Mental Health (WFMH).

Under the Germany's Nazi regime of the 1930s and '40s, Villinger acted as an expert in the government's T-4 Euthanasia Program.

On Social Welfare Education Day 1934, Villinger gave a speech on sterilization and described the reaction, fears and resistance of the boys involved.

He was involved in medical experiments on human beings and ordered thousands to their deaths during the Third Reich but supported Rev. Friedrich von Bodelschwingh's attempt to resist extermination of the mentally ill.

After World War II, Villinger continued his career in the Federal Republic of Germany and co-founded the Federal Ministry of Family, Youth and Health. He was honored by the German government.

Villinger attended the U.S. White House Conference on Children and Youth. In 1951, he became co-chairman of the WFMH Health and Human Relations Conference at Hiddesen-near-Detmold. In 1952, he was a member of a WFMH group on Educating the Public whose Annual Conference met in Brussels. In 1952, he was elected president of the German Association for Child and Youth Psychiatry, and in 1954 became the head of the medical department of Philipps University of Marburg.

In 1961, the German Federal Authorities announced their intent to try Villinger for his actions under the Nazi regime, but before he was brought to trial Villinger threw himself to his death off a mountain top near Innsbruck.

50.1 See also

- Ernst Rüdin
- Euthanasia
- List of Nazi doctors
- Nazi eugenics

50.2 References

- The Origins of Nazi Genocide

- In the Name of the People

- Medical and Psychological Effects of Concentration Camps on Holocaust Survivors

Chapter 51

Gerhard Wagner (physician)

This article is about the physician Gerhard Wagner. For other people of the same name, see Gerhard Wagner (disambiguation).

Gerhard Wagner (18 August 1888 in Neu-Heiduk, Prussian Silesia, now in Poland – 25 March 1939 in Munich) was the first Reich Doctors' Leader (*Reichsärzteführer*) in the time of Nazi Germany.

Born a surgery professor's son, he studied medicine in Munich and served as a doctor at the front in World War I (1914–1918). Among other things, he was awarded the Iron Cross, first class.

From 1919, Wagner ran his own medical practice in Munich, while also being a member of two *Freikorps* between 1921 and 1923, *von Epp* and *Oberland*. Just because of his Silesian origins, Wagner stayed on as leader of the Upper Silesia German Community Associations (*Deutschtumsverbände Oberschlesiens*). In May 1929, he switched to the NSDAP.

Dr. Wagner was co-founder and as of 1932 leader of the National Socialist German Physicians' Federation (NSDÄB), and also functioned from 1933 as a member of the Palatinate *Landtag*. A year later, in 1934, Wagner was ordered to the position of Reich Doctors' Leader. Moreover, he was "The Führer's Commissioner for National Health". By 1933, he had already become leader of the Main Office for National Health, and in 1936 came his appointment as that office's Main Service Leader (*Hauptdienstleiter*).

In December 1935, Wagner became leader of the *Reichsärztekammer* (Physicians' Chamber). At the 1936 Nuremberg Rally, he discussed the racial laws. As was typical of Nazi propaganda at this time, this was more in terms of the pure and growing race than the evil of the Jews.[1] A shift in his political career came in 1937 when he was promoted to SA Obergruppenführer. Meanwhile he was also commissioner for collegiate issues on Rudolf Hess's staff.

Wagner died quite young, at only 50. The cause of his sudden death is to this day unknown. His successor was Leonardo Conti.

Gerhard Wagner was jointly responsible for euthanasia and sterilization carried out against Jews and the handicapped, and showed himself at the Nuremberg Party Congress in 1935 to be a staunch proponent of the Nuremberg Laws, and thereby also of Nazi Germany's race legislation and racial politics. Under Wagner's leadership, the Nazi killing institution at Hadamar was established.

51.1   References

[1] "Race and Population Policy"

Chapter 52

Albert Widmann

Albert Widmann (8 June 1912 – 24 December 1986) was an SS officer and German chemist who worked for the Action T4 euthanasia program during the regime of Nazi Germany.

52.1 Early life

Widmann was born in Stuttgart. His father was a railroad engineer. Widmann studied at the Stuttgart Technical Institute, receiving his certificate in chemical engineering in 1936 and his doctorate in September 1938. Soon after, he was hired by Walter Heess, the chief of the Technical Institute for the Detection of Crime (*Kriminaltechnisches Institut der Sicherheitspolizei*, or KTI), who had previously employed Widmann as a temporary consultant. By 1940 Widmann had been promoted to chief of the KTI's section for chemical analysis.[1]

Widmann was not particularly involved in politics. However, in July 1933, as a student Widmann joined the National Socialist Motor Corps (*Nationalsozialistisches Kraftfahrkorps*, NSKK). He was admitted into the Nazi Party in May 1937. After Widmann joined the KTI, in December 1939 he was transferred from the NSKK to the SS with the rank of SS-*Untersturmführer* (second lieutenant).[1]

52.2 Action T4

Widmann became involved with Action T4 from its inception. Along with August Becker and Helmut Kallmeyer, he was one of the three chemists primarily involved with the program. Although Widmann was not directly employed by Action T4, he and his KTI office provided the program with the needed support services. Widmann took part in the early discussions about killing methods, participated in the first Brandenburg gassing experiment, tested gassing and dynamiting in occupied Bielorussia and, through KTI, obtained the necessary gas and poisons for T-4.

Widmann submitted the paperwork and obtained the carbon monoxide gas needed for the T4 killing centers to operate, as well as the "medicines" needed for killings in children's wards and "wild" euthanasia hospitals within the T-4 program. These wards were established in selected hospitals, eventually at least 22 throughout the German Reich, where doctors were recruited to kill infants sent to them. This was usually done by an overdose of common medication, supplied by Widmann. Over time the age limit moved from infants and children under three to older children and in some cases teenagers. Parents were deceived by local health authorities into believing that their children would receive special medical treatment. If they resisted, they could be threatened with loss of custody. An estimated 5,000 children had been murdered by this program by the end of the war.[2]

Widmann also shared his technological knowledge. While others in the T-4 program were in charge of supervising and administration, Widmann instructed and experimented with gassing techniques. In the early stages of T-4, Widmann discussed possible gassing methods with Viktor Brack to determine the best way to kill patients with gas. For example, Widmann suggested releasing gas into the hospital dormitories while the patients slept, but this idea was dismissed as

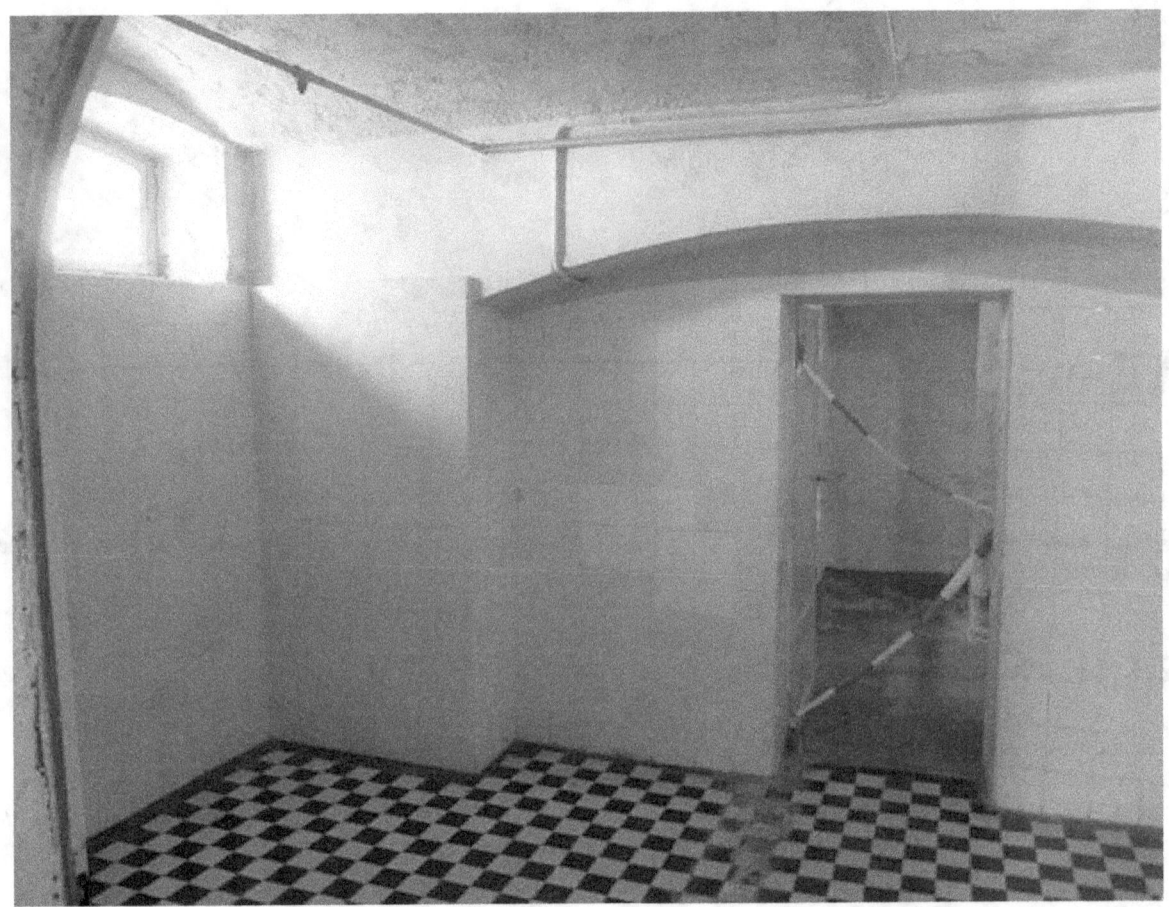

Gas chamber in Hadamar Euthanasia Centre

impractical. Widmann appeared at Brandenburg Euthanasia Centre to administer the first gassing experiment and teach the proper gassing method (for instance, how to measure the correct dose of carbon monoxide).[1][3] Others who attended the first gassing included Philipp Bouhler, Karl Brandt, Viktor Brack, Leonardo Conti and Christian Wirth as well as other officials and physicians from T4 headquarters in Berlin. Widmann visited other T-4 centers only when solutions to technical problems needed to be tested, such as, when the crematorium in Sonnenstein Euthanasia Centre did not function correctly. For Action T4, Widmann had tested gassing on animals before recommending it as the means to kill human beings.[1] One of the main goals of Widmann's work was to minimize the psychological impact that the killings bore upon the killers.[4]

With Arthur Nebe, commander of *Einsatzgruppe B*, and an unnamed explosives expert, Widmann experimented with dynamite as a means to kill patients, and also tested ways to pipe gas from a motor exhaust to the interior of a chamber:

In September 1941, *Einsatzgruppe B* was faced with the task of liquidating the patients of the lunatic asylums in the cities of Minsk and Mogilev. Nebe decided to find a simpler way for his men to kill the mentally diseased, other than by shooting them. He contacted Kripo headquarters and asked for their help in carrying out the killing of the insane with either explosives or poison gas. Dr. Widmann of the Criminal Police was sent to Nebe in Minsk, but before he left, Dr. Widmann discussed with the director of the Criminal Police Technological Institute, Dr. Heess, ways of using the carbon monoxide gas from automobile exhaust for killing operations in the East, based on the experience gained from the euthanasia program. Dr. Widmann took to Minsk 400 kgs of explosive material and the metal pipes required for the gassing installations.

Nebe and Dr. Widmann carried out an experimental killing using explosives. Twenty-five mentally ill people were locked into two bunkers in a forest outside Minsk. The first explosion killed only some of them, and it took much time and trouble until the second explosion killed the rest. Explosives therefore were unsatisfactory.

A few days later an experiment with poison gas was carried out by Nebe and Dr. Widmann in Mogilev. In the local lunatic asylum, a room with twenty to thirty of the insane was closed hermetically, and two pipes were driven into the wall. A car was parked outside, and one of the metal pipes that Dr. Widmann had brought connected the exhaust of the car to the pipe in the wall. The car engine was turned on and the carbon monoxide began seeping into the room. After eight minutes, the people in the room were still alive. A second car was connected to the other pipe in the wall. The two cars were operated simultaneously, and a few minutes later all those in the room were dead.[5]

Another source states that instead of adding a second car, the first car was replaced with a truck.[4] The idea to use gas was partly inspired by an incident involving Nebe. One night after a party Nebe had driven home drunk, parked in his garage and fell asleep with the car engine running. He had nearly died of carbon monoxide poisoning from the exhaust fumes.[4]

This engine exhaust testing inspired the development of gas vans. Back in Berlin, Reinhard Heydrich immediately set to work within the RSHA for the development of, in the words of Heydrich's subordinate Walter Rauff, a "more humane method of execution" than the *Einsatzgruppen* firing squads which had been used. When a prototype gas van was driven to KTI, Widmann explained to his young chemists that by adjusting the timing of the ignition, one could maximize the amount of poisonous carbon monoxide in the exhaust. Widmann further explained that firing squads on the eastern front could be spared.[6]

Some of Widmann's other experiments included testing poisoned ammunition on prisoners at Sachsenhausen concentration camp, which killed the subjects.

By 1944, he had been promoted to SS-*Sturmbannführer* (major). Problem solving was Widmann's specialty, and the kind of problem involved did not affect him. Widmann did not appear to be motivated by Nazi ideology, but rather saw himself as an expert determined to keep his job.[1]

After the war, Widmann was interned by U.S. occupying forces for several days before taking a job in a paint factory. He had worked his way up to chief chemist by the time of his arrest in January 1959. Apparently, Widmann ultimately served six years and six months in prison.

During his prosecution, Widmann was asked how Arthur Nebe's order to kill mental patients in Belarus was related to Nebe's and Widmann's supposed assignment there - antipartisan warfare. Widmann's response:

52.3   See also

- August Becker

52.4   References

[1] Friedlander, Henry (1995). *The Origins of Nazi Genocide: From Euthanasia to the Final Solution*. Chapel Hill, NC: University of North Carolina Press. pp. 209–210.

[2] Christopher Browning. *The Origins of the Final Solution : The Evolution of Nazi Jewish Policy, September 1939 – March 1942* (With contributions by Jürgen Matthäus), Lincoln : University of Nebraska Press, 2004. p. 190 ISBN 0-803-25979-4 OCLC 52838928

[3] Richard J. Evans (2009). *The Third Reich at War*, Penguin, p. 84. ISBN 978-1-59420-206-3

[4] Laurence Rees (2006). *Auschwitz: A New History*, Public Affairs, p. 53.

[5] Yitzhak Arad (1987). *Belzec, Sobibor, Treblinka: The Operation Reinhard Death Camps*, Bloomington: Indiana University Press, p. 10

[6] Christopher Browning. *The Origins of the Final Solution : The Evolution of Nazi Jewish Policy, September 1939 – March 1942* (With contributions by Jürgen Matthäus), Lincoln : University of Nebraska Press, 2004. pp. 355-356 ISBN 0-803-25979-4 OCLC 52838928

Chapter 53

Eduard Wirths

"Wirths" redirects here. For other people with this name, see Wirths (surname).

Eduard Wirths (4 September 1909 – 20 September 1945) was the Chief SS doctor (SS-Standortarzt) at the Auschwitz concentration camp from September 1942 to January 1945. Thus, Wirths had formal responsibility for everything undertaken by the nearly 20 SS doctors (including Josef Mengele, Horst Schumann and Carl Clauberg) who worked in the medical sections of Auschwitz between 1942–1945.

53.1 Early life

Eduard Wirths was born in Geroldshausen near Würzburg, Bavaria into a Catholic family with democratic Socialist leanings. His father served as a medical corpsman in the First World War and according to Dr. Robert Jay Lifton had emerged from the war "...in a depressed state with pacifist leanings, which were undoubtedly expressed in his (as one son put it) 'making doctors of us all...'" [1] Wirth's younger brother, Helmut, became a notable gynecologist (who later went to Auschwitz to visit his brother to participate in cancer experiments but claimed he left after only a few days on his brother Eduard's advice, due to a disagreement and because of his revulsion of the place[2]). According to Lifton "...Among the boys it was Eduard who came most under the father's influence in becoming meticulous, obedient, and unusually conscientious and reliable — traits that continued into his adult life. He never smoked or drank and was described as compassionate and "soft" in his responses to others..." [3] The Wirths family was not known to be anti-semitic or sympathetic to radical nationalist politics.

53.2 Nazi party membership

Eduard Wirths, however, became an ardent Nazi while studying medicine at the University of Würzburg (1930–35). He joined the Nazi Party and the SA in June 1933 and applied for admission into the SS in 1934. He entered the Waffen SS in 1939, saw action in Norway and the Russian Front and was classified as medically unfit for combat duty in the spring of 1942 after a heart-attack. Wirths then chose to undertake special training for Department leaders in Dachau Concentration Camp and served as chief SS psychiatrist in Neuengamme concentration camp during July 1942. Coincidentally, in 1942 Josef Mengele was also wounded at the Russian Front, pronounced medically unfit for combat, promoted to the rank of SS-Hauptsturmführer before being assigned to Auschwitz.

53.3 Auschwitz (1942-45)

Dr. Wirths was promoted to SS-Hauptsturmführer (captain) and appointed as chief camp physician[4] at Auschwitz in September, 1942. He was appointed on the basis of his reputation as a competent doctor and committed Nazi who would be capable of stopping the typhus epidemics that had increasingly affected SS personnel at Auschwitz.

At Auschwitz, Wirths was known to be protective of prisoner doctors and other prisoners doing medical work, to have improved conditions on the medical blocks and was remembered favourably by most prisoner doctors and other inmates who had contact with him. At the same time, Wirths in recommending Dr. Josef Mengele for promotion in August 1944, was able to speak of Mengele's "open, honest, firm … [and] absolutely dependable" character and "magnificent" intellectual and physical talents; of the "discretion, perseverance, and energy with which he has fulfilled every task … and … shown himself equal to every situation"; of his "valuable contribution to anthropological science by making use of the scientific materials available to him"; of his "absolute ideological firmness" and "faultless conduct [as] an SS officer" ; and personal qualities as "free, unrestrained, persuasive, and lively" discourse that rendered him "especially dear to his comrades".[5]

Rudolf Höss, the commandant of Auschwitz between 1940 and December 1943 is said to have held Wirths in particularly high regard. He is said to have remarked of Wirths that "During my 10 years of service in concentration-camp affairs, I have never encountered a better one." [6]

In 1943 Wirths' benevolent and kind concern for the well-being of Auschwitz inmates resulted in him receiving a Christmas card from Langbein a Jewish prisoner who worked with him, which contained the message "In the past year you have saved here the lives of 93,000 people. We do not have the right to tell you our wishes. But we wish for ourselves that you stay here in the coming year." It was signed: "One speaking for the prisoners of Auschwitz." The figure of 93,000 was the difference in mortality rate among prisoners from typhus in the year prior to Wirths' arrival.[7]

53.3.1 Prisoner experimentation

Wirths was involved in ordering medical experimentation, particularly in gynecological and typhus-related experimental tests. Wirths's primary research concerned pre-cancerous growths of the cervix. Dr. Wirths was also interested in the sterilization of women, by removing their ovaries through surgery or radiation. It is generally acknowledged that he himself never directly participated in such experiments but delegated their conduct to subordinates. The victims of these experiments were Jewish women who had been imprisoned in Block 10 of the main camp in Auschwitz.[8] Dr. E.W.J. Pearce, an Associate Professor of Obstetrics and Gynecology at the Truman Medical Center has made the following observation regarding Wirths' medical experiments: ". . . Wirths, without consent, photographed the cervices of women prisoners, then amputated the pictured cervices, and sent both photographs and specimens for study to Dr. Hinselmann of Berlin. Hinselmann was the physician who developed colposcopy.[9]

53.3.2 Selection of prisoners

Importantly, Wirths also asserted medical control of prisoner selections at the Auschwitz-Birkenau camp, which, prior to spring 1943, had been conducted by the camp commander and his subordinates. Wirths insisted upon taking his own personal turn in performing selections, which he could have deferred to physician subordinates. Witness testimony given at the Trial of Adolf Eichmann provided a useful insight into how the SS approached the issue of how to record the deaths of Auschwitz prisoners (this did not include those who had been immediately selected for gassing- their admission was simply not recorded in the death registers). Those who died while imprisoned at Auschwitz were always recorded as having died from natural causes and never from being executed or murdered.[10][11]

Wirths was promoted to SS-Sturmbannführer (major) in September 1944. Following the evacuation of Auschwitz in January 1945 he was transferred, along with many other former Auschwitz personnel, to the Mittelbau-Dora concentration camp in Thuringia. Wirths would again hold the post of chief camp physician until Mittelbau-Dora's evacuation in April 1945.

53.4   Capture and suicide

Wirths was captured by the Allies at the end of the war and held in custody by British forces. Later, on 20 September 1945, knowing that he would surely face trial for numerous war crimes, Wirths committed suicide by hanging.[12]

53.5   Summary of criminal career

Robert Jay Lifton has noted that

> ". . . Wirths was significantly immersed in Nazi ideology in three crucial spheres: the claim of revitalizing the German race and Volk; the biomedical path to that revitalization via purification of genes and race; and the focus on the Jews as a threat to this renewal, to the immediate and long-term "health" of the Germanic race. While Wirths did not absolutize these convictions in the manner of Mengele — they were in him combined with a strong current of medical humanism — his commitment to the Nazi cause was probably no less strong . . . "[13]

Perhaps illustrative of Wirths' commitment to medical 'leadership' was his tendency while at Auschwitz to drive about in a car flying a Red Cross flag as well as his enthusiasm for acting as a marriage counselor and personal adviser to other SS personnel. According to Helgard Kramer, Wirths ". . . first seized on a career as a military doctor and officer in the German elite troops of the SS, because he desperately wanted to become a member of the upper class; eventually to provide his future wife with a "decent marriage." To reach that goal he had to become a 'tough man'. . .".

53.6   See also

- The Holocaust
- Nazi human experimentation
- Josef Mengele
- Hans Münch

53.7   References

[1] Lifton: p. 385

[2] Lifton: p. 400

[3] Lifton, p. 385

[4] Naomi Baumslag, *Murderous Medicine: Nazi Doctors, Human Experimentation, And Typhus*, p.73, Greenwood Publishing Group.

[5] from "Beurteilung des SS Hauptsturmführers (R) Dr. Josef Mengele," 19 August 1949 (Berlin Document Center: Mengele)

[6] Lifton: p. 386

[7] Lifton: p. 389

[8] Hans-Joachim Lang: *Die Frauen von Block 10. Medizinische Experimente in Auschwitz.* Hamburg 2011, pp. 144–167.

[9] http://books.google.com/books?id=rB0yxE2WhWIC&pg=PA3&lpg=PA3&dq=colposcopy+Wirths+hinselmann&source=bl&ots=7cYPAlzM37&sig=HobpEVFkFIJqevsxRpGDTXwdpiU&hl=es-419&ei=AElJTdf1CoH98AaNwsirDg&sa=X&oi=book_result&ct=result&resnum=5&ved=0CEYQ6AEwBA#v=onepage&q=colposcopy%20Wirths%20hinselmann&f=false

[10] *The Trial of Adolf Eichmann*, Session 70 (Part 2 of 6)

[11] Eichmann trial - The District Court Sessions at www.nizkor.org

[12] "Memorial and Museum: Auschwitz-Birkenau". Retrieved 16 April 2009.

[13] Lifton, p. 412

- Hermann Langbein, (2004) *People in Auschwitz*. North Carolina: The University of North Carolina Press Chapel Hill & London in association with the United States Holocaust Memorial Museum.

- Dr. Robert J. Lifton, (1986) *THE NAZI DOCTORS: Medical Killing and the Psychology of Genocide*. New York: Basic Books.

- University of Linz: *SS-DOCTOR DR. EDUARD WIRTHS*

- Dr. E.W.J. Pearce, (1996) "Antigone: An Exercise in Medical Ethics" in *History and Philosophy of Medicine Newsletter* published by the University of Kansas Medical Centre.

- Transcript (in German) of the documentary Film (1975) "Dr. Eduard Wirths – Standortarzt von Auschwitz" by Dutch film makers Roland Orthel and others.

- Webster University, *Nazi Doctors & Other Perpetrators of Nazi Crimes*

Nazi Doctors at www.webster.edu

-

- Shoa.de - Eduard Wirths (1909-1945) at www.shoa.de

- Helgard Kramer, "The 'Doubled Self' of SS Doctors at Auschwitz Revisited" Paper presented at the 25th Annual Scientific Meeting of the International Society of Political Psychology (ISPP) in Berlin, July 16–19, 2002.

- *Healing-Killing Conflict: Eduard Wirths*

53.8 Text and image sources, contributors, and licenses

53.8.1 Text

- **Nazi human experimentation** *Source:* https://en.wikipedia.org/wiki/Nazi_human_experimentation?oldid=684795258 *Contributors:* The Anome, Patrick, IZAK, Skysmith, Tregoweth, Cgs, Vivin, Haukurth, Tpbradbury, Furrykef, Fifelfoo, Premeditated Chaos, Phthoggos, Kent Wang, Lupo, Barbara Shack, Rudolf 1922, Fastfission, Ich, Loui Da Boss, Varlaam, Alexdi, Darrien, Mateuszica, Wmahan, Seba~enwiki, Quandaryus, Antandrus, OverlordQ, Rdsmith4, Int19h, Ukexpat, Jayjg, Rich Farmbrough, KillerChihuahua, Bender235, CanisRufus, MBisanz, Jpgordon, Adambro, Meggar, Vortexrealm, Bbartlog, Sam Korn, Hooperbloob, Anthony Appleyard, GRider, Richard Harvey, Keenan Pepper, SlimVirgin, Water Bottle, NTK, Snowolf, Klaser, CaseInPoint, Fourthords, EAi, Shadowolf, Ghirlandajo, JALockhart, Cogito Ergo Sum, Reinoutr, TomTheHand, Apokrif, JRHorse, Snagari, Prashanthns, Bühler~enwiki, Graham87, BD2412, Kbdank71, Jclemens, Phoenix-forgotten, Rjwilmsi, SMC, Paj.meister, Tarc, Yamamoto Ichiro, Shultzc, Nihiltres, Nivix, Fragglet, AI, Elmer Clark, DuLithgow, Jrtayloriv, Alphachimp, Sairen42, CAD6DEE2E8DAD95A, Alec.brady, Jared Preston, VolatileChemical, YurikBot, RussBot, Gaius Cornelius, CambridgeBayWeather, Wimt, Thane, NawlinWiki, Kvn8907, Lexicon, Equilibrial, ScottyWZ, Derek.cashman, Nescio, Everyguy, Resigua, Wknight94, Jess Riedel, Mais oui!, H3rb, Some guy, Dan Atkinson, Bibliomaniac15, Sardanaphalus, Fightindaman, SmackBot, Gamnamu, Schyler, InverseHypercube, VigilancePrime, AndreasJS, Anastrophe, Delldot, Frymaster, William Case Morris, Kintetsubuffalo, Hmains, NickGarvey, Squiddy, Jake Larsen, Bluebot, Kingsbury, Dr bab, Hibernian, George Church, Mordantkitten, MaxSem, Mulder416, Sculpher, Amber388, Toko loko, Sbauman487, Rrburke, Edivorce, Midnightcomm, MartinRobinson, NoIdeaNick, Decltype, Nakon, Pwjb, The PIPE, BryanG, TheVikingRaider, Ohconfucius, John, Gobonobo, Peterlewis, BuckyRea, IronGargoyle, Mulletman500, MarkSutton, Slakr, Naevus, Waggers, Bassophile, HisSpaceResearch, Wizard191, Iridescent, Stringyflea, Pacerlaser, Courcelles, Tawkerbot2, Devourer09, GotPSP, CmdrObot, Wafulz, Sir Vicious, W guice, TheMightyOrb, Birdhurst, Shandris, Neelix, Malamockq, Cydebot, AniMate, Vinyanov, Palffy, Doug Weller, Nabokov, Optimist on the run, Nsaum75, SpK, Thijs!bot, Epbr123, Pajz, Deborahjay, N5iln, Marek69, His Ryanness, A3RO, Kaaveh Ahangar~enwiki, Srose, AntiVandalBot, Milton Stanley, Mengela, Desalvionjr, Webville, MikeLynch, HanzoHattori, JAnDbot, Tohru Honda13, Plm209, Andonic, Xeno, Cyningaenglisc, .anacondabot, Acroterion, Wasell, Plynn9, Seanette, Bongwarrior, VoABot II, No substitute for you, Hendrixjoseph, Swpb, Rh otherside cp, JRamlow, Froid, PIrish, Cgingold, Hamiltonstone, Allstarecho, Spellmaster, Teknomegisto, DerHexer, JaGa, Valerius Tygart, .V., NatGertler, MartinBot, Bonuscup98, El Krem, V-Man737, Ravichandar84, Bus stop, Nono64, J.delanoy, Pharaoh of the Wizards, Hodja Nasreddin, TomCat4680, BobEnyart, ElectricValkyrie, NewEnglandYankee, Juliancolton, Strig, Carlo V. Sexron, Jaimeastorga2000, AndreasJSbot, Signalhead, Malik Shabazz, Cireshoe, Agnelli.kate, Lear's Fool, Guardian Tiger, Kyle the bot, Philip Trueman, Zurishaddai, Agricola44, Jackfork, Seb az86556, Mannafredo, Retpyrc, Varoon Arya, StillTrill, Jack Naven Rulez, Onore Baka Sama, Joseph A. Spadaro, Falcon8765, Alectoris rufa, Enviroboy, Master of the Oríchalcos, Chickyfuzz14, Logan, Krautukie, Scottywong, Peter Fleet, Chronic Stoned Emo Ranger, Sonicology, Euryalus, Parhamr, Oda Mari, ZionWingmaster, Undead Herle King, JSpung, ZombieWacker, Lightmouse, Hobartimus, IdreamofJeanie, Svick, Msgv (usurped), USHMMwestheim, ClueBot, GorillaWarfare, The Thing That Should Not Be, Deviousbox, RashersTierney, Ryzic, Sw258, Boing! said Zebedee, Spy007au, Otolemur crassicaudatus, Pointillist, Excirial, Quercus basaseachicensis, Socrates2008, CrazyChemGuy, KC109, CowboySpartan, Mtsmallwood, Bulldog09, Noxia, Aitias, Versus22, Phxtri, Amareelussuria, Kamots, DumZiBoT, Crazy Boris with a red beard, Nathan Johnson, Stickee, Vlnnce, Ost316, Avoided, PhoenixMourning, Mifter, WikiDao, MystBot, Consensual Hysteria, On the other side, Thatguyflint, Gramy, Addbot, Some jerk on the Internet, Magus732, DougsTech, Bkmays, Jncraton, CanadianLinuxUser, Proxima Centauri, LaaknorBot, Veslatt, Debresser, Green Squares, Wall Screamer, Klay00, Ondewelle, Tide rolls, Lightbot, Ben Ben, Yobot, Kamagrian, Whatever404, Anonymous from the 21th century, AnomieBOT, VanishedUser sdu9aya9fasdsopa, Metalhead94, 1exec1, AdjustShift, Maxis ftw, Obersachsebot, 4twenty42o, Nasnema, Gilo1969, Ani medjool, ProtectionTaggingBot, Lectepreuve, FreeKnowledgeCreator, Surv1v4l1st, Kierzek, Luckyloma95, D'ohBot, HJ Mitchell, Benda2, Redrose64, Pinethicket, LinDrug, Yatzhek, Full-date unlinking bot, Apclass123, December21st2012Freak, Scythre, Vrenator, Gegenwind~enwiki, Tbhotch, Minimac, DARTH SIDIOUS 2, RjwilmsiBot, 7mike5000, Davejohnsan, Acather96, Tika bell, Dixtosa, Assayer, Tommy2010, Adrian Tofei, THEQUEEN99, ZéroBot, H3llBot, Wingman4l7, Jesanj, L Kensington, Zac, The Celestial City, ClueBot NG, Martin.Jares, Gilderien, Karl 334, Theopolisme, Helpful Pixie Bot, BG19bot, WikiTryHardDieHard, Ceradon, Wiki3Languages, Mertimer, Danielpublic, Altaïr, Harizotoh9, 93sandra, Ujaanthiny, RscprinterBot, Arigoldberg, Rlegends, YFdyh-bot, Ducknish, Douglas R. Skopp, Monochrome Monitor, Uhbooh, EduardoFernandez, Royalcourtier, Monkbot, Nonstopmaximum, Zeklandia, Prinsgezinde and Anonymous: 624

- **Wilhelm Beiglböck** *Source:* https://en.wikipedia.org/wiki/Wilhelm_Beiglb%C3%B6ck?oldid=667559971 *Contributors:* GCarty, Wernher, Dimadick, Lupo, Klemen Kocjancic, Cnyborg, Haham hanuka, Sherurcij, Plumbago, BanyanTree, Bühler~enwiki, GusF, BrainyBroad, Syrthiss, Crystallina, SmackBot, Nickhk, Martin8721, GoodDay, Jaellee, Ser Amantio di Nicolao, Tazmaniacs, Cydebot, AniMate, Thijs!bot, Mengela, HanzoHattori, Waacstats, Katharineamy, Thismightbezach, VolkovBot, TXiKiBoT, SieBot, Dawn Bard, Monegasque, Mtsmallwood, Good Olfactory, Addbot, Zorrobot, Yobot, Xqbot, GrouchoBot, Full-date unlinking bot, Jonkerz, RjwilmsiBot, Ripchip Bot, Bossanoven, ZéroBot, Helpful Pixie Bot, VIAFbot, KasparBot and Anonymous: 3

- **Block 10** *Source:* https://en.wikipedia.org/wiki/Block_10?oldid=672623347 *Contributors:* Alfa, Laurascudder, Kbdank71, Jclemens, Rjwilmsi, John, Stwalkerster, Cydebot, Alaibot, Natalie Erin, The Anomebot2, LedgendGamer, Omgitsmonica, Jklak, Davecrosby uk, Thistory2, Roland zh, Mtsmallwood, Addbot, VbCrLf, Sebastian scha., Ctruongngoc, D'ohBot, Trijnstel, Lotje, Diannaa, TjBot, H3llBot, Johannarebecca, Quick and Dirty User Account, FJS15, Dudenhofener, Lugia2453, Delta739 and Anonymous: 11

- **Franz von Bodmann** *Source:* https://en.wikipedia.org/wiki/Franz_von_Bodmann?oldid=688241475 *Contributors:* Keresaspa, Jeff5102, Cydebot, Waacstats, Deor, Addbot, RjwilmsiBot, Bossanoven, ÄDA - DÄP, KasparBot, TX6785 and Anonymous: 2

- **Karl Brandt** *Source:* https://en.wikipedia.org/wiki/Karl_Brandt?oldid=686361944 *Contributors:* 0, WojPob, Andre Engels, IZAK, GCarty, Schneelocke, Morwen, Wernher, Hadal, Lupo, MaGioZal, Andries, Karn, Catdude, Necrothesp, Karl-Henner, Creidieki, Klemen Kocjancic, D6, Eb.hoop, Haham hanuka, Storm Rider, Sherurcij, Bbsrock, Aka, Ebakunin, Boothy443, Woohookitty, Scriberius, Graham87, Kbdank71, Koavf, Olessi, Leithp, Nam, Bgwhite, Cornellrockey, Vuvar1, Jimp, Stephenb, Dake~enwiki, Syrthiss, Resigua, Nlu, Richardcavell, Gtdp, Bwiki, SmackBot, Eskimbot, Chris the speller, MalafayaBot, OrphanBot, Zazpot, Percommode, Andrew c, YegerMeister, Ser Amantio di Nicolao, ER MD, Peterlewis, Meco, Waggers, Ardavis, RCS, MaoMistikus, KnightLago, Cydebot, AniMate, CuteGargoyle, Otto4711, NorthernThunder, Visual kei, Aldis90, Thijs!bot, Mojo Hand, Massimo Macconi, Mengela, Smith2006, QuizzicalBee, Waacstats, Grandia01, Keith D, CommonsDelinker, LordAnubisBOT, Remember the dot, Useight, Retal, Thismightbezach, Sir Jelly Man, Broadbot, Hennap, Britzingen, SieBot, OberRanks, Nmadh, Monegasque, Maralia, Niceguyedc, Asmaybe, Mtsmallwood, Boleyn, Avi1111, Good Olfactory, Addbot,

Pelex, Eivindbot, LaaknorBot, Debresser, Numbo3-bot, Lightbot, Dreizung, Yobot, AnomieBOT, Jesi, Piano non troppo, MauritsBot, Xqbot, Oerlikonen, Omnipaedista, Vlastimil Svoboda, Joep01, Kierzek, Abductive, Moonraker, MastiBot, RjwilmsiBot, Bossanoven, Mamalala, Wik-itanvirBot, THEQUEEN99, Werieth, Fæ, ClueBot NG, Vincelord, Pefly123, Marcocapelle, Harizotoh9, BattyBot, ÄDA - DÄP, Douglas R. Skopp, VIAFbot, Jamesx12345, Bumblebritches57, Jamesmcmahon0, Obenritter, Pluperfectionist2, Kennethaw88, EurovisionNim, Skoppdr, Reb0118, KasparBot and Anonymous: 70

- **Bullenhuser Damm** *Source:* https://en.wikipedia.org/wiki/Bullenhuser_Damm?oldid=683842261 *Contributors:* The Anome, William Avery, Ineuw, Rich Farmbrough, Herzliyya, Woohookitty, FeanorStar7, Kbdank71, Marsoult, Hu12, Cydebot, Nabokov, Deborahjay, The Anomebot2, Rumiton, Falcon8765, Rontrigger, ImageRemovalBot, ClueBot, Iohannes Animosus, Flamenc, Cras26, WikHead, Addbot, Sebastian scha., Ondewelle, Lightbot, Roland.h.bueb, AnomieBOT, LilHelpa, Ulf Heinsohn, Shadowjams, NSH002, 7mike5000, EmausBot, John of Reading, Marrante, Cobaltcigs, Michaelerichards, Helpful Pixie Bot, Marcocapelle, 4Jays1034, Dexbot, Alayambo, Monkbot, Monopoly31121993 and Anonymous: 17

- **Max Clara** *Source:* https://en.wikipedia.org/wiki/Max_Clara?oldid=659404955 *Contributors:* Rjwilmsi, Cydebot, Waacstats, Aboutmovies, 28bytes, Scottywong, Brewcrewer, Addbot, Yobot, Citation bot, Gumruch, RjwilmsiBot, Bossanoven, ZéroBot, Gautehuus, Grosswardeyn, VIAFbot, Monkbot, KasparBot and Anonymous: 1

- **Carl Clauberg** *Source:* https://en.wikipedia.org/wiki/Carl_Clauberg?oldid=688241519 *Contributors:* Deb, Skysmith, GCarty, Schneelocke, Dimadick, Curps, Rparle, Radulf, Keresaspa, Klemen Kocjancic, Babelfisch, Rich Farmbrough, Bender235, Bobo192, ToastieIL, Dozzi, CaseInPoint, Fourthords, Stemonitis, JALockhart, Tellkel, Ekem, Akira625, Wikimike, Kbdank71, Avochelm, Sakkaro, Nam, Margos-bot~enwiki, DanMS, Zwobot, Arthur Rubin, Garion96, Blablabla, SmackBot, Squiddy, Kingsbury, Addshore, YegerMeister, Neelix, Cydebot, Otto4711, Thijs!bot, Mengela, HanzoHattori, Magioladitis, Waacstats, Nono64, Yonidebot, Aqwis, Thismightbezach, Deor, EvanCarroll, Mark v1.0, Broadbot, BOTijo, SieBot, Meinkampf~enwiki, Monegasque, USHMMwestheim, Jacurek, Excirial, Mtsmallwood, Addbot, Iron-holds, Debresser, Lightbot, Zorrobot, Luckas-bot, Yobot, ImperatorExercitus, Xqbot, Alexlange, J04n, Erik9bot, HRoestBot, Lotje, Alexandre Rongellion, RjwilmsiBot, Bossanoven, The name of any organization, Helpful Pixie Bot, Harizotoh9, Sourced much, BattyBot, YFdyh-bot, TheJJJunk, Dudenhofener, Zeeyanwiki, Douglas R. Skopp, VIAFbot, KasparBot, TX6785 and Anonymous: 34

- **Club cell** *Source:* https://en.wikipedia.org/wiki/Club_cell?oldid=687636731 *Contributors:* Alex.tan, Fuelbottle, DragonflySixtyseven, Jonathan Drain, Arcadian, Axl, Axeman89, Ceyockey, Kmg90, Jclemens, Rjwilmsi, Gaius Cornelius, Maristoddard, Thunderboltz, Jfurr1981, Gra-cenotes, Mrpark01, Mcstrother, MaxEnt, Cydebot, Mattbartek, Luke poa, Dawnseeker2000, STBot, Cd830, J.delanoy, Schnurrbart, Scotty-wong, SieBot, Daveeroy, Animeronin, ClueBot, Deviator13, Franamax, Addbot, 5 albert square, Filip em, Luckas-bot, Yobot, Addihockey10, Tagallyat, Gumruch, FrescoBot, Citation bot 1, Letdemsay, EmausBot, Jesse057, DarkArcher25, TyA, Yetiman9, ClueBot NG, Baseball Watcher, Frietjes, Helpful Pixie Bot, SharkinthePool, Jxs338, AvocatoBot, Dean Ulbrick, Iztwoz, Mattbroadhead, Monkbot and Anonymous: 32

- **Erwin Ding-Schuler** *Source:* https://en.wikipedia.org/wiki/Erwin_Ding-Schuler?oldid=659629476 *Contributors:* Folks at 137, Bender235, Grutness, Tswold, Cydebot, Magioladitis, Waacstats, Adamdaley, TXiKiBoT, Spy007au, MystBot, Addbot, Yobot, FreeRangeFrog, Anoth-erclown, DennisPeeters, RjwilmsiBot, Bossanoven, EmausBot, Marklinklaters, Helpful Pixie Bot, VIAFbot, Lekoren, KasparBot and Anony-mous: 3

- **Doctors of Infamy** *Source:* https://en.wikipedia.org/wiki/Doctors_of_Infamy?oldid=650988477 *Contributors:* Delirium, Black Falcon, Cy-debot, Shawn in Montreal, Maralia, Ad Orientem, Jackentasche and Filedelinkerbot

- **List of medical eponyms with Nazi associations** *Source:* https://en.wikipedia.org/wiki/List_of_medical_eponyms_with_Nazi_associations? oldid=663521520 *Contributors:* Rich Farmbrough, FT2, Jeodesic, Anthony Appleyard, Avenue, Ron Ritzman, Apokrif, Jclemens, Rjwilmsi, Tim!, Salix alba, TeaDrinker, Peterkingiron, Tony1, SmackBot, Mgiganteus1, Cydebot, Dream Focus, Furorimpius, Mark v1.0, Scottywong, Mjpresson, Yobot, Narthring, RjwilmsiBot, DexDor, S3819, Monkbot and Anonymous: 3

- **Feeder of lice** *Source:* https://en.wikipedia.org/wiki/Feeder_of_lice?oldid=641583725 *Contributors:* Bearcat, Piotrus, Art LaPella, Cromwellt, GregorB, Volunteer Marek, Bgwhite, RussBot, Lusanaherandraton, Maunus, Edgar181, Inwind, Malick78, France3470, Trfasulo, Sun Creator, Worldbruce, AnomieBOT, LauraHale, Kiefer.Wolfowitz, Seattle Jörg, RjwilmsiBot, EmausBot, John of Reading, Helpful Pixie Bot, Episeda, ChunkNugget, Monopoly31121993 and Anonymous: 4

- **Fritz Fischer (medical doctor)** *Source:* https://en.wikipedia.org/wiki/Fritz_Fischer_(medical_doctor)?oldid=661617752 *Contributors:* GCarty, Pigsonthewing, Lupo, Klemen Kocjancic, D6, JYolkowski, Jeltz, Fitzner, Kbdank71, Rjwilmsi, Koavf, Leithp, AI, Mhi, NiTenIchiRyu, Jm-chuff, Green Giant, Jkaharper, GiantSnowman, Cydebot, Otto4711, Thijs!bot, Mengela, HanzoHattori, Waacstats, MisterBee1966, Biologos, Alexbot, Mtsmallwood, MystBot, Good Olfactory, Addbot, Sebastian scha., Debresser, Lightbot, Zorrobot, Luckas-bot, Ykerzner, Xqbot, RedBot, Юрий Педаченко, RjwilmsiBot, Bossanoven, ZéroBot, Genealogy123, Mogism, VIAFbot, KasparBot and Anonymous: 8

- **Forgiving Dr. Mengele** *Source:* https://en.wikipedia.org/wiki/Forgiving_Dr._Mengele?oldid=671706153 *Contributors:* Paul Barlow, Ronz, Darkwind, Varlaam, Bender235, Holdek, SidP, Pegship, SmackBot, Gilliam, Chris the speller, Switchercat, Neelix, Cydebot, Brismile, Schuski, Wikid77, MarshBot, Kipholbeck, JNW, Karmela, Casperonline, JL-Bot, Nolesrock, Jmenton, Auntof6, Sonylad, Lightbot, Thisis4xtracredit, Full-date unlinking bot, Execjosh and Anonymous: 26

- **Karl Gebhardt** *Source:* https://en.wikipedia.org/wiki/Karl_Gebhardt?oldid=669519663 *Contributors:* GCarty, Wernher, Lupo, Necrothesp, Keresaspa, Cnyborg, Haham hanuka, Sherurcij, Mutt, Kbdank71, Rjwilmsi, Koavf, Nam, FlaBot, JdforresterBot, Chobot, YurikBot, Russ-Bot, Syrthiss, Arria Belli, Resigua, Nlu, Jmchuff, SmackBot, Neddyseagoon, AGK, Olaf Davis, Cydebot, AniMate, Meno25, Otto4711, Nottheking, Thijs!bot, Mengela, HanzoHattori, Nono64, Duch, Plasticup, DadaNeem, MisterBee1966, TXiKiBoT, Koalorka, All Hallow's Wraith, DragonBot, Alexbot, Mtsmallwood, Omerkhan1, Avi1111, Good Olfactory, Addbot, SpellingBot, Debresser, Lightbot, Luckas-bot, Yobot, DiverDave, AnomieBOT, Rubinbot, Citation bot, ArthurBot, MauritsBot, Xqbot, Tiller54, Kierzek, LucienBOT, Dinamik-bot, Di-annaa, RjwilmsiBot, Ripchip Bot, Bossanoven, EmausBot, Cacknbellz, Vincelord, Helpful Pixie Bot, ÄDA - DÄP, VIAFbot, Abiagiotaylor, OccultZone, Tadeusz Nowak, KasparBot and Anonymous: 22

- **Karl Genzken** *Source:* https://en.wikipedia.org/wiki/Karl_Genzken?oldid=660623808 *Contributors:* SimonP, DavidLevinson, Docu, GCarty, Wernher, Korath, DragonflySixtyseven, Klemen Kocjancic, Cnyborg, Haham hanuka, GRider, Sherurcij, Andrewpmk, Fitzner, Koavf, Leithp,

Syrthiss, SmackBot, Martin8721, Runcorn, Tazmaniacs, Tawkerbot2, Cydebot, AniMate, Thijs!bot, Mengela, HanzoHattori, Waacstats, MisterBee1966, McM.bot, Hozro, Monegasque, Mtsmallwood, JQ to you, Good Olfactory, Addbot, Lightbot, Rubinbot, Xqbot, Kierzek, Jonkerz, RjwilmsiBot, Bossanoven, Marrante, ZéroBot, Mrt3366, YFdyh-bot, ÄDA - DÄP, VIAFbot, Monkbot, KasparBot and Anonymous: 7

- **Julius Hallervorden** *Source:* https://en.wikipedia.org/wiki/Julius_Hallervorden?oldid=659404951 *Contributors:* Kenatipo, Rjwilmsi, Wctaiwan, Wolfmankurd, SmackBot, Cydebot, Waacstats, Scottywong, Addbot, Filip em, MastiBot, RjwilmsiBot, VIAFbot, Monkbot and KasparBot

- **Siegfried Handloser** *Source:* https://en.wikipedia.org/wiki/Siegfried_Handloser?oldid=681931855 *Contributors:* GCarty, Wernher, Klemen Kocjancic, Cnyborg, CheekyMonkey, Haham hanuka, Sherurcij, Fitzner, Sheynhertz-Unbayg, Kbdank71, Koavf, Olessi, FlaBot, Syrthiss, West Virginian, SmackBot, Colonies Chris, Bezapt, Cydebot, AniMate, Mojo Hand, Mengela, Waacstats, Bushcarrot, VolkovBot, Kernel Saunters, Oxymoron83, Mtsmallwood, Bilsonius, Good Olfactory, Addbot, H92Bot, SpBot, Yobot, Omnipaedista, Jake V, Юрий Педаченко, RjwilmsiBot, Bossanoven, ZéroBot, HumanNaturOriginal, YFdyh-bot, ÄDA - DÄP, OccultZone, HHubi, KasparBot and Anonymous: 4

- **Aribert Heim** *Source:* https://en.wikipedia.org/wiki/Aribert_Heim?oldid=690877375 *Contributors:* Magnus Manske, XJaM, William Avery, Skysmith, Haakon, Docu, WhisperToMe, Wernher, Carlossuarez46, Robbot, Moncrief, Rhombus, Fuelbottle, Lysy, Nunh-huh, Varlaam, Frencheigh, Edcolins, Sonjaaa, Gzuckier, Necrothesp, Ukexpat, Brianhe, MeltBanana, Bender235, Chairboy, Shanes, Nrbelex, Haham hanuka, Hooperbloob, Kvaks, Pedro Aguiar, Skyring, Richard Arthur Norton (1958-), Lapsed Pacifist, Canadian Paul, Kbdank71, Rjwilmsi, Koavf, Achtung~enwiki, Tswold, YurikBot, RussBot, Tdevries, Gaius Cornelius, GeeJo, Manxruler, NawlinWiki, Joshdboz, Yoninah, SM, JdwNYC, Adam Holland, Jrssystemsnet, BorgQueen, Petri Krohn, Bcastaneda, Fabian Boudville, Steve G~enwiki, Entheta, Narkstraws, SmackBot, John Lunney, Janawar, Verne Equinox, Wencer, Kintetsubuffalo, ThompsJohn, Canuck85, Anthonysenn, Bill Dawson, Sduplessie, Kaliz, Oatmeal batman, AltGrendel, OOODDD, Leoboudv, Detruncate, Mtmelendez, Evenfiel, ThurnerRupert, Tazmaniacs, Robofish, Thelongview, Charles-Martel, HisSpaceResearch, Iridescent, Joseph Solis in Australia, Gilabrand, Pudeo, Friendly Neighbour, Joegoodfriend, Cydebot, Poeticbent, Khatru2, Trident13, Nabokov, ITrate, CieloEstrellado, Thijs!bot, Yitzz2, Epbr123, JonEAhlquist, SGGH, Rodrigo Cornejo, JustAGal, Salavat, IrishPete, Yellowdesk, DagosNavy, HanzoHattori, Harryzilber, Matthew Fennell, Conspiration, Connormah, Autkm, Chris G, Lilduff90, Bus stop, CommonsDelinker, Alexb102072, Offæ, Swinquest, Wikieditor06, VolkovBot, Kanakukk, Nintendere, AlnoktaBOT, Davidwr, TXiKiBoT, Broadbot, Dirkbb, BOTijo, Cosprings, Gerakibot, PolarBot, Arbor to SJ, Offworlder, Lightmouse, Kumioko (renamed), DaddyWarlock, ImageRemovalBot, YSSYguy, Selecciones de la Vida, CiudadanoGlobal, All Hallow's Wraith, Kristamaranatha, Charlir91, Davidovic, Ktr101, Mtsmallwood, Muro Bot, BOTarate, DumZiBoT, CoolVin, Addbot, LaaknorBot, Barking1, AndersBot, Tide rolls, Abosaleh911, Luckyz, Lasy, Luckas-bot, Yobot, Tohd8BohaithuGh1, Gls20, Fishface42, AnomieBOT, Wüstenfuchs, TechBot, Jmundo, MerlLinkBot, Spellage, NSH002, Rapsar, Fixer88, MrX, RjwilmsiBot, Bossanoven, Sandmanisgod123, Mmm333k, Bassedan, Sreifa, Thargor Orlando, Noodleki, Andersonward, Manytexts, ClueBot NG, RJFF, Frietjes, BG19bot, Vale of Glamorgan, Harizotoh9, Z&N, Quasimodealert, Peacemaker67, Hmainsbot1, British Socialist, TwoTwoHello, VIAFbot, Lekoren, PMChi, LukeApple, TheUFE, Absolute98, KasparBot, Biggins1989, Rahagen and Anonymous: 145

- **Hans Heinze** *Source:* https://en.wikipedia.org/wiki/Hans_Heinze?oldid=662718731 *Contributors:* FeanorStar7, AI, Mark Schierbecker, BG19bot, Eustachiusz, KasparBot and Anonymous: 1

- **Kurt Heissmeyer** *Source:* https://en.wikipedia.org/wiki/Kurt_Heissmeyer?oldid=684563035 *Contributors:* Grutness, SmackBot, Hmains, Guruboy, Cydebot, Deborahjay, Blue Tie, Waacstats, Rontrigger, Denisarona, ImageRemovalBot, Dubmill, Addbot, Sebastian scha., Shadowjams, NSH002, Trijnstel, RjwilmsiBot, 7mike5000, Bossanoven, John of Reading, Cobaltcigs, ClueBot NG, ChrisGualtieri, ÄDA - DÄP, VIAFbot, Dog only nose, KasparBot and Anonymous: 4

- **Erich Hippke** *Source:* https://en.wikipedia.org/wiki/Erich_Hippke?oldid=662700910 *Contributors:* Renata3, TLSuda, Waacstats, Wgolf, MoohanBOT, MrScorch6200, RACHNEL1000, Aguilus, KasparBot and Anonymous: 1

- **August Hirt** *Source:* https://en.wikipedia.org/wiki/August_Hirt?oldid=687675572 *Contributors:* Media lib, Oaktree b, Zinnmann, Rich Farmbrough, Bender235, Longhair, Sherurcij, GregorB, Deansfa, Ashmoo, Kbdank71, Rjwilmsi, Valentinian, YurikBot, BOT-Superzerocool, SmackBot, Harald88, Dahn, Koubiak, The Wrong Man, RCS, Cydebot, Bluespaceoddity2, CFCF, DadaNeem, Twinchester, Paris75000~enwiki, Joseph A. Spadaro, Le Pied-bot~enwiki, Monegasque, Richard David Ramsey, Mtsmallwood, Good Olfactory, Addbot, H92Bot, Ctruongngoc, PimRijkee, SassoBot, Auntieruth55, FrescoBot, Rogriv, Cramyourspam, Lotje, RjwilmsiBot, 7mike5000, Bossanoven, WikitanvirBot, Werieth, Halfdrag, Helpful Pixie Bot, Divingpetrel, Sapere aude22, VIAFbot, Monkbot, Edelseider, KasparBot and Anonymous: 18

- **Waldemar Hoven** *Source:* https://en.wikipedia.org/wiki/Waldemar_Hoven?oldid=676741517 *Contributors:* GCarty, Wernher, Jmabel, Fifelfoo, Kent Wang, Klemen Kocjancic, Zscout370, Haham hanuka, Sherurcij, Kbdank71, Rjwilmsi, Koavf, FlaBot, Doc glasgow, YurikBot, MadMax, Neurotoxic, Syrthiss, Resigua, Nlu, SmackBot, Welkinridge, Hmains, Chris the speller, Newsmare, Bezapt, Michael David, ArglebargleIV, Ser Amantio di Nicolao, Cydebot, AniMate, Thijs!bot, Mengela, HanzoHattori, Epeefleche, Waacstats, MisterBee1966, Paris75000~enwiki, Jackismybestfriend, VolkovBot, BOTijo, Polbot, Richard David Ramsey, Drmies, Auntof6, Mtsmallwood, Good Olfactory, Addbot, Mootros, AndersBot, Luckas-bot, Vlastimil Svoboda, IP7869, Jun Nijo, Full-date unlinking bot, Pbrower2a, RjwilmsiBot, Bossanoven, WikitanvirBot, Gilderien, Vincelord, Quote54, ÄDA - DÄP, KasparBot and Anonymous: 13

- **Jewish skeleton collection** *Source:* https://en.wikipedia.org/wiki/Jewish_skeleton_collection?oldid=688375038 *Contributors:* Secretlondon, Woohookitty, Mandarax, Peterlewis, Drlegendre, Cydebot, Lonenut2000, Eilish99, CommonsDelinker, TomCat4680, Boneyard90, Socrates2008, Addbot, Prairieplant, AnomieBOT, Dirk Mahsarski, JackieBot, Alexlange, Briony Coote, Omnipaedista, FrescoBot, NSH002, Lotje, 7mike5000, EmausBot, ClueBot NG, Austrianbird, Kim Traynor, Jckrgn600, Virago250, Dudenhofener, Grzegornadolski, Pincrete, Burning-Bright-in-the-Night, Hashi0707 and Anonymous: 25

- **Emil Kaschub** *Source:* https://en.wikipedia.org/wiki/Emil_Kaschub?oldid=642088976 *Contributors:* Grutness, Mangojuice, Kbdank71, FlaBot, Maunus, Hmains, Ser Amantio di Nicolao, Cydebot, Otto4711, DagosNavy, Waacstats, Kudpung, Firth m, Mtsmallwood, Addbot, Debresser, Luckas-bot, Yobot, Tea with toast and Anonymous: 1

- **Josef Klehr** *Source:* https://en.wikipedia.org/wiki/Josef_Klehr?oldid=659656253 *Contributors:* Kbdank71, Rjwilmsi, SmackBot, Soarhead77, GiantSnowman, Cydebot, AniMate, Biruitorul, WilliamH, Ericoides, Waacstats, MisterBee1966, Signalhead, Omegastar, WOSlinker, BotMultichill, Binksternet, Iohannes Animosus, Mtsmallwood, Baszkiewicz, Addbot, Vejvančický, Yobot, Materialscientist, Wroman, MerlLinkBot, DrilBot, RjwilmsiBot, Bossanoven, Vincelord, Helpful Pixie Bot, ÄDA - DÄP, VIAFbot, Monkbot, KasparBot and Anonymous: 2

- **Hans Wilhelm König** *Source:* https://en.wikipedia.org/wiki/Hans_Wilhelm_K%C3%B6nig?oldid=688241900 *Contributors:* Timrollpickering, RadioFan, Deor, OberRanks, Unbuttered Parsnip, Addbot, Bossanoven, ÄDA - DÄP, Beroniq91, KasparBot, TX6785 and Anonymous: 2

- **Eduard Krebsbach** *Source:* https://en.wikipedia.org/wiki/Eduard_Krebsbach?oldid=679695966 *Contributors:* Halibutt, Kbdank71, Rjwilmsi, Bgwhite, Nlu, SmackBot, Hmains, Ceplm, Cydebot, Waacstats, Fallschirmjäger, MisterBee1966, Thismightbezach, Kumioko, Auntof6, Alexbot, Mtsmallwood, Addbot, Yobot, GrouchoBot, LittleWink, 7mike5000, Bossanoven, GoingBatty, Frietjes, Vincelord, ÄDA - DÄP, Loose eel, KasparBot and Anonymous: 3

- **Johann Kremer** *Source:* https://en.wikipedia.org/wiki/Johann_Kremer?oldid=681569062 *Contributors:* Frecklefoot, Skysmith, Klemen Kocjancic, Maclean25, PWilkinson, Grutness, SlaveToTheWage, Kbdank71, Fnorp, Dysmorodrepanis~enwiki, SmackBot, HeartofaDog, Gilliam, Bluebot, Stevenmitchell, Vanisaac, Cydebot, AniMate, Thijs!bot, HanzoHattori, QuantumEngineer, Goral~enwiki, STBotD, Mtsmallwood, Good Olfactory, Addbot, Luckas-bot, Yobot, FrescoBot, Full-date unlinking bot, RjwilmsiBot, 7mike5000, Bossanoven, EmausBot, AvicAWB, Karl-Friedrich Boerne, ÄDA - DÄP, VIAFbot, Michaela.constant, Пробегающий, KasparBot and Anonymous: 11

- **Elisabeth Marschall** *Source:* https://en.wikipedia.org/wiki/Elisabeth_Marschall?oldid=656725141 *Contributors:* Kbdank71, Nlu, Rms125a@hotmail.com, SmackBot, Cydebot, AniMate, Magioladitis, Waacstats, Thismightbezach, Polbot, Brewcrewer, Mtsmallwood, SilvonenBot, MystBot, Good Olfactory, Addbot, Apothecaryrose, Luckas-bot, Yobot, Citation bot, RjwilmsiBot, Bossanoven, Helpful Pixie Bot, ÄDA - DÄP and Anonymous: 3

- **Josef Mengele** *Source:* https://en.wikipedia.org/wiki/Josef_Mengele?oldid=690238649 *Contributors:* AxelBoldt, Vicki Rosenzweig, Mav, The Anome, Danny, William Avery, SimonP, Shii, Mintguy, Olivier, Kchishol1970, D, Paul Barlow, Pit~enwiki, Kwertii, Dominus, Taras, IZAK, 6birc, Paul Benjamin Austin, Bplotter, Ahoerstemeier, Angela, Nahum, Marco Krohn, Error, Whkoh, Sugarfish, Evercat, Jengod, RodC, Reddi, Pladask, WhisperToMe, Zoicon5, ThomasStrohmann~enwiki, Tpbradbury, Maximus Rex, Furrykef, LMB, Zero0000, Wernher, Joy, Olathe, Johnleemk, Davidmaxwaterman, Owen, Dimadick, Kizor, Moncrief, Yelyos, Modulatum, Chris Roy, Mirv, Bertie, Gidonb, Hadal, Jsonitsac, Rege~enwiki, JackofOz, Wereon, Profoss, Fuelbottle, Kent Wang, Ruakh, Lupo, HaeB, Hcheney, Xanzzibar, Lysy, Yacine~enwiki, Fennec, Nikodemos, Barbara Shack, Philwelch, Tom harrison, Folks at 137, Fastfission, Everyking, Koifish, Gamaliel, Xinoph, Get-back-world-respect, Pascal666, AlistairMcMillan, Elmindreda, Sidar, Jackol, Nlaporte, Wmahan, Adenosine, Pinnecco, CryptoDerk, Sonjaaa, Antandrus, Beowulph, Loremaster, MylesCallum, Jossi, MacGyverMagic, Oneiros, DragonflySixtyseven, Rlquall, Bk0, Sam Hocevar, Creidieki, Neutrality, Joyous!, Michael L. Kaufman, TJSwoboda, Magnum1, Dcandeto, Klemen Kocjancic, Syvanen, Adashiel, Trevor MacInnis, Canterbury Tail, Gcanyon, Clubjuggle, Tasiel, Mike Rosoft, D6, Sdrawkcab, Jayjg, RedWordSmith, An Siarach, Discospinster, Rich Farmbrough, Sargant, Pie4all88, Kooo, Ivan Bajlo, Mjpieters, Antaeus Feldspar, GregoryWeir, MarkS, Bender235, Terrapin, Flapdragon, Kaisershatner, Johnh, Shrike, Twilight (renamed), Kwamikagami, Kross, Shanes, Wesman83, Percederberg, Jpgordon, Dom Lochet, Bobo192, DanielNuyu, Gatta, Smalljim, Meggilyweggily, Viriditas, Xevious, Vortexrealm, JeR, Ziggurat, Of~enwiki, Maxl, Haham hanuka, Benbread, Leifern, Petdance, Alan Isherwood, Phils, Jumbuck, Alansohn, JYolkowski, Anthony Appleyard, Sherurcij, MoO, Philip Cross, Rd232, Supine, DrBat, Ricky81682, Xanxz, Andrew Gray, Ashley Pomeroy, Lectonar, Gaurav1146, Bigjarom, MpegMan, Hohum, Snowolf, Melaen, Bbsrock, Binabik80, Msclguru, Randy Johnston, Mcmillin24, Dave.Dunford, Reaverdrop, Alai, Czolgolz, Duplode, Richard Weil, Dismas, Hijiri88, A D Monroe III, Richard Arthur Norton (1958-), Mel Etitis, OwenX, Woohookitty, Spamguy, Berti, LOL, Tomnason1010, MrWhipple, Zealander, MONGO, Kelisi, Terence, Optichan, Wayward, Toussaint, Gimboid13, Class316, Jordan Yang, Raybechard, Slugworth, Palica, Dynamax, Mirddes, Mandarax, RichardWeiss, Jebur~enwiki, Ashmoo, Graham87, Magister Mathematicae, Cuchullain, Qwertyus, Bunchofgrapes, CheshireKatz, Sjakkalle, Lhademmor, Rjwilmsi, Nightscream, Hitssquad, Rogerd, Panoptical, Ikh, Stephonovich, PatrickSaucy, JHMM13, Staecker, Sdornan, Feydey, Soakologist, Tawker, Sakkaro, UriBudnik, S Chapin, Mcauburn, CQJ, Boccobrock, Driscoth, Olessi, Sango123, Cassowary, Yamamoto Ichiro, Ansbachdragoner, Leithp, Disembodied, FlaBot, Vespertine27, Naraht, Ian Pitchford, RobertG, CalJW, Gtamber, Twipley, Who, Fragglet, AI, Lilmul123, Flowerparty, Blaster009, RexNL, Gurch, Eric Winesett, Quuxplusone, Wongm, Maustrauser, Kernitou, Manufracture, Chobot, Knobme3, Antilived, Jaraalbe, DVdm, VolatileChemical, Hall Monitor, Digitalme, Gwernol, The Rambling Man, YurikBot, Noclador, Phil Wardle, Tommyt, Sceptre, A.S. Brown, Hairy Dude, JarrahTree, RussBot, Xoloz, FrenchIsAwesome, Jtkiefer, Peter S., Anonymous editor, Witan, Farside6, Splash, Yllosubmarine, GusF, BillMasen, Dotancohen, Million Little Gods, Gaius Cornelius, Imladros, Wimt, Manxruler, NawlinWiki, Thomas E. Goodwin, G.G., Wiki alf, Mipadi, Obarskyr, NW036, Grafen, Jaxl, ONEder Boy, DavidMarsh, Dureo, Irishguy, Nick, Hybrid1486, Aaron Brenneman, Sir48, Trollderella, Azazell0, PhilipC, GeorgeC, Epa101, DGJM, Sirlearnsalot, Karl Meier, AdelaMae, CDA, DeadEyeArrow, Psy guy, Caspian, Tyler Mitchell, Essexmutant, Acetic Acid, Speedoflight, Phenz, Superluser, FF2010, Show no mercy, Ninly, Joshmaul, Bayerischermann, Flyerhell, Rms125a@hotmail.com, .cosme., Wiki brah, GraemeL, JoanneB, Fram, Arislan, HereToHelp, Anclation~enwiki, Spliffy, Curpsbot-unicodify, Kungfuadam, Dystopianray, Carlosguitar, DVD R W, Entheta, Fightindaman, SmackBot, Hux, Khaosaming, Slashme, InverseHypercube, KnowledgeOfSelf, Ma8thew, Chazz88, Hr2, Ze miguel, Unyoyega, Pgk, Korossyl, Tchernobog, Geno-Supremo, Anastrophe, Vanished user fij2093ju5mf8j23romsg, Jihiro, Mdd4696, Veesicle, Cessator, Kintetsubuffalo, Cheezisyum21, Master Deusoma, Robsomebody, SmartGuy Old, Moralis, Marktreut, JFHJr, Gilliam, Phizzy, Hmains, Bluenile, JorgePeixoto, Squiddy, GeorgeBuchanan, Scatr99, Xchrisblackx, SlimJim, Persian Poet Gal, MK8, Razwww, Canuckofithaca, Hibernian, Sadads, Colonies Chris, Gracenotes, Mordantkitten, Royboycrashfan, Zsinj, Chwilliam, Tsca.bot, Can't sleep, clown will eat me, DLCinMaine, Ww2censor, Rrburke, Spout, Addshore, Mr.Z-man, Celarnor, Phaedriel, Krich, Gabi S., Iapetus, Cybercobra, Nakon, Riff Raff, Aelffin, Dreadstar, Netofunk, Batman2005, EricSpokane, PStatic, The PIPE, Parrot of Doom, Where, Mwelch, Pilotguy, Kukini, Ohconfucius, Bouncingmolar, Blahm, YegerMeister, Esrever, Nishkid64, Rory096, Ser Amantio di Nicolao, Seelie, RASAM, JohnnyRuin, AmeriCan, JzG, AlanD, Sanya, Aplomado, Kuru, John, Carnby, Nowhy, Mcshadypl, Tazmaniacs, Iglew, Ocanter, Jefe619, RootBeerKisses, CPMcE, Pat Payne, Fleft, Linnell, Heini~enwiki, Kransky, Anand Karia, Fernando S. Aldado~enwiki, A. Parrot, JHunterJ, MarkSutton, Agathoclea, Penguify, Slakr, Werdan7, Noah Salzman, ILorbb, Jimmy Pitt, Mbisgaier, Stizz, Rorschach12, Meco, Vr, Ryulong, Lenn0r, Hu12, ThuranX, Tpalkki, Nonexistant User, HisSpaceResearch, Walton One, Gregory Benoit, Vocaro, Gopchristian, Redneck bigdog, Xchorusxromancex, Newyorkbrad, Pacerlaser, Courcelles, GiantSnowman, Wilhelm Wiesel, Eluchil404, LonelyPilgrim, JoannaSerah, Tawkerbot2, Andy120, Nitinblr, Ehistory, Daedalus969, TORR, Aizhen, Betaeleven, CmdrObot, Tanthalas39, Ale jrb, Wafulz, Sir Vicious, W guice, Maester mensch, Unottakeacrziichance, Xous, KnightLago, Dgw, OMGsplosion, Birdhurst, WeggeBot, Shizane, Neelix, Dthdc4, Proskauer, MrFish, Hemlock Martinis, Josephano, Multi-fauceted, Multifauceted, Kribbeh, Michfan2123, Cydebot, PeterPan23, Abeg92, PDTantisocial, Reywas92, Treybien, Jammy simpson, Anna manana, Wiknik, Wordbuilder, Lugnuts, Trident13, Schrodingers Mongoose, DumbBOT, Gulivar, Justincop, Knifeboy3, AJMW, JodyB, Iss246, Instaurare, PamD, Satori Son, Rab V, Trueblood, FanOfDegrassi, Thijs!bot, Epbr123, Supparluca, Smee, Mojo Hand, WilliamH, Hesperides, MsMojoRising, Massimo Macconi, Dead-Inside, Griffjam, Nirvana77, Philippe,

Microeconomia, Dawkeye, Big Bird, WhaleyTim, Robert Ham, Dlh15, Sean William, Afabbro, MachoCarioca, Cladeal832, AntiVandal-Bot, BokicaK, Yonatan, Mengela, Seaphoto, QuiteUnusual, Bigtimepeace, Shirt58, Tomakaangus, Smith2006, AaronY, Dr who1975, James steeth, Fayenatic london, Doc cadence, MECU, Mr. Yooper, Gohnarch, MikeLynch, DagosNavy, Ser4ph, HanzoHattori, JAnDbot, Do-gru144, The penfool, MER-C, Stephencraigen, Amoruso, Instinct, Kerror, Bostonboy3, Chicagoboy3, Plm209, Andonic, Hut 8.5, Meeowow, Pj44300, Cf014i6283, Acroterion, Waitsian, Magioladitis, Connormah, Dodo19~enwiki, Bennybp, Bongwarrior, VoABot II, Weebiloobil, Ishikawa Minoru, Liverpool Scouse, JNW, Cypher056E, Aquinate~enwiki, Morbid Angel83, Sojourner001, Waacstats, Twsx, Tokul, Froid, ChristinaDunigan, Hekerui, Catgut, Animum, Cgingold, 28421u2232nfenfcenc, Trevgreg, Spellmaster, Jonesl84, Cliché guevara, Grimgerde, Smartings, ShaunProm, Cdecoro, PsyMar, MartinBot, SolitaryWolf, RapaNui75, Quickmythril, Rockerdude716, B33R, Timoteostewart, Coo-liorobert, RFM57, Nooddawgg, Rettetast, Mitch.sc, InnocuousPseudonym, Birdie, SeeYa32, Bus stop, R'n'B, CommonsDelinker, Nono64, LittleOldMe old, Lilac Soul, Chipdukes, Tgeairn, Dinkytown, RockMFR, J.delanoy, Jahanas, DrKay, Trusilver, Hlnodovic, Parp555, Bo-gey97, Sp3000, Rsreston, Uncle Dick, STANE, Hodja Nasreddin, Octopus-Hands, Jahredtobin, TomCat4680, EH74DK, Andy5421, Being blunt, Katalaveno, LordAnubisBOT, JayFout, Andrej Kvasnica, Dexter prog, ElectricValkyrie, Congram, AntiSpamBot, ChainSuck-Jimmy, HiLo48, GhostPirate, Alexb102072, Hut 6.5, NewEnglandYankee, Cadwaladr, Taxico, DadaNeem, SJP, Thesis4Eva, Maidenslayer, Macar-rones, JHeinonen, T3hllama, Prhartcom, KylieTastic, Barfunkle, Cometstyles, DarkSaber2k, Jimokay, The great rd, Namekal, Dmx100, Misha-Pan, Ja 62, AndreasJSbot, CA387, Scottydude, Nattfodd, Xiahou, Idioma-bot, Fr33kman, Wikieditor06, Sam Blacketer, Malik Shabazz, Deor, 28bytes, VolkovBot, CWii, Coolman19876545, Zell IW, Himmler14meensmyage, ABF, Viral Slayer, Holme053, Mesmacat, AlnoktaBOT, Gab.popp, Dom Kaos, Toddy1, Philip Trueman, Sağlamcı, Mcjohnz, TXiKiBoT, KevinTR, Vipinhari, CrashingWave, Hayden5650, Rei-bot, Zizibo, Charley sweeney, Doglover2352, Awsemo426, Steven J. Anderson, Cicaneo, Iowamutt, Corvus cornix, SGT141, Gorgon5555, Hoo Hoo Howie!, Familienoriginalbenutzer~enwiki, Josephabradshaw, Jimmybuffet5, Rumiton, Emre43, Pegaroo88, Madhero88, Captain-gup, Doug, Gustav Lindwall, Silent52, Plutonium27, TheLoverly, Kittenlvr, Ivanushka~enwiki, Falcon8765, Piratedan, Anna512, Burntsauce, BOTijo, Insanity Incarnate, Northfox, Sarevok1, Krautukie, MetalA, Anickle060193, Chergles, Dusti, OberRanks, OGOL, Caulde, Moon-riddengirl, Scarian, Morcus, Schizodelight, Dawn Bard, Karaboom, Wadey4, AFrayMo~enwiki, Quasso, Dinlo juk, BlackSlivers, Mjiadzki, Calabraxthis, Til Eulenspiegel, Oda Mari, Sue Wallace, Monegasque, Strodie, JSpung, Jocedun, Oxymoron83, Jack1956, Antonio Lopez, Harry~enwiki, Steven Crossin, Senor Cuete, Ks0stm, Alex.muller, WacoJacko, Ahangar-e-Gaz, Joaopchagas2, Seventh Ares, JohnSawyer, Spitfire19, Mariaflores1955, MadmanBot, Janggeom, Cyfal, Pinkadelica, Richard David Ramsey, Canglesea, Shlimozzle, Kanonkas, Isthatyou-johnwayneisthisme, Explicit, Steve, RegentsPark, Kobi13, ClueBot, Foxj, The Thing That Should Not Be, All Hallow's Wraith, Rodhullandemu, General Epitaph, Rise Above the Vile, Sierenia, Maru-Spanish, Drmies, Kamix, Pucko67~enwiki, Boing! said Zebedee, OfficeBoy, BANZ111, Otolemur crassicaudatus, Trivialist, Klazno4, Oswego Palomar, Arunsingh16, Puchiko, JustinClarkCasey, Brewcrewer, Dreamspeaker, Ex-cirial, Socrates2008, Jusdafax, Aliasfoxtrot, Jammy0002, John Nevard, Nsmb2, Lartoven, MacedonianBoy, Renzo Grosso, SaneSerenity, Jumanji656, M.O.X, Mtsmallwood, Razorflame, Nicholasweed, 6afraidof7, Polly, Another Believer, John Paul Parks, Thingg, Lindberg, Hell-stomper, Aitias, Clippership, Cajunsauce, Versus22, Berean Hunter, Shamanchill, DumZiBoT, Finalnight, InternetMeme, Fastily, Spitfire, Jthughes01, Jdellaro, WillOakland, Doc9871, Shakalooloo Doom, PL290, Truetom, Paragon of Arctic Winter Nights, Mrthomas333, Ar-taxerxes, Kaiwhakahaere, Rexroad2, Shahinrani, Julystana77, RomanSoldier9001, Ktmrider628, Chasnor15, Addbot, Cheka92, Shaunrobert-smith78, Willking1979, Manuel Trujillo Berges, Some jerk on the Internet, Signthis, Ave Caesar, SnoopleCats, CATMANDOOOOO, Binary TSO, Magus732, VbCrLf, Blethering Scot, Bkmays, Ronhjones, SHarold, PlumCrumbleAndCustard, GD 6041, Menne12345, CanadianLin-uxUser, Fluffernutter, Zanzibar666, Ka Faraq Gatri, Orange Carrot, Benjomania, Ebaumsworlddotcom001, Download, Glane23, Debresser, SteveLaino, Favonian, Setwisohi, Theking17825, Tide rolls, Luckas Blade, Marksdaman, Ben Ben, Legobot, Luckas-bot, Yobot, Discourseur, Fraggle81, Donfbreed, Evans1982, The Earwig, Reenem, Matanya, Mr T (Based), Hadding, IW.HG, BeBoldInEdits, Magog the Ogre, Anony-mous from the 21th century, AnomieBOT, Mike Hayes, Hairhorn, Peril, Crecy99, RandomAct, Materialscientist, Eeems, E2eamon, Eumolpo, Keystoneridin, Clark89, Quebec99, Gsmgm, FreeRangeFrog, Xqbot, Zad68, Sionus, St.nerol, Alexlange, Capricorn42, Baseballjarrett, Weath-ergirl123, Jsharpminor, Tyrol5, Srich32977, WotWeiller, Vasant56, Horroroftheteenagelobstercello, J04n, C+C, REVUpminster, Alumnum, Omnipaedista, Anotherclown, Mvaldemar, NOLA504ever, Zeldakitten, Doulos Christos, Zzzlugnut, Gtamob69, Thatdoodwithglasses, Peliri-rojo778, E0steven, 🔲, X-ponerd20, Erik9, Mjasfca, ProfessorThompson, Green Cardamom, Dan6hell66, Hemuln, Accretianboy, FrescoBot, Facefartmaster, NAKALAK, Surv1v4l1st, Kierzek, Tobby72, Rrrick333, Tobetheman, KMFDM Fan, Super soaker15, HJ Mitchell, CHARG-ERLEVANI, Ghouse78, Weetoddid, Pxos, Citation bot 1, RaveDog, DrilBot, Alonso de Mendoza, Tinton5, Wikitanvir, VenomousConcept, Cramyourspam, NFSreloaded, Wusha, Vrenator, Thesniperremix, Dcs002, Cassianto, Reaper Eternal, Ktlynch, Diannaa, ThinkEnemies, Tb-hotch, Stianh22, DARTH SIDIOUS 2, RjwilmsiBot, Bento00, Bossanoven, Beyond My Ken, Polylepsis, Immunize, Dadaist6174, Nerissa-Marie, GoingBatty, Smitty1337, Bt8257, Tommy2010, TEHodson, Wikipelli, Mikemacdee, BurtAlert, Cogiati, Illegitimate Barrister, Bongo-ramsey, Fæ, Josve05a, Countess of Landsfield, ElationAviation, Anir1uph, AOC25, Dunblas, Davisdigi, Laelius Linguae, Drcjel, Icehouse-Cover, Ikemanfow, Wingman417, Jonathan Snack, Gratkkk, Usb10, Ego White Tray, Mystichumwipe, Razzattack, Mcc1789, AxMan11, 19thPharaoh, Brutal Adept, Winnipeger16, ClueBot NG, Serasuna, FourLights, WPWWHH1488, Jkta97, Slartibartfastibast, Crassybassy, Joetlawrence2004, Goochgooch, Widr, PaoloNapolitano, Pudge MclameO, LucasNHall, Jjmax5, StrawberryGURL, Helpful Pixie Bot, Aten-staedt, Newyork1501, LiLKingDog, Calabe1992, Jackdawson1970, Hengist Pod, Lowercase sigmabot, BG19bot, Arnavchaudhary, MariceEt-tlinCaro, Meepiemcmeep, Julien16, Msaunier, Neil Gibbons, MusikAnimal, Kendall-K1, Badon, AwamerT, Virago250, Piguy101, Inves-tigativeReporter, J R Gainey, Lolo7890, Slushy9, Jorgealamilla, Glacialfox, Hoiguy, Loudmoner, Masonfreemason, Echolima47, Trishawiki, Alexandra Golda, Vanished user lt94ma34le12, Fraulein451, Jimw338, Calebgeske, Mediran, Tandrum, Bardrick, Ekren, Lindsla, ÄDA -DÄP, Dexbot, Mogism, DJ-Joker16, Cuddyc, UselessToRemain, Dirk Küchmeister, Edmond Honda, VIAFbot, Zakr07, 93, Silverback2173, BrokenArticlesLOL, Isaacshackleford, BirgittaMTh, Beppo911, Epicgenius, Mr. Watson (before the phd), Figfoe89, Marchino61, Comp.arch, Prokaryotes, Pietro13, Hitcher vs. Candyman, Jonas Vinther, Marcest19xx, MCarsten, Elmeanopeno, Filedelinkerbot, Signthis1, Gfdsasd, Liz-zles86, TridiaChaplain, Youngdrake, Peralta2305, Cirflow, Lux ex Tenebris, KasparBot, TX6785 and Anonymous: 1507

- **Joachim Mrugowsky** *Source:* https://en.wikipedia.org/wiki/Joachim_Mrugowsky?oldid=660620067 *Contributors:* GCarty, Wernher, Ha-ham hanuka, Sherurcij, Fitzner, A D Monroe III, Kbdank71, Koavf, Leithp, FlaBot, Jared Preston, Syrthiss, Arria Belli, Nlu, SmackBot, AaronRichard, MooseMan1342, Jac16888, Cydebot, AniMate, Barticus88, Mengela, Waacstats, VolkovBot, TXiKiBoT, BOTijo, Mone-gasque, Alexbot, Mtsmallwood, Leia, SilvonenBot, Good Olfactory, Addbot, Lightbot, Omnipaedista, Hushpuckena, Jonkerz, RjwilmsiBot, Bossanoven, ZéroBot, VIAFbot, Tiddle the pips, KasparBot and Anonymous: 5

- **Herta Oberheuser** *Source:* https://en.wikipedia.org/wiki/Herta_Oberheuser?oldid=690209354 *Contributors:* Liftarn, IZAK, Ahoerstemeier, Kingturtle, Schneelocke, David.Monniaux, Owen, Lupo, HaeB, Edsanville, Kate, D6, Guanabot, Aranel, Fitzner, Kbdank71, Rjwilmsi, FlaBot,

- **Ludwig Stumpfegger** *Source:* https://en.wikipedia.org/wiki/Ludwig_Stumpfegger?oldid=660346158 *Contributors:* Paul Barlow, GCarty, PBS, Wyss, Necrothesp, Rich Farmbrough, Chowells, Sherurcij, ProhibitOnions, Mutt, BD2412, Kbdank71, Rjwilmsi, Olessi, Tswold, Elmer Clark, RussBot, Arria Belli, Resigua, CWenger, SmackBot, David Kernow, Hmains, Chris the speller, TheGeck0, Ser Amantio di Nicolao, Zeraeph, Kransky, Wheeltapper, Brownlee, Cydebot, Hydraton31, Jackyd101, AniMate, Cnhardman, Thijs!bot, Barticus88, Edwardx, Escarbot, Tishers, Desertsky85451, Pzg Ratzinger, Magioladitis, Waacstats, FruitMonkey, MisterBee1966, Thismightbezach, TXiKiBoT, Mrzubrow, Mkpumphrey, Dirkbb, Politics rule, Flyer22 Reborn, SallyForth123, Joao Xavier, Mtsmallwood, Avi1111, Addbot, Lightbot, Luckas-bot, AnomieBOT, C2equalA2plusB2, ArthurBot, Brad101AWB, Kierzek, Ver-bot, Trappist the monk, RjwilmsiBot, Bossanoven, WikitanvirBot, Bahavd Gita, IluvatarBot, ÄDA - DÄP, VIAFbot, Captainmad, Kotjap, KasparBot and Anonymous: 19

- **Alfred Trzebinski** *Source:* https://en.wikipedia.org/wiki/Alfred_Trzebinski?oldid=688242146 *Contributors:* Kbdank71, Manxruler, Nlu, SmackBot, Iridescent, Tsf, Ryanjo, Cydebot, Tec15, Otto4711, Nabokov, Hypnosadist, Almanacer, Waacstats, Ekki01, MisterBee1966, Thismightbezach, Deor, Monegasque, Plastikspork, Mtsmallwood, Addbot, Sebastian scha., Debresser, Yobot, PMLawrence, GODKING OF ICE CERBERUS WERE-GARURUMON, Citation bot 1, RjwilmsiBot, Bossanoven, DASHBot, Marrante, SporkBot, Toshio Yamaguchi, Frietjes, Pippi553, ÄDA - DÄP, VIAFbot, Monkbot, KasparBot, TX6785 and Anonymous: 17

- **Carl Værnet** *Source:* https://en.wikipedia.org/wiki/Carl_V%C3%A6rnet?oldid=667274690 *Contributors:* Necrothesp, Holdek, Geschichte, Wtmitchell, Stephan Leeds, Twthmoses, Kbdank71, BorgHunter, Rjwilmsi, Ecelan, Valentinian, YurikBot, Friedfish, Manxruler, Kisch, Shawnc, T. Anthony, Garion96, SmackBot, Squiddy, Rex Germanus, Sounirvalice, Wuzzy, Tazmaniacs, Pudeo, CmdrObot, Cydebot, AniMate, Treybien, Otto4711, Nsaum75, Kingstowngalway, Qwerty Binary, Waacstats, Broadbot, StAnselm, Knorpel, Fadesga, Saddhiyama, Mtsmallwood, Skoojal, MystBot, Addbot, Debresser, Luckas-bot, Yobot, AnomieBOT, Rockypedia, Chuckiesdad, Wikignome0529, Amaury, Kierzek, Meishern, Garrythefish, Alec Fischer, TobeBot, Lukaschek, RjwilmsiBot, Bossanoven, Exok, ZéroBot, ClueBot NG, Helpful Pixie Bot, BG19bot, MisterMorton, Griot-de, Delotrooladoo, VIAFbot, O revolucionário aliado, Buyers remorse, KasparBot and Anonymous: 21

- **Werner Villinger** *Source:* https://en.wikipedia.org/wiki/Werner_Villinger?oldid=670073755 *Contributors:* Edward, Irmgard, Rebrane, Darwinek, Pearle, Kbdank71, Exeunt, AI, BirgitteSB, SmackBot, Robth, DavidCooke, Keith-264, Cydebot, AniMate, Jammy simpson, Otto4711, Mengela, Nono64, Mark v1.0, BOTijo, Rjd0060, Straightway, Mtsmallwood, Gennarous, Addbot, Magus732, LaaknorBot, Debresser, Lightbot, SoiledDishcloth, Pflastertreter, RjwilmsiBot, Bossanoven, Furor Teutonicus, Decathlete, VIAFbot, OccultZone, KasparBot and Anonymous: 2

- **Gerhard Wagner (physician)** *Source:* https://en.wikipedia.org/wiki/Gerhard_Wagner_(physician)?oldid=660247898 *Contributors:* Dimadick, Donarreiskoffer, Kelisi, Kbdank71, Rjwilmsi, Olessi, Str1977, RussBot, SmackBot, Colonies Chris, Neddyseagoon, Cydebot, Goldfritha, Otto4711, Doug Weller, Barticus88, HanzoHattori, Nono64, Deor, Richard David Ramsey, De728631, Niceguyedc, PixelBot, Mtsmallwood, Addbot, Debresser, Lightbot, Yobot, Kierzek, HRoestBot, Full-date unlinking bot, RjwilmsiBot, Bossanoven, ZéroBot, AvicAWB, Pehazet, Morgis, Decathlete, VIAFbot, Lekoren, KasparBot and Anonymous: 6

- **Albert Widmann** *Source:* https://en.wikipedia.org/wiki/Albert_Widmann?oldid=687332591 *Contributors:* Cydebot, Waacstats, Gr8opinionater, AnomieBOT, Materialscientist, Kierzek, Bossanoven, EmausBot, ÄDA - DÄP, Loose eel, KasparBot and Anonymous: 3

- **Eduard Wirths** *Source:* https://en.wikipedia.org/wiki/Eduard_Wirths?oldid=688242235 *Contributors:* Skysmith, Dimadick, Jokestress, Keresaspa, Rich Farmbrough, ToastieIL, Woohookitty, Tabletop, Kbdank71, FlaBot, Blaster009, Volunteer Marek, Agamemnon2, Closedmouth, SmackBot, C.Fred, Hmains, Squiddy, Kingsbury, Hgrosser, Michael David, Cydebot, AniMate, Otto4711, Nabokov, AJMW, Epbr123, WilliamH, Klepas, Escarbot, Mengela, HanzoHattori, Gavia immer, Magioladitis, Waacstats, Jackson Peebles, EyeSerene, Alro, Dexter prog, Plasticup, DadaNeem, MisterBee1966, DH85868993, Deor, Abberley2, Brenont, Typritc, Monegasque, Bernd Michael Uhl, Polbot, Panyd, Mtsmallwood, Spitfire, Addbot, Some jerk on the Internet, Sebastian scha., LaaknorBot, Debresser, Luckas-bot, Yobot, AnomieBOT, Ulric1313, Alexlange, Kierzek, LucienBOT, Jun Nijo, My very best wishes, Full-date unlinking bot, RjwilmsiBot, Bossanoven, ZéroBot, Robartinc, Mystichumwipe, ClueBot NG, Scanner man, Dudenhofener, ÄDA - DÄP, ColonelHenry, VIAFbot, DavidLeighEllis, Comp.arch, JLHicks, KasparBot, Jdh1234, TX6785 and Anonymous: 38

53.8.2 Images

- **File:66935A.jpeg** *Source:* https://upload.wikimedia.org/wikipedia/commons/5/51/Child_survivors_of_Auschwitz.jpeg *License:* Public domain *Contributors:* USHMM/Belarusian State Archive of Documentary Film and Photography http://collections.ushmm.org/search/catalog/pa14532 *Original artist:* Alexander Voronzow and others in his group, ordered by Mikhael Oschurkow, head of the photography unit

- **File:Aribert_Heim.jpg** *Source:* https://upload.wikimedia.org/wikipedia/en/8/8c/Aribert_Heim.jpg *License:* Fair use *Contributors:* Immediate source: www.Standard.co.uk *Original artist:* Historical portrait

- **File:Auschwitz-Birkenau_Hauptgebäude.jpg** *Source:* https://upload.wikimedia.org/wikipedia/commons/c/ce/Auschwitz-Birkenau_Hauptgeb%C3%A4ude.jpg *License:* CC BY-SA 3.0 *Contributors:* Own work *Original artist:* Diether

- **File:Auschwitz_Mengele_Block_10.jpg** *Source:* https://upload.wikimedia.org/wikipedia/commons/e/e5/Auschwitz_Mengele_Block_10.jpg *License:* GFDL *Contributors:* Own work *Original artist:* VbCrLf

- **File:BU_003749.jpeg** *Source:* https://upload.wikimedia.org/wikipedia/commons/7/7d/BU_003749.jpeg *License:* Public domain *Contributors:* This is photograph BU 3749 from the collections of the Imperial War Museums. *Original artist:* Malindine E G (Capt) No 5 Army Film and Photographic Unit, British Army

- **File:Balkenkreuz.svg** *Source:* https://upload.wikimedia.org/wikipedia/commons/1/1f/Balkenkreuz.svg *License:* Public domain *Contributors:* German Junkers Ju 52 Messerschmitt Me-262

Own work and also based on Page 49 of

Original artist: David Liuzzo

- **File:Dachau_cold_water_immersion.jpg** *Source:* https://upload.wikimedia.org/wikipedia/en/4/4c/Dachau_cold_water_immersion.jpg *License:* Fair use *Contributors:*

  Taken from: Hanauske-Abel, Hartmut M. "Not a Slippery Slope or Sudden Subversion: German Medicine and National Socialism in 1933." *BMJ: British Medical Journal* 313(7070): 1453-1463. 7 December 1996. The journal does not claim ownership of the copyright. *Original artist:* ?

- **File:Edit-clear.svg** *Source:* https://upload.wikimedia.org/wikipedia/en/f/f2/Edit-clear.svg *License:* Public domain *Contributors:* The *Tango! Desktop Project. Original artist:*

  The people from the Tango! project. And according to the meta-data in the file, specifically: "Andreas Nilsson, and Jakub Steiner (although minimally)."

- **File:Elisabeth_Klein.jpg** *Source:* https://upload.wikimedia.org/wikipedia/commons/e/e1/Elisabeth_Klein.jpg *License:* Public domain *Contributors:*

- http://www.holocaust-history.org/hirt/ *Original artist:* Unknown

- **File:Esclapius_stick.svg** *Source:* https://upload.wikimedia.org/wikipedia/commons/7/7a/Esclapius_stick.svg *License:* Public domain *Contributors:* No machine-readable source provided. Own work assumed (based on copyright claims). *Original artist:* No machine-readable author provided. Melian assumed (based on copyright claims).

- **File:Escola_Bullenhuser_Damm.jpg** *Source:* https://upload.wikimedia.org/wikipedia/commons/5/50/Escola_Bullenhuser_Damm.jpg *License:* CC BY-SA 3.0 *Contributors:* Own work *Original artist:* flamenc

- **File:Flag_Schutzstaffel.svg** *Source:* https://upload.wikimedia.org/wikipedia/commons/3/33/Flag_Schutzstaffel.svg *License:* Public domain *Contributors:* Flag Schutzstaffel.gif: <a href='//commons.wikimedia.org/wiki/File:Flag_Schutzstaffel.gif' class='image'><img alt='Flag Schutzstaffel.gif' src='https://upload.wikimedia.org/wikipedia/commons/thumb/1/1c/Flag_Schutzstaffel.gif/18px-Flag_Schutzstaffel.gif' width='18' height='12' srcset='https://upload.wikimedia.org/wikipedia/commons/thumb/1/1c/Flag_Schutzstaffel.gif/27px-Flag_Schutzstaffel.gif 1.5x, https://upload.wikimedia.org/wikipedia/commons/thumb/1/1c/Flag_Schutzstaffel.gif/36px-Flag_Schutzstaffel.gif 2x' data-file-width='324' data-file-height='216' /></a> *Original artist:* NielsF

- **File:Flag_of_Austria.svg** *Source:* https://upload.wikimedia.org/wikipedia/commons/4/41/Flag_of_Austria.svg *License:* Public domain *Contributors:* Own work, http://www.bmlv.gv.at/abzeichen/dekorationen.shtml *Original artist:* User:SKopp

- **File:Flag_of_Denmark.svg** *Source:* https://upload.wikimedia.org/wikipedia/commons/9/9c/Flag_of_Denmark.svg *License:* Public domain *Contributors:* Own work *Original artist:* User:Madden

- **File:Flag_of_German_Reich_(1935–1945).svg** *Source:* https://upload.wikimedia.org/wikipedia/commons/9/99/Flag_of_German_Reich_%281935%E2%80%931945%29.svg *License:* Public domain *Contributors:* Own work *Original artist:* Fornax

- **File:Flag_of_Germany.svg** *Source:* https://upload.wikimedia.org/wikipedia/en/b/ba/Flag_of_Germany.svg *License:* PD *Contributors:* ? *Original artist:* ?

- **File:Flag_of_Germany_(3-2_aspect_ratio).svg** *Source:* https://upload.wikimedia.org/wikipedia/commons/8/86/Flag_of_Germany_%283-2_aspect_ratio%29.svg *License:* Public domain *Contributors:* Own work *Original artist:* User:Mmxxxxxxxx

- **File:Flag_of_the_German_Empire.svg** *Source:* https://upload.wikimedia.org/wikipedia/commons/e/ec/Flag_of_the_German_Empire.svg *License:* Public domain *Contributors:* Recoloured Image:Flag of Germany (2-3).svg *Original artist:* User:B1mbo and User:Madden

- **File:Flag_of_the_NSDAP_(1920–1945).svg** *Source:* https://upload.wikimedia.org/wikipedia/commons/c/cf/Flag_of_the_NSDAP_%281920%E2%80%931945%29.svg *License:* Public domain *Contributors:* Original PNG version created by de:Benutzer:Kookaburra with the name "Bild: Flag Germany 1933.png" in de.wikipedia; uploaded to the Wikimedia Commons by User:Guanaco, later converted to SVG by User:Rotemliss and later modified by other Wikimedia Commons people. *Original artist:* ?

- **File:Folder_Hexagonal_Icon.svg** *Source:* https://upload.wikimedia.org/wikipedia/en/4/48/Folder_Hexagonal_Icon.svg *License:* Cc-by-sa-3.0 *Contributors:* ? *Original artist:* ?

- **File:Fritz_Fischer_KZ-Arzt.jpg** *Source:* https://upload.wikimedia.org/wikipedia/commons/a/a9/Fritz_Fischer_KZ-Arzt.jpg *License:* Public domain *Contributors:* http://www.ushmm.org/uia-cgi/uia_query/photos?hr=null&query=kw163389 *Original artist:* USHMM, courtesy of Hedwig Wachenheimer Epstein

- **File:George_Lincoln_Rockwell.jpg** *Source:* https://upload.wikimedia.org/wikipedia/commons/b/bc/George_Lincoln_Rockwell.jpg *License:* Public domain *Contributors:* Freedom of Information Act material, NPRC *Original artist:* United States Navy

- **File:Gerh_Rose.jpg** *Source:* https://upload.wikimedia.org/wikipedia/commons/4/40/Gerh_Rose.jpg *License:* Public domain *Contributors:* USHMM [Photograph #07324] *Original artist:* USHMM, courtesy of Hedwig Wachenheimer Epstein

- **File:Gerhard_Rose_during_the_Doctors_Trial.jpg** *Source:* https://upload.wikimedia.org/wikipedia/commons/a/aa/Gerhard_Rose_during_the_Doctors_Trial.jpg *License:* Public domain *Contributors:* Image from the USHMM, courtesy U.S. National Archives. *Original artist:* Unknown

- **File:Hadamar_012.JPG** *Source:* https://upload.wikimedia.org/wikipedia/commons/6/6f/Hadamar_012.JPG *License:* CC BY 3.0 *Contributors:* Own work *Original artist:* Frank Winkelmann

- **File:Hans-Reiter.jpg** *Source:* https://upload.wikimedia.org/wikipedia/commons/d/df/Hans-Reiter.jpg *License:* CC BY-SA 4.0 *Contributors:* Own work *Original artist:* Ahmed H Elbestawey

- **File:Helmut_Poppendick.jpg** *Source:* https://upload.wikimedia.org/wikipedia/commons/c/cd/Helmut_Poppendick.jpg *License:* Public domain *Contributors:* USHMM [Photograph #07322] *Original artist:* USHMM, courtesy of Hedwig Wachenheimer Epstein

- **File:Herta_Oberheuser.jpg** *Source:* https://upload.wikimedia.org/wikipedia/commons/6/68/Herta_Oberheuser.jpg *License:* Public domain *Contributors:* ? *Original artist:* ?

- **File:Rod_of_Asclepius2.svg** *Source:* https://upload.wikimedia.org/wikipedia/commons/e/e3/Rod_of_Asclepius2.svg *License:* CC BY-SA 3.0 *Contributors:* This file was derived from: Rod of asclepius.png
  Original artist:

- Original: CatherinMunro

- **File:Rudolf_Brandt_(SS-Mitglied).jpg** *Source:* https://upload.wikimedia.org/wikipedia/commons/b/b6/Rudolf_Brandt_%28SS-Mitglied% 29.jpg *License:* Public domain *Contributors:* http://www.ushmm.org/uia-cgi/uia_doc/photos/1175?hr=null *Original artist:* USHMM, courtesy of Hedwig Wachenheimer Epstein

- **File:SS-Hauptsturmführer_Collar_Rank.svg** *Source:* https://upload.wikimedia.org/wikipedia/commons/4/4b/SS-Hauptsturmf%C3%BChrer_ Collar_Rank.svg *License:* CC BY-SA 3.0 *Contributors:* Own work *Original artist:* Mintz l

- **File:SS-Obersturmbannführer.svg** *Source:* https://upload.wikimedia.org/wikipedia/commons/c/cd/SS-Obersturmbannf%C3%BChrer.svg *License:* CC BY-SA 2.0 fr *Contributors:* Own work *Original artist:* Rama

- **File:SS-Sturmbannführer_collar.svg** *Source:* https://upload.wikimedia.org/wikipedia/commons/0/09/SS-Sturmbannf%C3%BChrer_collar. svg *License:* CC BY-SA 3.0 *Contributors:* Own work *Original artist:* Mintz l

- **File:Scientist.svg** *Source:* https://upload.wikimedia.org/wikipedia/commons/0/03/Scientist.svg *License:* CC-BY-SA-3.0 *Contributors:* Own work *Original artist:* Viktorvoigt

- **File:Selection_Birkenau_ramp.jpg** *Source:* https://upload.wikimedia.org/wikipedia/commons/8/89/Selection_Birkenau_ramp.jpg *License:* Public domain *Contributors:* Yad Vashem. The album was donated to Yad Vashem by Lili Jacob, a survivor, who found it in the Mittelbau-Dora concentration camp in 1945. *Original artist:* Unknown. Several sources believe the photographer to have been Ernst Hoffmann or Bernhard Walter of the SS

- **File:Sergio_de_Desimone.jpg** *Source:* https://upload.wikimedia.org/wikipedia/en/5/5f/Sergio_de_Desimone.jpg *License:* ? *Contributors:* http://blog.edidablog.it/files/Image/il%20raglio%20del%20prof/desimone.jpg *Original artist:*
  Unknown

- **File:Siegfried_Handloser_NS-Arzt.jpg** *Source:* https://upload.wikimedia.org/wikipedia/commons/1/1d/Siegfried_Handloser_NS-Arzt.jpg *License:* Public domain *Contributors:* http://www.ushmm.org/uia-cgi/uia_doc/photos/1178?hr=null *Original artist:* USHMM

- **File:Speaker_Icon.svg** *Source:* https://upload.wikimedia.org/wikipedia/commons/2/21/Speaker_Icon.svg *License:* Public domain *Contributors:* No machine-readable source provided. Own work assumed (based on copyright claims). *Original artist:* No machine-readable author provided. Mobius assumed (based on copyright claims).

- **File:Stefan_Krikl-01.jpg** *Source:* https://upload.wikimedia.org/wikipedia/commons/3/32/Stefan_Krikl-01.jpg *License:* CC BY-SA 2.0 *Contributors:* Portrait /closeup/, one of several: Dr.Carl Clauberg "The beast" *Original artist:* stefan krikl from Orange County, USA

- **File:Strasbourg_Hôpital_civil_plaque_institut_anatomie.jpg** *Source:* https://upload.wikimedia.org/wikipedia/commons/c/c4/Strasbourg_ H%C3%B4pital_civil_plaque_institut_anatomie.jpg *License:* CC BY-SA 3.0 *Contributors:* Own work *Original artist:* <a href='//commons. wikimedia.org/wiki/User:Ctruongngoc' title='User:Ctruongngoc'>**Photo Claude TRUONG-NGOC**</a>

- **File:Struthof.PNG** *Source:* https://upload.wikimedia.org/wikipedia/commons/2/22/Struthof.PNG *License:* GFDL *Contributors:* No machine-readable source provided. Own work assumed (based on copyright claims). *Original artist:* No machine-readable author provided. Edelseider assumed (based on copyright claims).

- **File:Text_document_with_red_question_mark.svg** *Source:* https://upload.wikimedia.org/wikipedia/commons/a/a4/Text_document_with_ red_question_mark.svg *License:* Public domain *Contributors:* Created by bdesham with Inkscape; based upon Text-x-generic.svg from the Tango project. *Original artist:* Benjamin D. Esham (bdesham)

- **File:Translation_to_english_arrow.svg** *Source:* https://upload.wikimedia.org/wikipedia/commons/8/8a/Translation_to_english_arrow.svg *License:* CC-BY-SA-3.0 *Contributors:* Transferred from en.wikipedia; transferred to Commons by User:Faigl.ladislav using CommonsHelper. *Original artist:* tkgd2007. Original uploader was Tkgd2007 at en.wikipedia

- **File:User_icon_1.svg** *Source:* https://upload.wikimedia.org/wikipedia/commons/0/04/User_icon_1.svg *License:* Public domain *Contributors:* Ripped directly from the Tango project's System-users.svg by bdesham. *Original artist:* Benjamin D. Esham (bdesham)

- **File:WP_Josef_Mengele_1956.jpg** *Source:* https://upload.wikimedia.org/wikipedia/commons/1/19/WP_Josef_Mengele_1956.jpg *License:* Public domain *Contributors:* Gerald Astor: "The last Nazi - The Life and Times of Dr. Josef Mengele", p. 206. D.I. Fine, 1985 *Original artist:* Anonymous photographer, not identified anywhere

- **File:Waldem_Hoven.jpg** *Source:* https://upload.wikimedia.org/wikipedia/commons/2/2a/Waldem_Hoven.jpg *License:* Public domain *Contributors:* USHMM Photograph #07319, courtesy of Hedwig Wachenheimer Epstein *Original artist:* U.S. Military Government for Germany

- **File:Weigl-Lwow.jpg** *Source:* https://upload.wikimedia.org/wikipedia/en/e/e7/Weigl-Lwow.jpg *License:* ? *Contributors:* Profesor Rudolf Weigl at the National Museum of Przemyśl Land (*Muzeum Narodowe Ziemi Przemyskiej*) reproduced by Stanisław Kosiedowski from the originals. *Original artist:* ?

- **File:Wiki_letter_w_cropped.svg** *Source:* https://upload.wikimedia.org/wikipedia/commons/1/1c/Wiki_letter_w_cropped.svg *License:* CC-BY-SA-3.0 *Contributors:*

- Wiki_letter_w.svg *Original artist:* Wiki_letter_w.svg: Jarkko Piiroinen

- **File:Wikiquote-logo.svg** *Source:* https://upload.wikimedia.org/wikipedia/commons/f/fa/Wikiquote-logo.svg *License:* Public domain *Contributors:* ? *Original artist:* ?

- **File:Wikisource-logo.svg** *Source:* https://upload.wikimedia.org/wikipedia/commons/4/4c/Wikisource-logo.svg *License:* CC BY-SA 3.0 *Contributors:* Rei-artur *Original artist:* Nicholas Moreau

53.8.3 Content license

www.ingramcontent.com/pod-product-compliance
Lightning Source LLC
Chambersburg PA
CBHW081443170526
45166CB00008B/2302